P9-CJV-239

CANCER: THE BEHAVIORAL DIMENSIONS

Cancer:
The Behavioral
Dimensions

Edited by

J. W. Cullen, B. H. Fox, and R. N. Isom

National Cancer Institute
National Institutes of Health
U.S. Department of Health, Education, and Welfare
Bethesda, Maryland

Raven Press ■ New York

Raven Press, 1140 Avenue of the Americas, New York, New York 10036

1976

Made in the United States of America

International Standard Book Number 0-89004-104-0
Library of Congress Catalog Card Number 75-43192

Dedication

This book is dedicated to:

MYRON R. KARON, M.D.
(February 27, 1932, to November 16, 1974)

pediatric oncologist and humanitarian, whose deep under-
standing of oncology and careful application of behavioral
principles in the management of his patients exemplified the true
embodiment of medicine and behavioral sciences.

Foreword

There now exists an abundance of knowledge about cancer, and we continually add to what we know. But a store of knowledge alone will never conquer cancer. In order to apply it to cancer control, we must learn how to encourage constructive health-related behavior among both the public and health professionals. The conference which produced this volume was assembled to gather and assess what we understand about the behavioral sciences as they relate to cancer management and to strengthen the interest of behaviorists in this chronic disease. Activities such as this conference exemplify the strong commitment of the Division of Cancer Control and Rehabilitation to the motivational and behavioral aspects of chronic disease control. By bringing together professionals in the field to compare notes about the best existing knowledge, we intend to establish a base of knowledge from which we can proceed to help those at risk. This volume provides to all those concerned about potential and actual cancer patients greater understanding and perspective from which will evolve a more comprehensive approach to cancer management.

The Division of Cancer Control and Rehabilitation has been mandated within the National Cancer Institute to ensure that cancer research results are translated into use. The strategy for translating cancer findings into effective control programs includes intervention activities extending to all stages of cancer care. At present, the vast majority of the efforts of cancer-oriented medical and allied health professionals are devoted to diagnosis and treatment of symptomatic cancer patients, in whom the chances of cure are slimmest. But as has been true of most diseases that have been controlled or eliminated, prevention offers the greatest hope for the control of cancer.

The majority of all cancers are preventable and result from exposure to environmental carcinogens. Reducing or eliminating cigarette smoking, altering dietary habits, reducing overexposure to sunlight, and controlling occupational hazards are examples of how behavioral modification could effect meaningful cancer prevention. Groups such as those at high risk because of medical, social, or economic factors require special attention. If prevention programs are to succeed, not only must people modify their destructive behavior, but health professionals who so influence the public must also change their attitudes and practices.

Human behavior plays a vital role in preventive health care. People normally want to stay healthy, but may dread cancer, fear the medical system, suffer from indifference, lack information about services available, or not understand the utility of screening procedures. Those with suspicious symptoms may delay seeking diagnosis. And yet one out of every six cancer deaths could be prevented by earlier diagnosis and treatment. Overcoming these barriers to good health habits is a behavioral problem, not a medical one.

For persons who develop cancer and for health professionals who must deal with cancer patients, the importance of morbidity and mortality statistics pales in comparison to the disease itself. Health professionals are not immune to the fear, the frustrations, the denial, and the guilt that cancer may cause. In order to help their patients in the best way possible they must learn to deal with these feelings. For the patient, life may be precarious and therefore ever more precious. Whether the course of the patient's disease calls for rehabilitation or for continuing care, the nature of that care is important.

The medical community has traditionally fought merely to keep the cancer patient alive as long as possible. As we learn better how to do this, the ramifications of treatment of the patient assume equal importance. Where there has existed inadequate follow-up care, the goal now is a complete rehabilitation program for the patient and his family. The physician may feel that he is providing the best service through radical treatment without realizing that he may also be giving the patient a new set of physical and psychological problems with which to deal. Therefore, rehabilitation must begin at the point of diagnosis as an integral part of the care process to avoid dehumanization of the patient.

A revised look at psychosocial rehabilitation is just one aspect covered in this volume. It has produced a broad look at the state of the art, which must only serve as a beginning. We do not question the value of assessing our current knowledge and exploring what we must know. But beyond such assessment we must learn how to practice techniques for effectively changing behavior to assure that people take the best care of themselves and that they take advantage of the best care available. Then we will have done our utmost to arrest the threat of cancer.

Diane J. Fink, M.D.
*Director, Division of Cancer Control
and Rehabilitation*

Preface

Part of the Congressional mandate presented to the National Cancer Institute under the authority of the National Cancer Act of 1971 was to develop and implement a coordinated national effort to reduce cancer incidence, morbidity, and mortality in the United States. Organizationally, within the Office of the Director of the National Cancer Institute, the Cancer Control Program was instituted as one arm in the offensive to achieve this objective. In 1974 the Cancer Control Program was expanded and elevated to divisional status, becoming the Division of Cancer Control and Rehabilitation (DCCR).

The goal of the cancer control component of the National Cancer Institute is to identify, field test, evaluate, demonstrate, and promote the widespread application of the available and new methods for reducing the incidence, morbidity, and mortality from cancer. The strategy to achieve this goal is defined in terms of the three major intervention areas of (1) prevention, (2) detection, diagnosis, and pretreatment evaluation, and (3) treatment, rehabilitation, and continuing care. Implementation of this strategy is effected through a number of individual, operational programs. The efforts within each of these programs are characterized by the following types of activities:

1. Identification of new methods, knowledge, and techniques that may be applicable to control activities. These activities involve close monitoring of the progress of research efforts and potential results, surveys to identify proven, practical knowledge and techniques, and data collection efforts to compile available information directly applicable to control activities.

2. Field testing of potential control knowledge and techniques in limited community field trials to determine their potential for widespread community usage. This effort provided an orderly transition from Phase III, clinical research trials, to community usage.

3. Evaluation of potentially useful control knowledge and techniques to determine their effectiveness, practicality, acceptability, impact on the disease, and economic or cost benefits prior to embarking on costly, wide-scale community demonstration and promotion efforts.

4. Demonstration of effective, practical, control knowledge and techniques in large-scale, community environments that are geographically widespread and demographically diverse to provide the public and health professionals with first-hand knowledge of the utility and effectiveness of the demonstrated knowledge and techniques and to provide the basis for continued community support of the efforts.

5. Promotion of demonstrated, effective, practical knowledge and techniques to assure their rapid, widespread utilization in all areas of the nation.

Cancer is a complex, chronic disease that has an impact on the potential and actual patient, the patient's family, multiple health care professionals, and society as a whole. In addition to its purely medical dimension, there are also behavioral dimensions. Consequently, in the mission of the Division of Cancer Control and Rehabilitation, attention is also being paid to the social, economic, and psychological impact of the disease on society in general and the patient and his family in particular. Indeed, it was the judgment of those advisory bodies who recommended and government planners who decided what the role of the Division should be in attempting to achieve the objectives of the National Cancer Act, that all aspects of the disease, including the behavioral, must be considered in the war on cancer. Since information relating to the behavioral aspects of cancer is scarce and certainly not available as a unified resource, it was imperative for those responsible for carrying out the national directive of the Division of Cancer Control and Rehabilitation to determine what was available; and it was considered important to promote an interaction between behaviorists and other health professionals who deal with cancer and cancer patients on a daily basis. To accomplish this goal, the Division of Cancer Control and Rehabilitation held a conference in San Antonio in January of 1975 on "Cancer Control and the Behavioral Sciences." The objectives of this conference were:

I. To determine the state-of-the-art of the behavioral sciences as they relate to chronic disease in general and cancer in particular;
II. To strengthen interest among behaviorists toward applying their knowledge and skills to chronic disease, particularly cancer; and
III. To provide the staff of the National Cancer Institute and more particularly the Division of Cancer Control and Rehabilitation with information and perspective so that a more comprehensive approach to the management of cancer would be possible under the guidelines and mandate of that Division.

It was anticipated that Objective I would materialize from the content developed during the conference. Objective II was also expected to be partially achieved during the conference when the participants interfaced with each other and would later be more fully achieved when the ideas presented were published and reached a larger audience whose health interests were primarily the behavioral aspects of the disease. Achievement of Objective III was expected to result from an integration of the state-of-the-art disclosed at the conference with program goals of the National Cancer Control Program.

This monograph is a record of the proceedings from this conference. It is composed of invited papers by noted experts in communications, epidemiology, health administration, health education, nursing, oncology, psychiatry, psychology, public health, sociology, and social work. It also contains a critical examination of their ideas in the form of chapters from invited respondents as well as

considerable audience response and discussion. It should also be noted that
included among the speakers and in the audience were cancer patients—some
professional, some lay.

This monograph, then, represents a concerted attempt to unite those subspecialties of medicine and behavior whose daily professional activities are addressed
to all aspects of cancer management. It is categorically asserted that any potential
benefits will only follow from such a union.

When Drs. Fox, Isom, and I first started to plan this conference, and by
extension this monograph, we agreed that there were behavioral considerations
that required discussion across all aspects of the cancer management continuum.
Consequently, the conference program included three major sessions: (1) Health
Care Behavior, (2) Communications, and (3) Coping with Cancer. With each of
these sessions we have tried to focus attention on the purveyors of cancer
management, its potential and actual recipients, and the system within which each
of these two target populations interdigitate.

In the process of planning for and holding the conference from which this
monograph proceeded, we used and appreciated the advice and experience of
many people. These included Dr. Diane Fink, Director of the Division of Cancer
Control and Rehabilitation, the members of the Cancer Control and Rehabilitation
Advisory Committee, the Executive Committee of the National Cancer Institute,
many officers of the American Cancer Society, Dr. R. Lee Clark, the staff of the
Division of Cancer Control and Rehabilitation and, in particular, Dr. Margaret
Edwards, Dr. George Jay, JRB Associates, Inc., and my secretary, Ms. Dorothy
Jones.

I would also like to express my special thanks to the other two editors, Dr.
Bernard Fox and Dr. Ruby Isom, whose cooperation and wisdom over many
hours of planning, execution, and editing were and will be the greatest harbingers
of the success of this venture.

Joseph W. Cullen, Ph.D.*
National Cancer Institute
National Institutes of Health
Bethesda, Maryland 20014

---

*Present address: Deputy Director, UCLA Cancer Center, Los Angeles, California 90024.

Contents

**Role of the Health Care System in Affecting the
Attitudes and Behavior of Practitioners and Patients**

Communication

**Mass Communications: An Evaluation
of Its Impact and Discussion of How It Could
Be Used More Effectively in Changing Health Behavior**

Coping with Cancer
Confronting the Diagnosis

Living With Cancer:
Adjustments of Patients and Practitioners
to the Consequences of Cancer

The Terminal Patient

Cancer: The Behavioral Dimensions, edited by J. W. Cullen, B. H. Fox, and R. N. Isom. Raven Press, New York © 1976.

Psychologic Reactions of Patients and Health Professionals to Cancer

R. Lee Clark

M. D. Anderson Hospital and Tumor Institute, University of Texas, Houston, Texas 77025

The President of the International Union Against Cancer, Professor Pierre Denoix, opened the XI International Cancer Congress in Florence, Italy, with a plea directed to authors and journalists throughout the world to "...bid them to abandon 'cancer' as a dramatic motif and a term that denotes terror and tragic inevitability. Eliminate the false connotations from your writing and you will have made an incalculable contribution to the campaign we are waging, together, against this disease—since you will have helped to reduce the unjustified terror that the inept use of this word tends to perpetuate."

Perhaps we need to examine why the word cancer strikes fear into the minds of many, but not at all in the minds of others such as chronic, long-term cigarette smokers who inhale smoke as deeply as always while reading the abundant warnings of the dangers of developing not only lung cancer but also heart and other lung diseases.

Many authors, examining this problem of fear at the mention of cancer, have theorized and made suggestions regarding some of the reasons:

1. Cancer can occur silently, without warning, until the skills of the physician are no longer adequate to save the life.
2. Cancer is not confined to the original site but spreads silently to any body tissue if not checked.
3. For centuries, nothing could be done to arrest the course of cancer after an early period of growth, particularly for those cancers that were not evident externally.
4. Cancer deprives the rest of the body tissues of nutrients, causing wasting of these tissues while it thrives.
5. Advanced cancer often causes intractable pain, often not responsive to available narcotics and analgesics.
6. Cancer causes an attitude of hopelessness in many people, including many physicians, leading to abandonment of cancer patients by those who should be supportive.
7. Often the diagnosis of cancer and the type is unsure, and inadequate therapy

may be administered until metastasis has occurred.

8. Therapy is often mutilative and deprives the patient of familiar self-image, independence, and perhaps of a means of livelihood.
9. The etiologies of many types of cancer are not known.
10. The patient has little or no personal control over the disease process; that is, even if he gives full cooperation to his physician, there can be no guarantee that the therapy will be successful.

PHYSICIAN ATTITUDES

Statements, often made publicly, such as this one made by August Bier (1861–1949), the German surgeon, were essentially true but certainly not reassuring to the public: "There is a tremendous literature on cancer, but what we know for sure about it can be printed on a calling card."

In his book, *The Spontaneous Regression of Cancer,* the Canadian pathologist and bacteriologist William Boyd (1885–   ) (1) presented the general attitude when he eloquently wrote:

> When we think of cancer in general terms we are apt to conjure up a process characterized by a steady, remorseless and inexorable progress in which the disease is all-conquering, and none of the immunological and other defensive forces which help us to survive the onslaught of bacterial and viral infections can serve to halt the faltering footsteps to the grave.

Although we have made more progress in acquiring knowledge about cancer in the last 25 years than in the entire previous history of humanity, unfortunately there are too many physicians still practicing medicine and teaching in medical schools whose medical philosophies include these defeatist attitudes regarding cancer therapy. Many physicians see so few cancer patients in their medical careers that they find no need to keep abreast of what is available for the diagnosis and treatment of cancer. Too many general surgeons consider their knowledge adequate to perform cancer surgery and thus deprive their patients of a truly curative procedure possible only through adjunctive use of radiotherapy and/or chemotherapy.

We could be more optimistic about the eventual demise of pessimism regarding cancer therapy among our physicians and nurses if medical and nursing students were informed about the new and effective therapeutic tools now available for the control and cure of cancer to encourage and challenge them to consider it a curable disease. Studies such as that done by E. C. Easson (2) in 1967 on the problem of pessimism among general practitioners and medical and nursing students, however, reveal that this is not true. Generally, students still see predominantly terminal cases on charity wards for whom most or all hope has been forfeited and who are receiving merely palliative therapy until death ensues.

There is a strong and understandable propensity for physicians in any medical specialty to concentrate on the presenting medical problem and its solution rather than on the patient as a person. It is agreed that for busy physicians confronted daily with large numbers of medical problems, there seems to be minimal time for dealing with the psychological needs of their patients. Many physicians believe that because they chose not to specialize in psychology or psychiatry, they should not be expected to be very knowledgeable regarding psychological subtleties. Most of them receive little or no exposure to the basic concepts of human psychology or behavioral sciences during any phase of their medical training. These attitudes, although understandable if one assumes that physicians are obligated to see as many patients as possible each day, because there is a chronic shortage of physicians, and because some treatment is better than no treatment at all, are untenable if one accepts the age-old medical tradition that a true physician is obligated to treat the whole patient—the person—not just an organ or a system.

It was known by physicians long before Freud's contribution to the world that a patient's emotional status can directly affect both the course of a disease and the effectiveness of the therapy. To move progressively away from this concept in the name of specialization, to ignore the effect of the psyche on the soma except in the specialties of psychology and psychiatry, is in great measure to refute the entire tradition of medicine as a "healing art" as well as a collection of reparative sciences.

Nowhere is this need for physicians to be actively concerned with the emotional well-being of their patients better exemplified than in the field of oncology, and particularly in pediatric and adolescent oncology. Numerous studies have been done, and are discussed in this volume, by individuals far more expert in these matters than I, regarding the many facets of human reaction to cancer—reactions of patients, family members, nursing personnel, physicians, rehabilitation specialists, social workers, volunteers, and so on.

PATIENT ATTITUDES

But what of individual patient reactions to seeking diagnosis and accepting it once it is made, of agreeing to initial therapy, and of cooperating with the physician through long-term therapy and follow-up examinations?

Cobb (3) conducted a study at the M. D. Anderson Hospital between 1951 and 1954 to determine why patients did or did not delay in seeking a diagnosis of suspected cancer, and why they refused therapy or detoured to nonmedical sources or quacks for treatment once the diagnosis was made. Factors involved were as follows.

1. *Sociocultural background*—Was there a family history of cancer, what were the cultural or ethnic attitudes toward cancer for those immediately surrounding peers, and also such factors as sex, age, occupation, source of income, financial status, and educational and religious backgrounds.

2. *Site of the lesion*—Often it was not considered sufficiently serious to seek help unless the initial lesion could be seen, felt, or it impaired function, and the growth rate was so slow that psychological adaptation to the lesion occurred; in addition, fear of surgical loss of a limb, breast, part of the face, or sexual function contributed to delay or rejection of therapy and resort to nonsurgical quackery.

3. *Cancer education or experience*—Often, even with awareness of the American Cancer Society's 7 warning signals, individuals delayed seeking diagnosis out of the fear of inevitable death; in addition, previous relationships with members of the medical profession were important—those physicians who had rejecting personalities, or who had previously treated a family member for cancer and had taken the attitude, following the failure of their initial therapeutic attempt, that "nothing more can be done" were not consulted.

4. *Fear* (the most potent single factor)—In addition to the above-mentioned fears regarding surgical mutilation, fears of extended suffering and pain, financial devastation, fate of dependents (e.g., small children, invalid parents), abandonment by a repelled spouse were factors.

5. *Patient's personal evaluation of the problem*—If the patient decided the lesion was benign or believed it couldn't be serious because there would be accompanying pain, there was delay.

6. *Management of cancer following diagnosis and before therapy*—If a physician made an incorrect diagnosis and began ineffectual therapy, or vacillated in the decision about how and when to treat the patient, of if the physician was not optimistic and supportive regarding the intended therapy, quacks were often consulted because they invariably were supportive and exuded optimism regarding the success of therapy. It has been estimated that $50 million is spent annually in the United States on cancer quackery (4).

Many additional studies, such as those reviewed in *Cancer Medicine* by Holland and Frei (5), revealed many of the reasons that the potential successes of oncologists are thwarted and made more difficult. Potential success in the treatment of cancer can also be affected by the attitudes of oncologically trained health personnel.

PSYCHOLOGICAL SUPPORT OF CANCER PATIENTS

Diagnosis

Once a diagnosis of cancer is made, the manner in which the physician tells the patient of the diagnosis is critical. Because of the present emphasis on patients' rights in medical situations and the legal requirement of informed consent, if experimental procedures are to be employed, there is little justification for not telling a patient of the diagnosis of cancer, as was frequently done in the past. If the physician is honest and sincerely optimistic regarding the planned therapy, the patient's ability to cope emotionally with the diagnosis will be much better than if the physician seems indifferent, unsure, or frankly pessimistic.

Even if the patient has disseminated cancer and curative therapy is negated, the physician's assurance that his palliative efforts will be directed toward physical comfort during the remaining time and toward death without pain, will reassure the patient and convey the message that his life as an individual will be respected right up to the time of death—that he need not fear abandonment by those caring for him. It is important for physicians to lay a foundation for a possible long-term relationship with the patient, and they should avoid premature speculation that might cause alarm or give the patient false hopes. Most patients are less fearful if they know what to expect. At the initial and subsequent meetings the patient should be allowed to ask questions. Honest answers by the physician, stated in understandable terminology, will reassure the patient and reduce anxieties. The physician should enumerate hopeful possibilities, if not for cure, then for the possibility of new therapies showing promise and for long-term remissions. If there will likely be impairment of function or loss of a body part, the patient should be told in advance. If it is necessary for cure or for reduction of later complications, the patient will probably consider the loss worth whatever gains are made.

Problems of Concurrent Noncancerous Medical Conditions

Psychological problems are elicited not only by the diagnosis of cancer, but are often compounded by the presence, particularly in patients over 50 years of age, of degenerative diseases such as cerebrovascular disease, diabetes, heart diseases, and so forth. These diseases must be medically managed concurrently with the cancer, and often the necessary, sometimes life-threatening procedures for cancer cure must be compromised or are affected by the presence of these other disease entities. Superimposed on these almost overwhelming problems are the realities of compromised nutrition of the patient and concurrent debilitation, often a direct result of the cancer therapy. In such cases, active concern for the psychological trauma inflicted by these multiple conditions and therapies may be essential for the maintenance of the patient's will to live.

Once a patient has agreed to undergo cancer therapy, in his own mind he may surrender most or all of his former security. The patient is forced to substitute uncertainty of the future for self-assurance, perhaps unemployment for a steady, predictable income, and financial threat for solvency; suffer disfigurement or pain; risk the possibility of dissolution of the family unit and an uncertain future for the members of this unit; lose social status and recognition as an independent individual; and forego many of the other things that represent security, such as a familiar and comforting home environment, if hospitalization is necessary.

Postcurative Therapy Anxiety

Even if curative therapy has been completed, the patient will experience some anxiety regarding the potential for rehabilitation, if needed, and regarding the possibilities of recurrence, particularly at the periodic follow-up examinations. If signs of recurrence appear, the patient may be more devastated than at the initial diagnosis, and care should be taken to help the patient accept the further therapeutic plans because there is great danger at this time that some patients will begin to "doctor shop" or seek hope from quackery.

The physiatrist or rehabilitation expert should be part of the initial team of clinicians making decisions about therapeutic strategy. Rehabilitation, emotional and physical, should begin immediately, so that the patient and family members present during hospitalization will be familiar with prostheses and will be well along the way toward psychological and physical adjustment by the time the patient is dismissed from the hospital.

Progressive Disease

For those patients who experience progression of disease despite therapy, depression can be expected, and efforts to point out an appreciation of what they had in the past and the little joys of the present may help alleviate some of the sadness and depression. The knowledge that life offers no certainty of a future to any person, whether he has cancer or not, and that the only future any of us truly has is the present moment, which *was* the future, helps many people achieve a different perspective.

When physicians are faced with the knowledge that the cancer can no longer be controlled, a number of things can be done to reassure the patient that interest is not flagging. For instance, the type of narcotic being used for pain can be changed; an electrolyte imbalance can be corrected; the physician can strive for an improvement in nutrition; physical therapy can be instituted when it can be tolerated; an addition of a tranquilizer might be reinforcing to the patient; an ulcerating, malodorous lesion can be kept meticulously clean; a therapy may be instituted that may have shown poor results in the past but will do no further harm and might reassure the patient that interest in his welfare is still active. If the patient is willing, the staff psychiatrist or a chaplain may give spiritual assistance, although the physician should avoid the temptation to delegate the entire responsibility of the patient to them. Often, frank discussions of death by the patient with someone he trusts will result in a lessening of the need for pain medication, and he might begin to sleep better at night. It will be helpful to all to achieve an attitude of "cooperation with the inevitable" (6). The knowledge that they have done the best they can should be sufficient reward for physicians.

Anxieties Related to Cancer in Children

Children with cancer are generally incapable of fully understanding why they must undergo painful procedures and debilitating and unpleasant therapy. A large part of the burden falls on the parents, who must bear up under the knowledge that their children are unable to understand why their previously loving parents are now allowing these frightening and painful things to happen and are not protecting them from harm. Parents also often experience guilt feelings because they did not suspect the presence of cancer and seek therapy sooner, probably increasing their child's chances for survival.

Parents begin to experience grief almost at the moment of diagnosis of cancer in their child. Most often the grief stems from a personal feeling of loss and can be incapacitating and actually harmful to the child. It is very important for parents to gain sufficient perspective to control their personal grief and concentrate on loving, reassuring support of the ill child, who looks to them for comfort and some confidence that what is being endured is really done for their own benefit. Opportunities for more mutuality and a new type of loving closeness are frequently experienced between parents and child during these difficult experiences.

Many physicians believe small children should not be told in advance of therapy procedures to avoid anticipatory anxiety, but many parents have found that their children respond better and accept the inevitability of the procedures when they are informed in advance of what to expect. It seems more difficult for many children to continually cope with painful or frightening surprises. There is disagreement about whether or not a parent should be in the treatment room. The essential aspect is whether the parents can exercise sufficient emotional control to avoid conveying the attitude that they wish to protect the child from the medical care team, who are collectively responsible for the unpleasantness. The child must sustain a feeling of confidence that the medical team is trying to help. The persons most likely to assist in helping the child feel this confidence are the parents. For the parents, the belief that not only their own child might benefit, but that other children will also, helps them accept, in the event of the death of their child, that it was not all in vain.

Psychologically, these experiences can split a family asunder or can strengthen the relationships as understanding and maturation occur. A key figure during these events is the primary physician. If he or she is willing to answer questions, volunteer information and friendly encouragement, and show sympathetic concern for the feelings of the child and parents, all are strengthened.

PSYCHOLOGICAL NEEDS OF ONCOLOGICALLY TRAINED HEALTH PERSONNEL

Fortunately, some of the younger physicians are optimistic about the potential success of cancer therapy and accept the diagnosis as a challenge to their skills. For these physicians and for oncologists, the interest and optimism are much easier to maintain for the earlier stages of cancer, but become progressively more difficult for advanced cancer, cancer that is not responding to therapy, and particularly for terminal disease. The physician treating these cases must be aware that it is difficult for humans, especially those dedicated to helping their fellow human beings, to accept failure with equanimity. The feeling of failure is likely first to be turned inside the physician in the form of self-anger for not having sufficient knowledge and skill to succeed, which often inspires feelings of inadequacy. The anger or frustration may then be turned outwardly toward the patient for not seeking help sooner, for not giving the physician a "fighting chance" to succeed, or for being disappointed that the physician cannot restore health. This anger and frustration experienced by physicians is rarely expressed overtly but may take the forms of cold, impersonal professionalism, or progressive abandonment of the patient. The physician may prefer to concentrate his efforts on patients who can benefit from his skills.

These attitudes are destructive to the patient and to the physician, because there is danger that gradually the physician's self-confidence will erode or his internalized anger will decrease his efficiency. With a change in perspective, achieved through honest evaluation of his own emotional responses, discussion with other medical personnel, and most particularly with the other members of the team caring for the patient in question (nurses, other physicians, technologists), he will be able to accept as sufficient challenge his palliative efforts to keep the patient comfortable and functioning at some level. The rewards are different, but each patient values his own life and can be grateful and friendly toward other individuals who also value it.

All members of the medical team should ventilate their feelings among themselves—honestly confess their feelings of frustration, grief, or even hostility toward some patients—and thereby sustain a sufficient emotional balance to be able to convey a relaxed, confident, concerned attitude to patients.

It is important that psychologists and psychiatrists be considered essential members of the cancer care team. Their special training in assisting individuals, medical and nonmedical, to understand their own emotional responses and achieve insight into the attitudes of others is invaluable to all involved in these complex relationships.

As Stehlin and Beach (6) expressed in a publication presenting a cancer surgeon's point of view, the relationship of cancer physicians and their patients should be open and honest and "sustained by hope within a framework of reality." He stressed that "incurable" and "hopeless" are not synonymous—that incurability is a state of the body, and hopelessness is a state of the mind. One can have or be treating an incurable cancer but maintain a hopeful attitude toward the time remaining and what can be learned about the disease, oneself, and others.

PSYCHOLOGICAL TRAINING IN CLINICAL CANCER INSTITUTIONS

Approximately 25 years ago, an effort was begun at the M. D. Anderson Hospital to establish a psychology program specifically designed for a cancer research hospital (7). The aims were service, research, and training.

In 1951 a clinical psychologist, Dr. Beatrice Cobb, joined the research medical staff under the supervision of the Department of Medicine. Her activities were under the guidance of an interdisciplinary advisory council made up of physicians, a psychiatrist, a sociologist, and another psychologist. Her assignments were to conduct research on cancer patient behavior and attitudes, and to determine the possible areas of service and research. After 17 months, Dr. Cobb made recommendations to utilize psychologists for service, following adequate medical training courses, to assist and enhance the acquisition of insight into the special problems faced in a cancer research hospital. The program was to supplement the medical efforts to alleviate stress and, thereby, to help in the management of cancer patients. In addition, a training program was instituted to provide research experience for the psychology trainees to prepare them for research careers. The program was continued until 1958, at which time Dr. Cobb accepted a position with another university. It became progressively difficult to sustain the program due to a number of factors, and the training activities were finally discontinued.

I believe that such programs are of inestimable value, and that support of similar programs in cancer centers throughout the country should be seriously considered.

REHABILITATION

In summary, it is clear that we as oncologists have been so busy attempting to save lives or stave off the most devastating aspects of widespread cancer that we have neglected to help our patients adjust to the emotional trauma of cancer, cancer therapy, and the change in status and altered habitus when our therapeutic efforts are successful. Now that we are saving more lives and obtaining long-term remissions, which make normal life possible for significant periods, we are obligated to make further efforts to help this return to life be a quality experience.

Specific areas in which beginnings have been made and expanded programs can be initiated immediately are in aiding patients who have undergone mastectomies, limb amputations, and head and neck surgery with resultant mutilation that cannot always be totally repaired by plastic surgery, laryngectomies, colostomies, and other procedures requiring external stomas. The need has been so great that in desperation, patients have joined together to help themselves, as evidenced by such groups as the Reach to Recovery, the Candlelighters, Make Each Day Count, and other groups that were self-initiated and then perhaps underwritten by such larger groups as the American Cancer Society.

Rudolf Virchow (1821–1902), the great German pathologist, stated in his treatise, *Disease, Life and Man* (8), that:

> Medicine is a social science in its very bone marrow...No physiologist or practitioner ought ever to forget that medicine unites in itself all knowledge of the laws which apply to the body *and the mind*.

REFERENCES

1. Boyd, W. *The Spontaneous Regression of Cancer,* Charles C Thomas, Springfield, Ill. (1966).
2. Easson, E. C. Cancer and the problem of pessimism. *CA, 17:*7–14 (1967).
3. Cobb, B. A. Why 20 patients went to quacks. *Med. Economics, 32:*123–138 (1954).
4. Allman, D. B. Financial cost of caring for the cancer patient. In *The Physician and the Total Care of the Cancer Patient,* American Cancer Society, Inc., New York (1962).
5. Holland, J. F., and Frei, E. III (eds.): *Cancer Medicine,* Chapter 16, Lea & Febiger, Philadelphia (1973).

6. Stehlin, J. S., Jr., and Beach K. H. Psychological aspects of cancer therapy: A surgeon's viewpoint. *JAMA, 197*:100–104 (1966).
7. Cobb, B. A., Clark, R. L., Jr., Howe, C. D., and Trunnell, J. B. A psychology program in a cancer research hospital. *Tex. Rep. Biol. Med., 12*:30–38 (1954).
8. Virchow, R. *Disease, Life and Man: Selected Essays,* Stanford University Press, Stanford, Calif. (1958).

Cancer: The Behavioral Dimensions, edited by J. W. Cullen, B. H. Fox, and R. N. Isom. Raven Press, New York © 1976.

The Psychosocial Epidemiology of Cancer

Bernard H. Fox

National Cancer Institute, National Institutes of Health, Bethesda, Maryland 20014

One useful definition of epidemiology of a disease is its study in relation to the attributes of the group of persons in whom it occurs and their environment. The main purpose of epidemiology is to discover the causes or promoters of disease, but testing of preventive or ameliorating public health measures is also an important objective (1). We distinguish primary and secondary prevention. The first means preventing the disease; the second means the halting or slowing of progression of the disease and preventing and reducing unwanted sequelae (2). I stress primary prevention, whereas others in this volume deal more with the latter.

The psychosocial epidemiologist is interested in social and personal characteristics and behavior as conditions associated with higher and lower risk of cancer and its consequences in a given population. However, because the bulk of cancers about whose etiology we have a fair-to-good idea involve these conditions as part of the etiologic picture, it is hard to separate them from associated environmental or biological conditions. Nevertheless, the main psychosocial variables can be organized coherently into subcategories and some judgments can be made about them in terms of prevention. Certain fundamental principles apply in most, if not all cases. First, the association of a condition with increased risk of cancer does not imply that it produces or contributes to that risk, although it may. Second, the mere presence of the condition with such increased risk in one or several studies does not imply that wherever the condition is found the risk will likewise be increased. The increase may be conditional on the presence of other variables. Third, for any variable, the discovery of increased risk implies either greater susceptibility of the host or increased exposure to a carcinogen and sometimes both—regardless of amount, concentration, or time. And last, the value of examining psychosocial variables associated with the appearance or progression of cancer lies in the possibility of preventing that appearance or slowing that progression. Hence we look for high- and low-risk groups in the hope of finding successful countermeasures. Where the etiologic hypothesis is broadly accepted, the problem ceases to be of concern to the epidemiologist investigating etiology; at that point the hypothesis-testing and countermeasures-testing roles are involved.

Table 1 lists many conditions and behaviors that have been examined in relation to the appearance and outcomes of cancer—both increased and decreased risks.

TABLE 1. *Conditions associated with cancer*

Conditions	Range of confidence[a]	Site[b]
I. What people are, or what happens to them personally.		
A. Psychological characteristics		
1. Personality	3–4	Nonspecific
2. Transient or newly occurring states		
a. Mental illness, especially schizophrenia	4	Nonspecific
b. Depression	4	Nonspecific, pancreas, blood
c. Neurologic symptoms	3–4	Nonspecific
d. Specific life stresses		
(1) Hypotheses: low male hormone; high blood corticosteroids; conditioned immunosuppression	4	Stomach, nonspecific
(2) Experimental stress in animals	3–4	Nonspecific
B. Physical characteristics		
1. Somatotype	4	Nonspecific
2. Specific body dimensions		
a. Structure	4	Breast, nonspecific
b. Obesity	3	Endometrium
c. Height and weight	3–4	Breast, cervix
3. Hair color	4	Breast
4. Complexion and eye color	1–3	Skin
C. Congenital and genetic traits		
1. Age at menarche	3	Cervix, breast
2. Age at menopause	4	Breast
3. Family history of cancer	1–4	Breast, various nonspecific
4. Congenital deficiency or abnormality	1–4	Various
D. Other diseases and pathology		
1. E.g., cirrhosis of liver, skin keratoses, kidney or bladder stones	2–4	Various
2. Traumata, scars, burns	2–4	Skin, esophagus
3. Communicable diseases	2–4	Bladder, blood
4. Irritation of tissues	3–4	Nonspecific
E. Demographic and social characteristics		
1. Sex	1	Various
2. Age	1	Nonspecific
3. Socioeconomic level	1–4	Nonspecific
4. Marriage	2–4	Breast, cervix
5. Race	1–4	Various, nonspecific
6. Religion	1–4	Various
7. Ethnicity	1–4	Various
8. Geographic location		
a. World (ozone, ultraviolet)	1–4	Various
b. Country, region	1–4	Various
c. Urban-rural	1–4	Various
d. Rainfall	4	Nonspecific, esophagus
9. Culture	2–4	Nonspecific
II. What People Do to Themselves		
A. Habits		

Conditions	Range of confidence[a]	Site[b]
1. Drinking	1	Mouth, throat, larynx, liver, esophagus
2. Tobacco use		
a. Smoking, chewing, snuff-dipping	1–3	Lung, mouth, throat, larynx, esophagus, bladder
3. Coffee	4	Nonspecific
4. Marihuana	4	Nonspecific
5. Narcotics (reduced risk)	4	Cervix
B. Customs and cultural behavior		
1. Cultural behaviors		
a. The sun cult	2	Skin
b. Breast feeding	4	Breast
c. Age at marriage	2–4	Breast, cervix
d. Size of family	4	Leukemia
e. Circumcision	2–4	Penis, cervix
f. Sick pets	4	Leukemia
g. Eating habits	4	Esophagus
2. Hygiene		
a. Washing, douching	4	Cervix
b. Mouth cleanliness	4	Oral
c. Trichomonas infection	1–3	Cervix
3. Intercourse		
a. Early, several partners	1–3	Cervix
b. Many other variables	2–4	Cervix
III. Diet		
A. Natural components and lacks		
1. Amount eaten	2–4	Nonspecific
2. Fat, protein	4	Colorectal
3. Vitamin deficiencies	3	Esophagus, other
4. Carcinogens	2–4	Various
B. Processing effects		
1. Refined foods and lost bulk	3–4	Colorectal
2. Preservatives and colorants	3–4	Nonspecific
3. Purification of water	4	Various
IV. What Is Done to People		
A. Environmental pollution		
1. Pesticides, herbicides	4	Liver, nonspecific
2. Air pollution	2–4	Lung, nonspecific
3. Water pollution	4	Nonspecific
4. Ionizing radiation	1–4	Leukemia, thyroid, other
B. Occupation		
1. Carcinogen known		
a. Some examples: X-ray, uranium, asbestos, arsenic, polyvinyl-chloride, certain organic compounds, sun, benzo[a]pyrene	1–4	Various
2. Dangerous nonbehaviors	2–3	Various
C. Possible iatrogenic effects		
1. Drugs	1–4	Various
2. X-ray—therapy and diagnosis	1–4	Various

Conditions	Range of confidence[a]	Site[b]
3. Irritation by prosthetics	3–4	Various
4. Immunosuppression (e.g., transplantation medication)	1–4	Various
5. Errors in diagnosing precancerous states	2–4	Various
6. Tonsillectomy	4	Hodgkin's disease

[a] Range of confidence that the condition is associated with higher or lower risk of cancer (personal judgment): (1) certain, (2) high to moderate, (3) moderate to low, (4) suspicion or not enough data.

[b] Site(s) that has been associated with the variable.

The found relationship is not necessarily the true relationship. Many categories overlap, perforce, but each variable has arbitrarily been assigned to one main category. For example, hair color has been placed under physical characteristics, but it is clearly a genetic trait also. Obviously the list is not complete. Also, not all variables noted have consistently been found to be related to the occurrence of cancer. In some the found relationship is clearly zero, and in some there is considerable disagreement about the relationship. I have tried to indicate a range of confidence in the observed associations.[1] For each variable the most relevant cancer sites are also noted.

The list of psychosocial variables given in Table 1 describes conditions that have been reviewed in association with cancer. It is given in an attempt to show the large variety of variables with psychosocial components that have been suspected to have epidemiological relevance to cancer—some merely as associated conditions that might provide potential etiologic leads, such as age, sex, religion, marital state; and others as possible causes of increased risk, such as excessive eating, or as possible causes of reduced risk, such as eating less without mineral or vitamin deficiency.

Table 1 lists only possible associates of cancer; it does not imply causation. It falls to the person considering behavior change for preventive purposes to follow the general hints of the table and to determine the consensus about whether the high-relationship variables are also causes of cancer. If so, the question of possible behavior change for prevention can then be faced.

The estimates of confidence that the condition is associated with higher or lower risk of cancer are meant to include a range within a category, since the full description of each category would be too lengthy. For example, it is generally believed that schistosomiasis among Egyptian fellahin produces high risk of bladder cancer (see Table 1, I.D. 3.). There is only a suspicion that mononucleosis increases risk of certain blood cancers; some believe that there is no association

---

[1] These are obviously personal judgments about confidence, since such opinions are not always expressed by authors. Particularly, they do not necessarily reflect the official views of the National Cancer Institute.

at all. These two facts lead to the mixed entry 2–4 for the communicable diseases category.

It would not be possible here to address each of the variables individually. However, I would like to discuss specifically the variables of personality and mental illness, to give some idea of the variety of views to be found in the psychosocial area. One cannot feel great confidence in the aggregate evidence that some personality types are more prone to get cancer than others. Most studies dealing with this question compared patients and noncancerous patients or well people. The implication of many of these authors, and often their explicit inference from the data, is that the observed personality differences existed before the cancer was found. This conclusion is subject to grave question without strong validating data, preferably prospective. People with cancer or those who suspect they may have it are subject to minor and major changes in outlook, recollection (4,5), mood, feeling, and capability, due to the cancer itself. For example, frank neurologic defects are associated with a substantial proportion of patients [17 to 38% reported for certain cancer types (6)], both through metastases and through the primary lesion; perceptual changes with cancer have been noted (7); depression and other psychic (aside from neurologic) symptoms often accompany some cancers (8–11). Many chemotherapeutic agents are neurotoxic (12,13). But even when cancer patients and others are successfully distinguished before the examiner knew their disease status (14, partially, 15,16), this only verifies the fact that in some dimensions based on mood, recollection, or test performance, cancer patients differed from noncancerous patients. It is true that common threads of earlier personal loss or social trauma and poor emotional outlet seem to run through certain studies showing such differences (17). Negative findings arise now and then, for example (18), and certain review articles do not arouse enthusiasm about support for the hypothesis (19,20).

Anterospective studies showing personality differences or unusual family relationships years before the cancer became evident (21,22) are perhaps more convincing, but they too need to be verified. [Indeed, one such attempt is now in progress (23)]. The difficulty is that these anterospective studies (21,22) are not true prospective studies, but are types of retrospective study, in that the person studied is chosen because of the presence of cancer, and the earlier test or interview results of cancer and control patients are then compared. Only in the necessary and important elimination of effect of cancer on test results are they superior to the others. The most definitive study, choosing people on the basis of the personality factor and determining success in predicting cancer, has not been done. It is, truly, a most difficult type of research.

What does all this mean for prevention? First, I have discovered only two estimates of the relative probability that certain personality characteristics are present in cancer patients compared to others: 2.5 and 1.4 times the probability for the respective controls, who were presumably representative of the population (16,21). If it were established that such internal conditions were truly associated with greater risk of cancer, one of the ways such conditions could be used would now be open to study—investigating what bodily or external conditions were different in this group (not necessarily caused by the personality difference), which allowed the group to be at greater risk. The epidemiologic hypothesis-tester and the biologic investigator would then be called to the search.

The important question of personality differences leading to smoking or not smoking is too complicated to discuss here, but if one could easily distinguish such people, the principle of attention to high-risk people applies directly.

Is mental illness associated with greater or lesser risk of getting cancer? Claims have been made (24) and suspicions voiced (25) that mental illness, or at least schizophrenia, protects against cancer. At least three reviews have been made (20,26,27) and the evidence is fairly strong against the hypothesis. The actual rates found can be explained on the basis of statistical and circumstantial conditions whose effect on reported cancer mortality is well known. One promising hypothesis, which has not been well investigated, is that the mentally ill with paranoid features may be at greater risk than others.

Rather than discuss each of the remaining variables in the same way, perhaps it would be valuable to point out some of the theoretical and practical aspects of cancer control associated with such behavior-based variables. What features of cancer bear on successful cancer control?

The sequence of tissue states in carcinogenesis is normal, minor cell transformation or dysplasia, more advanced premalignancy, clear local malignancy, and metastasis or spread of the cancer to other organs. Sometimes there is regression from a later to an earlier state. The best-known examples are regression from minor cervical dysplasia to normalcy, and from leukoplakia to normalcy, fairly well-documented phenomena (28,29).

Occasionally, more advanced states will also regress (30). Aside from these, since the progression is forward, detecting a tissue abnormality will be helpful to the degree that one can stop or reverse the progression. If a condition or behavior is known to increase risk of getting cancer, it is clearly advantageous, even before any cell abnormality appears, to prevent the first appearance of that abnormality, or delay that appearance if it cannot be prevented. Also, if a condition or substance produces or promotes cancer, usually the more the exposure the greater the chance of cancer. Often prevention is easier when it is possible to have direct access to the tissue involved, either for inspection or tissue-sampling purposes. Thus we know about the progression, in a small proportion of cases of leukoplakia (white patches on mucous membrane), to cancer by direct inspection and tissue sampling. Similarly, we can sample cells from the cervix by the Papanicolaou test and observe conditions that will be followed by cancer in a certain small proportion of patients. Or we can carry out a colorectal examination and check for the presence of villous polyps, which are also followed by cancer in a certain proportion of individuals. In the cases of occult precancer the problem is very severe.

The list of psychosocial variables given in Table 1 was not organized into a hierarchy of immediacy, but theoretically it could be, and if one were planning an overall attack on the problem, it might be worth doing. This hierarchy of closeness to causation applies to most diseases. We can hypothesize about possible immediate causes [e.g., ingestion of aflatoxin, a known carcinogen (31)]; possible intermediate causes [e.g., drinking beer contaminated by aflatoxin among some Africans (32)], and possible distant causes (e.g., the agricultural environment and tribal development of specific ways of life that led to making and drinking such beer). In this triplet behavioral causes are sometimes immediate; for example, the former chronic use of metal warming-boxes next to the abdomen among some groups in Japan as a source of skin cancer (3). Usually, however, behavioral causes are intermediate or distant, which is both an advantage and a disadvantage. The transmittal of effect from remote to immediate causes can easily be diffused along its path, thus yielding a lesser relationship of remote causes to the disease; on the other hand, a larger variety of countermeasures can usually be applied to the series of remote causes.

A process of combining risk factors to alert people to the need for detection tests has been carried out by Dr. Daniel Miller, Strang Clinic, New York. He has set down a combination of variables, each of which was associated with an increased risk of breast cancer, and specified the degree of watchfulness to be exercised when a woman had any of the various combinations. That is, he specified in a flow chart how often and what kind of periodic examinations should be done for each relevant combination (33). In effect, he assigned implied probabilities of getting breast cancer to the various combinations. The elements were presence or absence of nipple discharge, pain, mass or lump, former endometrial cancer, former breast cancer, breast cancer in female relatives, and age over 35 or 45. There is no reason that a similar procedure could not be done for primary prevention for each of the cancer sites. In some, we would have no success at all, since we are unaware of changeable behaviors that can affect the chances of getting the disease (e.g., brain cancer). In others, we could be more successful. For example, for oral cancer we would study the drinking patterns, smoking patterns, appearance of mouth lesions, age, diet, and eating habits. It may not be possible to arrive at a number that one could swear by, but surely a ball-park figure of increased risk could be derived. For many cancers, this kind of procedure is not out of the question.

A note on payoff is appropriate here. It is my impression that, except for lung cancer, public information and education efforts have focused mainly on detection. I am sure that very few parents, for example, know the important factors that accompany greater risk of cervical cancer in their daughters, namely, early sex experience and multiple partners. Perhaps if they knew, they would be less permissive about the relaxed sexual mores which seem to be more common among the young persons in our society. Already the Finns have witnessed an increase in cervical erosion in women under 20 whose sex experience started very early (34). Such erosion is associated with greater risk of cancer. How many people know that smoking is associated with increased risk not only of lung cancer, but also bladder, mouth, larynx, and esophagus (35)? How many employees or employers for that matter, know that exposure to certain materials, usually at work, increases risk of cancer 20 to 40 times (36)?

There is extensive literature on the effect of amount and type of diet on cancer incidence and survival among animals. It has been repeatedly verified (37,38) that a clearly low caloric diet without mineral or vitamin deficiency leads to longer life in mice and rats, ranging from a 10 to 50% increase in lifespan. The clear reduction of cancer incidence observed in these animals was an important contributor to that extended lifespan. If it were to be shown that this finding also applies to humans, we might have a very important aid in the war against cancer. At least as important from a behavior change point of view, if verified in humans, is the finding (39) that lifespan in these animals was extended no matter when the reduced intake began. Of course, the later the start of reduced intake, the less the increase in lifespan.

As each new finding appears where behavior change can reduce the risk of cancer, three things should be done. First, the value of assigning high priority to a verifying study should be estimated. Usually the main components of this will be: (1) the probable success of the countermeasure if a control program is entered into, (2) the payoff associated with the program, that is, how many cases of the disease would be prevented. Assuming a high priority, the second action should be to undertake the verifying study. Is the original finding valid? And (3), if so, active countermeasures should be initiated.

A good example could be the recent finding that among children (40) and adults (41) with leukemia, more families of such patients had sick cats or birds in the household than did well families. There was no difference for well pets. This is as yet a very preliminary finding, but it is susceptible to very concrete action, dependent on verifying the finding, determining whether sick pets cause greater cancer risk, and finally on payoff as described above.

One might ask what conditions associated with higher risk of cancer could be changed so as to lower that risk by some kind of behavior. We can define two kinds of behavior—doing something and not doing something. Those behaviors that involve nonaction are difficult to deal with because they may involve major conflict of goals. For example, when a doctor fails to carry out a screening test during an examination, can the doctor be held accountable if the patient came in with a particular complaint and is examined for that complaint? If there are precancer tests that involve procedures which the doctor will find patients reluctant to undergo (e.g., proctoscopy), how much of an attempt at convincing can we demand of the doctor? How much nonbehavior, for example, failure of some high-risk factory workers to wear masks, is due to ignorance? How much by doctors is due to ignorance? There are some nonbehaviors that might be corrected if appropriate effort was made, either by rules or by education.

The other side of the coin, doing something, is no less a problem. First, people and institutions have to be convinced about the value of the desired behavior. Then they have to carry out the behavior. Inevitably there will be conflicts of priority. But failure to take any preventive measures is not defensible. We have clear evidence of success of such efforts in the decline of smoking among British doctors and the average decline in cigarettes smoked per person in this country, starting at about the time the first Surgeon General's Report on Smoking and Health was released. We have seen a remarkable regular increase in the number of women having Pap smears.

Table 2 describes those characteristics from Table 1 where I felt that one's behavior could alter the risk of cancer to a greater or lesser degree if the characteristic contributed to the cause of cancer. Every one of the conditions listed was assumed to influence appearance of cancer. That assumption, of course, is not necessarily true. For example, we can only speculate that marihuana may be carcinogenic, since all we know now is that chronic users have been found to have lowered cell-mediated immunosuppressive capability (42).

TABLE 2. Conditions associated with personal characteristics or behavior that could be changed by various agents[a]

Condition	Behavior by			
	Individual	Physician	Government	Industry
Psychological characteristics				
0[b] Life stresses	x			x
Physical characteristics				
?[b] Obesity	x			
Other diseases and pathology				
?-+ Communicable diseases	x	x	x[c]	
0 Tissue irritation	x			
Habits				
+[b] Drinking	x	x		
+ Smoking, chewing, snuff	x	x	x	x
0-? Marihuana	x	x		
Customs and culture				
+ Sun cult	x	x		
0 Age of marriage	x			
0 Eating habits	x	x		
0 Living habits	x			
? Personal hygiene	x			
+ Intercourse, age of initiating, multiple partners	x			
Diet, natural components				
+ Amount eaten	x	x		
? Fat, protein	x	x		
+ Severe vitamin deficiency	x	x		
? Mineral deficiency	x	x		
0 Carcinogens (e.g., aflatoxin)			x	x
Diet, processing effects				
? Refined foods and lost bulk	x	x	x	x

Condition	Behavior by			
	Individual	Physician	Government	Industry
? Preservatives and coloring			x	x
? Water purification			x	x
Environmental pollution				
0-? Pesticides (home use, industry)	x		x	x
? Air pollution (tires, exhaust, factories)	x[d]		x	x
? Water pollution (tires, exhaust, factories, purification)	x[d]		x	x
? Excessive radioactivity			x	x
Occupation				
+ Known carcinogens			x	x
+ Dangerous nonbehaviors (not wearing masks, careless contact with radioactive materials)	x			x
Possible iatrogenic effects				
+[f] Carcinogenic drugs		x		x[e]
+ X-ray therapy and diagnosis		x		
? Prosthetics		x		
+[g] Immunosuppression (e.g., from transplantation medication)		x		
+ Errors in detecting and diagnosing precancerous sites		x		

[a] All the entries, both categories and judgments, reflect personal views and are not necessarily official views.

[b] + implies that a clear-cut improvement in cancer risk could be achieved

? implies that a questionable amount of improvement could be achieved

0 implies that behavior change would affect cancer risk little or not at all or that behavior change is very difficult to bring about.

[c] For example, damming up the Nile increased schistosomiasis, which probably increased the risk of later bladder cancer.

[d] The individual contributes in the sense that driving is a part of our current life style, our current civilization.

[e] By educating physicians.

[f] The most prominent known examples involve drugs used much less today than formerly.

[g] If this results from treatment of a life-threatening disease, how should the doctor decide?

A proper and productive team including a psychosocial epidemiologist, economist, health systems planner, public health educator, medical education specialist, union health administrator, and relevant others is clearly needed. Assuming that behavior will affect an etiologic agent, the task elements of the team are: to examine the probable result of each of the various behavior changes (including institutional and governmental policy, and economic, medical, and individual behaviors) on incidence and mortality associated with various types of cancer; to explore the possibilities of bringing about each behavior change; to determine what it would take and how much change could be brought about for each of them; to determine the priorities of making the investment and effort; and finally to proceed if it is worthwhile. We must always keep in mind, of course, the problem of balancing the profit associated with prevention and the cost associated with worry by many people if they discover their greater risk.

The bottlenecks facing effective prevention are well known: conflict between priorities, decision making in the face of opposing objectives and uncertainty, and limits on time, money, and available professionals. But in sum, if my judgment is correct, the picture that emerges is not so grim as it appeared earlier, and many real preventive possibilities exist.

REFERENCES

1. Lilienfeld, A. M., Pedersen, E., and Dowd, J. E. *Cancer Epidemiology: Methods of Study,* The Johns Hopkins Press, Baltimore, 1967.
2. Clark, D. W. A vocabulary for preventive medicine. In Clark, D. W., and MacMahon, B. (eds.): *Preventive Medicine,* Little, Brown & Co., Boston, 1967.
3. Treves, N., and Pack, S. T. The development of cancer in burn scars. *Surg. Gynecol. Obstet.,* 51:749–782 (1930).
4. Rosenthal, I. Reliability of retrospective reports of adolescence. *J. Consult. Clin. Psychol.,* 27:189–198 (1963).
5. Haggard, E., Brekstad, A., and Skard, A. On the reliability of the anamnestic interview. *J. Abnorm. Psychol.,* 61:311–318 (1960).
6. Newman, S. J., and Hansen, H. H. Frequency, diagnosis and treatment of brain metastases in 247 consecutive patients with bronchogenic carcinoma. *Cancer,* 33:492–496 (1974).
7. George, R. W. Cancer and other disorders related to certain perceptual tests. *Percept. Mot. Skills,* 30:155–161 (1970).
8. Paal, G. Zur Bedeutung psychischer Befunde für die Frühdiagnose von Hirntumoren. (The significance of psychological findings for early diagnosis of brain tumors.) *Schweiz. Arch. Neurol. Neurochir. Psychiatr.,* 97:135–143 (1966).
9. Brain, W. R., and Norris F. (eds.): *The Remote Effects of Cancer on the Nervous System,* Grune & Stratton, New York, 1965.
10. Richardson, E. P., Jr. The neurologic effects of cancer. In Holland, J. R., and Frei, E. III (eds.): *Cancer Medicine,* Lea & Febiger, Philadelphia, 1973.
11. Fras, I., Litin, E. M., and Pearson, J. S. Comparison of psychiatric manifestations in carcinoma of the pancreas with those in some other intra-abdominal neoplasms. *Am. J. Psychiatry,* 123:1553–1562 (1967).
12. Weiss, H. D., Walker, M. D., and Wiernik, P. H. Neurotoxicity of commonly used antineoplastic agents, Part I. *N. Engl. J. Med.,* 291:75–81 (1974).
13. Weiss, H. D., Walker, M. E., and Wiernik, P. H. Neurotoxicity of commonly used antineoplastic agents, Part II. *N. Engl. J. Med.,* 291:127–133 (1974).
14. Stavraky, K., Psychological factors in the outcome of human cancer. *J. Psychosom. Res.,* 12:251–259 (1968).
15. Schmale, A. H., and Iker, H. P. The effect of hopelessness and the development of cancer. *Psychosom. Med.,* 28:714–721 (1966).
16. Kissen, D. M. The significance of personality in lung cancer in men. In Bahnson, C. B., and Kissen, D. M. (eds.): Psychophysiological aspects of cancer. *Ann NY Acad Sci.,* 125:820–826 (1966).
17. Bahnson, C. B., and Kissen, D. M. (eds.): Psychophysiological aspects of cancer. *Ann NY Acad. Sci.,* 125:775–1055 (1966).
18. Krasnoff, A. Psychological variables and human cancer: A cross-validation study. *Psychosom. Med.,* 21:221–295 (1959).
19. Weir, J. *Psychosomatic Research in Cancer.* Prepublication draft. George Williams Hooper Foundation for Medical Research, University of California, San Francisco, 1972. By permission.
20. Perrin, G. M., and Pierce, I. R. Psychosomatic aspects of cancer. *Psychosom. Med.,* 21:397–421 (1959).

21. Hagnell, O. The premorbid personality of persons who develop cancer in a total population investigated in 1947 and 1957. In Bahnson, C. B., and Kissen, D. M. (eds.): Psychophysiological aspects of cancer. *Ann. NY Acad. Sci.*, 25:846–855 (1966).

22. Thomas, C. B., and Duszynski, K. R. Closeness to parents and the family constellation in a prospective study of five disease states: suicide, mental illness, malignant tumor, hypertension and coronary heart disease. *Johns Hopkins Med. J.*, 134:251–270 (1974).

23. Weir, J. Personal communication. George Williams Hooper Foundation for Medical Research, University of California, San Francisco, 1975.

24. Rassidakis, N. C., Kelepouris, M., Goulis, K., and Karaiossefidis, K. Malignant neoplasms as a cause of death among psychiatric patients. *Int. Ment. Health Res. Newsletter*, 14:1 (1972).

25. Sackler, A. M. Does schizophrenia protect against cancer? *Hosp. Tribune* (Jan. 1, 1973), p. 20.

26. Scheflen, A. E. Malignant tumors in the institutionalized population. *Arch. Neurol.*, 66:145–155 (1951).

27. Fox, B. H., and Howell, M. A. Cancer risk among psychiatric patients: A hypothesis. *Int. J. Epidemiol.*, 3:207–208 (1974).

28. Koss, L. G. Significance of dysplasia. *Clin. Obstet. Gynecol.*, 13:873–888 (1970).

29. Klein, E., Burgess, G. H., and Helm, F. Neoplasms of the skin. In Holland, J. F., and Frei, E. III (eds.): *Cancer Medicine*, Lea & Febiger, Philadelphia, 1973.

30. Everson, T. C. Spontaneous regression of cancer. *Ann. NY Acad. Med.*, 114:721–735 (1964).

31. Shank, R. C., Bhamarapravati, N., Gordon, J. E., and Wogan, G. N. *Food Cosmet. Toxicol.*, 10:171–179 (1972). Dietary aflatoxin and human liver cancer. IV. Incidence of primary liver cancer in two municipal populations of Thailand.

32. International Agency for Research on Cancer, 1970. Reported by Muir, C. S. Geographical Differences in Cancer Patterns. In Doll, R., and Vodopija, I. (eds.): *Host Environment Interactions in the Etiology of Cancer in Man*. WHO/IARC Sci. Publ. 7 (1973).

33. Miller, D. G. Preventive medicine by risk factor analysis. *JAMA*, 222:312–316 (1972).

34. Punnonen, R., Gronroos, M., and Peltonen, R. Increase of premalignant cervical lesions in teenagers. *Lancet*, ii:949 (1974).

35. *The Health Consequences of Smoking. A Report to the Surgeon General*, 1971. U.S. Dept. of Health, Education, and Welfare, U.S. Govt. Print. Off., Washington, D.C.

36. Enterline, P. E. Respiratory cancer among chromate workers. *J. Occup. Med.*, 16:523–526 (1974).

37. Tannenbaum, A. Nutrition and cancer. In Hornberger, F. (ed.): *Physiopathology of Cancer*, 2d ed., Harper & Row, New York, 1959.

38. Ross, M. H., and Bras, G. Tumor incidence patterns and nutrition in the rat. *J. Nutr.*, 37:245–260 (1965).

39. Ross, M. H. Length of life and caloric intake. *Am. J. Clin. Nutr.*, 25:834–838 (1972).

40. Bross, I. D. J., and Gibson, R. Cats and childhood leukemia. *J. Med. (Basel)*, 1:180–187 (1970).

41. Bross, I. D. J., Bertell, Sister Rosalie, and Gibson, R. Pets and adult leukemia. *Am. J. Public Health*, 62:1520–1531 (1972).

42. Peterson, B. H., Graham, J., Lemberger, L., and Dalton, B. Studies of the immune response in chronic marihuana smokers. *Pharmacologist*, 16:259 (1972). (Abstract)

Delay Behavior in Breast Cancer Screening

Raymond Fink

*Department of Research and Statistics, Health Insurance Plan of Greater New York,
New York, New York 10022*

Progress toward mass screening for early breast cancer detection will probably move forward in some areas of development, whereas other areas may move more slowly. We are aware of the potential for such programs from the results reported thus far from the breast cancer screening research program of the Health Insurance Plan of Greater New York (HIP). This study shows that periodic screenings involving the use of mammography and clinical breast examinations significantly reduce mortality from breast cancer (1). Technical advances in mammography equipment and the potential for screening procedures that reduce radiation exposure provide additional encouragement for the progress of breast cancer screening.

There remains, however, a number of significant issues that must be addressed to assure successful screening for this disease in a broad population and on a systematic basis. These include the frequency with which screening for breast cancer is most effective and the extent to which the costs of currently available screening methods draw on the financial and medical resource requirements for the care of other important health problems. Of particular relevance to these meetings are those issues relating to population participation in breast screening programs and the follow-up of positive findings detected on screening.

Opportunities to look at several of these considerations are available through some of the research and health action programs in the HIP. HIP is a prepaid, comprehensive medical-care program in which, at present, about 750,000 members are served by 28 multispecialty medical groups located in the five boroughs of New York City and in Nassau and Suffolk Counties on Long Island. HIP membership includes a broad spectrum of ethnic and socioeconomic groups. About half of the present membership includes employees of the government of the City of New York and their families. Membership also includes federal and state government employees and their families, and enrollees from union groups outside of government service. Enrollment through Medicaid constitutes 8% of the HIP membership and about 9% is through Medicare. HIP members, in return for a premium, are entitled to receive comprehensive medical care from physicians associated with the affiliated medical groups. Coverage is for preventive, diagnostic, and therapeutic services in the office, home, or hospital.

This report attempts to bring into perspective some of the findings of HIP research programs as these relate to specific issues of population participation in screening programs and to follow-up care for positive findings detected on screening. Several of these studies have introduced procedures which are aimed at maximizing response to health screening programs and which follow patients through the process of receiving health care based on these programs. Documentation of procedures used in contacting persons eligible for screening enables identification of the characteristics of participants and nonparticipants in these programs, and of the extent of their continued involvement in regular screenings. Some information is also available describing the process through which care is received following the detection of breast problems.

SOME RESEARCH ISSUES IN SCREENING FOR BREAST CANCER

Screening for breast cancer and, indeed, screening for cancer in other sites have some specific requirements that may not be applicable to other screening programs. Among these, for example, is the need for regularly spaced repetitive screening, rather than single efforts, although the issue of the interval between screens is not settled. Follow-up on positive screening observations by more closely spaced screening intervals or through the close personal observation of a physician is also a characteristic of screening for breast cancer. Another is the need for special X-ray and possibly other expensive equipment that generally requires centralized screening sites, although there are some successful mobile screening units. These requirements and other characteristics of breast disease call for a review of those issues of participation relating specifically to screening for breast disease, and those having broader applicability to screening for other disease and to the utilization of health services generally.

Some of the research issues we may wish to examine have been reviewed extensively in a range of health care settings, while others have barely been the subject of speculation. For example, there is developing substantial literature on some of the demographic factors associated with participation in preventive health care programs, and to a lesser extent on some of the attitudinal correlates (2). The relationship between participation in preventive health care programs and other health behavior is less well documented, however. Related to the latter is the question of the extent to which the phenomenon of self-selection for participation in screening programs is related to concern with a specific disease or concern for one's health in general.

Some of the data examined in this report are based on the special research opportunities offered in the setting of a prepaid group practice with a well-defined population base. These include the extent to which direct contact with target population individuals can increase response rates and influence the characteristics of the population screened. Also examined is the relationship between population characteristics and participation in repetitive screenings.

The greater part of the data presented here is based on findings of the HIP Mammography Study, a breast cancer screening research program started in 1963. Another source of data is the HIP study of the role of thermography in mass breast cancer screening. While the latter study is in an earlier stage of development than the mammography study and screenings are now under way, some of its contrasts offer useful insights.

HIP MAMMOGRAPHY STUDY

Design

In December 1963, in cooperation with 23 of its medical groups, HIP launched a large-scale screening program to determine whether periodic breast cancer screening with mammography and clinical examination holds promise for lowering mortality from breast cancer in the female population. Two stratified random samples of about 31,000 women, aged 40 to 64, were selected, one designated as the "study" group, the other as the "control" group. Study group women were offered an initial screening examination and three follow-up examinations at annual intervals, except for women found to have breast conditions requiring earlier follow-up.

Examinations were given at the medical group center where the women were enrolled, and 65% of the study women were examined at the intial screening examination. Women who did not have the initial screening examination were not asked to participate in the annual reexaminations. Attempts early in the study to involve nonparticipants in the initial examination in subsequent annual screenings brought too few of these into the program to justify the considerable effort required to gain their participation.

All women who came for examination were interviewed on various subjects including demographic characteristics, history of breast problems, and family history of cancer. A 20% random sample of examined women were further questioned about their prior health behavior and about their views on a number of health topics. A more brief interview was conducted among a random sample of nonparticipating women with listed telephones. Information on participation in the first examination is based on interviews with 1,125 women who had initial examinations during the first study year, and 633 telephone interviews with nonparticipants. Information on participation in the annual examinations is based on interviews with 3,232 examined women in the 20% sample during the full study period. Many of the findings described below which bring together earlier reports of this study, and study details, including research methods used, may be found in these sources (3,4).

Contacting Women

To achieve a reasonably high rate of response for the study group, direct letter and telephone contacts were used. Two weeks before a woman was scheduled to be examined she was informed by letter of the study and asked to make an appointment through the use of an enclosed postal card giving a choice of appointment hours. When the postal card was returned, she received in reply another postal card confirming the appointment and reminding her of the date and time. Women not responding to the first mailing received a second letter with appointment card, and telephone calls were made to women not responding to mail requests. The one-fourth of the study group without telephones were contacted only by mail. Women who failed to keep appointments were telephoned, and about 60% of these were eventually examined. Similar procedures were followed for the reexaminations.

Study women with at least the initial examination were classified into three major categories according to the effort required to gain their participation. These were: the "minimal effort group," women requiring only one mailing; the "secondary effort group," women who, after they had failed to appear for a scheduled examination, required either additional letters to gain their participation or who required a single contact after a missed appointment; and the "repeated effort group," women for whom telephone calls were required or for whom repeated attempts were made to reschedule examinations after failure to keep an appointment.

Results of Contacts

Among all women in the study sample both examined and not examined, 47% were in the "minimum effort group", 7% in the "secondary effort group", 10% in the "repeated effort group", and 35% were nonparticipants.[1] More than one-fourth of the examined women would not have participated had contact efforts been limited to one or two letters.

When compared with nonparticipants, participating women tended to be younger, better educated, more likely to be Jewish, and less likely to be Catholic. During the year preceding the breast screening examination participants were more likely to have seen an HIP physician. Participants were more likely than nonparticipants to be concerned about the possibility of having cancer and to report specific symptoms associated with cancer.

Increased contact efforts tended to have some small influence on the overall characteristics of the examined population, and while there were some large differences between the "minimum" and "repeated" groups, most differences were not large. Those requiring "repeated" efforts were more likely than the "minimum" group to be Catholic, foreign born, and low users of medical services generally. These "reluctant" respondents were also less likely to be

---

[1]Mammography study data reported here are based on the sample interviewed on special study questionnaires and may differ from total study findings due to sampling variability.

involved in the medical care programs of their medical groups as measured through their self-reports on the use of nongroup physicians and on whether they regarded a medical group physician as their sole family doctor. Those requiring repeated efforts were less likely than the others to report symptoms of or concern about cancer. The groups did not, however, differ significantly on age, marital status, ethnic background, income, or most recent occupation. There was also no difference in time required to travel to their medical group.

Contact Effort and Participation in Annual Examinations

Sixty percent of those who participated in the initial examination also had the three subsuquent annual examinations for breast cancer. Only 12% had the initial examination alone and another 12% the initial and one annual examination. In the "minimum" group 67% had all four examinations compared with 50% in the "secondary" group and 38% in the "repeated" group. Of particular significance is that even in the group requiring the most effort to bring into the study initially, that is, the "repeated" group, 56% had either three or four examinations.

In general, many of the variables differentiating between those having the full series of examinations and those who did not, also characterized the differences between participants and nonparticipants in the initial examination. Thus, the same population groups who participate tend to remain in the program through the full set of examinations. On the other hand, the participation of more than half the "repeated" group in three or four examination marks some success in involving those initially reluctant to do so in a set of repetitive examinations over several years.

The test of the value of involving those requiring additional efforts in breast screening programs is the extent to which breast cancer is detected in this group and the effect of early intervention resulting from the screening program. Present evidence indicates that involving the reluctant participant in breast cancer screening contributes to detection at a stage of development of the disease which improves its prognosis. First, rates of detection on screening are about the same for the "minimum" group as for those requiring greater efforts. In addition, in both "minimum" and 'secondary" groups, the proportions of those diagnosed on screening or between screenings with no axillary node involvement was the same—about 62%. Among study nonparticipants there were only 40% with no axillary node involvement.

Some Further Observations on Nonparticipants

Additional insights into reasons for nonparticipation in the breast cancer screening program come from study observations comparing causes of death among study participants and nonparticipants. From mail survey and death records

5 years after entry into the study, it was found that while the total mortality rate was the same for both groups, mortality from all causes other than breast cancer was considerably greater among nonparticipants than among participants (nonparticipants, 77.4 deaths per 10,000; participants 41.5 deaths per 10,000). The major contribution to this difference was in the category "circulatory system" (nonparticipants, 38.0 deaths per 10,000; participants, 16.7 deaths per 10,000). These observations, taken togehter with survey response differences between participants and nonparticipants, provide further insights into reasons for nonparticipation. Nonparticipants were considerably more likely to agree with the following statements than participants: "I only take X-rays and check-ups for sicknesses which I might actually have," and "My doctor already knows all my health conditions without my having to take any more special tests." It would thus appear that one operating factor in the self-selection process may have been greater concern among nonparticipants with diseases other than breast cancer.

RESPONSE RATE COMPARISONS IN CENTRALIZED AND DECENTRALIZED SETTINGS

As noted earlier, Mammography Study screening examinations were conducted in the medical groups where women received their usual medical care. In addition, the medical groups are often selected by HIP members because they are conveniently located near their homes. In planning the Mammography Study it was anticipated, partly because of this, that a response rate of 65% could be achieved. There is presently under way in HIP another study on the use of thermography, a rapid heat-radiation technique in mass screening for early breast cancer detection. Methods for contacting women in the Thermography Study are substantially the same as those used in the Mammography Study, and a random sample of women age 45 through 64 years is being contacted through these procedures for the first of two examinations to be given at 2-year intervals. A total of 20,000 women will receive the initial examination and be contacted for the biennial examination.

A major difference between the two studies is that screening in the Thermography Study is being done in three centralized hospitals in the New York City area. This is necessary because the high cost of the required study equipment makes direct medical group involvement financially unfeasible. It was expected from the beginning that the response rate in this study would be in the 40 to 50% range, and at the time when 2,853 had been contacted for participation, utilizing the full set of contact procedures, 44% had been examined. Although this preliminary response rate is substantially lower than in the Mammography Study, it has been observed that nearly three-fourths of those who are screened participate in response to a minimal contact only, and that additional contact efforts are needed to achieve response rates suitable for study requirements (see Table 1). This fact appears to confirm the expectation that removal of screening from women's usual source of medical care reduces response rates.

TABLE 1. *Participation in initial breast cancer screening examination and effort required to gain participation in medical group and in centralized hospital programs*

	Study site			
	Medical group[a]		Central Hospital	
Effort required	Study group sample (%)	Participant sample (%)	Study group sample (%) [b]	Participant sample (%) [c]
Participants	65	100	44	100
Minimum	47	73	33	74
Secondary	7	11	4	10
Repeated	10	16	7	16
Nonparticipants	35	—	56	—
Total number of participants	4,972	3,232	2,853	1,255

[a] Based on data from a 20% sample of women contacted in the HIP Mammography Study.
[b] Includes all women in the HIP Thermography Study initially contacted during the period from December 1, 1973 through February 28, 1974, and for whom all contact efforts were completed. This does not include women contacted but for whom efforts were not exhausted by the cutoff date of October 1, 1974.
[c] Includes all women examined by September 3, 1974.

FROM BIOPSY RECOMMENDATION TO BIOPSY

One of the uncharted areas in our understanding of the process of cancer care is patient movement through the medical care system following a recommendation of biopsy by a physician. For the most part, interest in receiving medical care for specific health problems has centered on the speed with which medical care is sought once a person has detected a symptom (5). Screening programs introduce the elements of the medical care system and physician judgement into the patient's movement toward medical care, and these will, of course, heavily influence patient decision and action in the course of seeking this care.

Even in the relatively closed system of a prepaid, medical group practice, the steps from biopsy recommendation to surgery are often not direct. In the HIP Mammography Study the processing of screening reports by a study staff includes confirmation of positive observations by more than a single physician and then notification of positive findings to the medical group physician responsible for the patient's care. To assure rapid movement of patients in the screening program with positive findings, a special study staff worked with medical group physicians in bringing these patients to early diagnostic work-up where recommended.

The physician responsible for the patient's care also enters into the decision process, of course. The physician may choose to act very quickly on a biopsy recommendation, or to defer action pending further observations.

The patient may or may not choose to act quickly once informed that the breast screening indicates the need for medical attention. Some women sought second opinions from surgeons outside of HIP, and study staff provided these physicians with screening information, including mammograms when needed. Women with

TABLE 2. *Elapsed months between biopsy recommendation based on screening by result and source of recommendation, HIP mammography study*

Elapsed months	Total	Radiological only		Clinical only [a]		Both		Total	
		Con-firmed (%)	Benign (%)	Con-firmed (%)	Benign (%)	Con-firmed (%)	Benign (%)	Con-firmed (%)	Benign [a] (%)
Less than 2 months	72	50	53	92	79	93	83	78	71
Two months or more, less than 4 months	19	34	36	7	12	4	17	15	20
Four months or more	9	16	11	2	10	3	—	7	10
Total %	100	100	100	101	101	100	100	100	101
Total no. of biopsies	649	44	159	59	333	29	25	132	517

[a] Does not notal 100% because of rounding.

breast problems recommeded for biopsy may wish to defer this, and in some cases there were refusals to permit surgery.

For this report, information on the total process of moving toward biopsy in the screening program is limited to variables reflecting those parts of the process associated with physicians' decisions. Some of this information is presented here to lift the curtain on the total transition to surgery.

A total of about 1,000 women were recommended for biopsy as a result of initial or follow-up breast screenings. It is known that from 98 to 99% consulted a physician concerning these recommendations. About 80% of the recommendations were confirmed by physicians providing care, and four out of five went to surgery. Among those who did not go to surgery, the failure was largely due to physician preference for keeping the patient under further observation before going to surgery. Information continues to be obtained by the study staff about these patients.

Information is presented here on the elapsed time between the biopsy recommendation and surgery for 649 women who went to biopsy on the basis of a screening recommendation (Table 2). The date of a biopsy recommendation is defined here as the examination that culminated in a biopsy recommendation. In many cases this recommendation was made some time after the screening date when a positive finding was reported. Women were often placed under closer observation by the study staff or the physicians, and a biopsy recommendation may not have been made immediately following screening. Women with suspicious finding on screening may have been recalled 3 months later, for example, and a biopsy recommended at that time. [Note: This method of measuring elapsed time between recommendation and biopsy should be distinguished from procedures used to measure lead time gained in breast cancer detection using mammography and a clinical examination of the breast. The baseline data used in measuring lead time is the date of screening when any positive finding called a woman to the study group's attention even if it did not result at that time in a recommendation for biopsy (6).]

Seventy-two percent of the biopsies based on screening evidence were performed within 2 months of the recommendation, and an additional 20% were performed in 2 to 4 months following the recommendation. Elapsed time from recommendation to biopsy differed somewhat according to the outcome of the biopsy and according to whether the recommendation was based on radiological or clinical evidence. Seventy-eight percent of the biopsies resulting in a confirmed breast cancer were performed within 2 months of the recommendation, and 71% of the benign cases received surgery within this length of time. Biopsies based on clinical recommendations were more likely to be performed within 2 months of the recommendation than those based on radiological readings. Among women with confirmed cancers, 92% of the biopsies based on clinical recommendations were performed within 2 months, and 50% of the biopsies based on radiological recommendations were performed within this elapsed time, while another 34% were done 2 to 4 months following the recommendation. These differences may be largely due to the additional steps required to bring to biopsy positive findings based on radiological evidence. The elapsed time between physician visit and biopsy was increased by the time it takes to complete study procedures for reading mammography films and to transmit findings to the provider of care. Clinically based recommendations were often made by the physician, who also had the responsibility for the surgical care of the patient.

These findings suggest that part of the delay in reaching biopsy may be related to how the physician providing medical care regards the recommendation of the Mammography Study physician. Surgeons considering a biopsy recommendation appear more willing to act on a palpable mass than on the kinds of lesions often revealed through mammography. Moreover, it should be recalled that this study was conducted during a period when the use of mammography for breast cancer screening was untested and when some hesitation about performing biopsies on this evidence alone might be expected.

DISCUSSION

The HIP Mammography Study employed a continuous process in which multiple efforts were made to involve the target population of women in the initial and annual examinations, and to bring those with positive findings to medical care. Increased efforts to contact women resulted in a 65% response rate, about one-third higher than what might have been reached through the minimal efforts of one or two letters. Similar efforts brought 60% of those who had the initial screening into the full set of three additional annual screenings, and 78% had at least one additional screening.

It was observed that women in higher socioeconomic groups and women more involved with the HIP medical care system were more likely than others to participate in the initial screening, findings in conformity with those of other studies of participation in preventive health examinations (7). It was also noted that the same characteristics of those participating initially also described those who tended to have the annual examinations, although there was a fair return rate among women in the lower socioeconomic group as well.

Strategies that would maximize response rates to screening programs for breast cancer must take into account the accessibility of the screening facilities and population characteristics as well. The HIP Thermography Study is currently screening women in three hospital centers in New York rather than in HIP medical groups, to maximize the use of the equipment needed for the program. This resulted in the "trade-off" of a lower anticipated response rate for the screenings. It is not now known how this will alter response rates among different socioeconomic groups. Also in the Mammography Study, while distance from the medical group was unrelated to efforts required to gain participation in the initial examination, there was a relationship between distance from the center and participation in annual examinations.

Involvement of population groups on a broad base is a complex problem. Of particular difficulty for solution is how to obtain participation rates from low-income groups. Research evidence identifies as a possible major factor in the low medical care utilization among this group the low use of preventive health services (8). Outreach programs have had some success in bringing to regular medical attention those with chronic health conditions (9), but preventive health service programs appear to present different problems for involving the poor.

Finally, with regard to strategies for involving population groups in mass screening, the identification of high-risk groups would be promising if such groups were readily known and identifiable. Appeals can be concentrated on these high-risk groups urging their participation, and self-selection for screening among this group would be desirable. Regrettably, for breast cancer there is no set of variables offering a high degree of sensitivity and specificity (10). Should such variables be identified, questionnaires and health histories fashioned according to current survey research techniques would be of considerable value in bringing these groups to the attention of screeners.

We have had only limited views of how the medical system operates in bringing medical care to persons with health problems diagnosed through screening. The use of cohort studies following patients through the system of care is of great value for observing this process. Cases detected on screening bring into play actions of both patient and providers of care. We know little about the "bargaining" process that may take place in those circumstances.

Research techniques are now available that would allow the documentation of steps in the process from designation of a target population, through repetitive examinations, and through the treatment process, with measurements of treatment outcomes. Involved is a combination utilizing medical records, vital records, and survey reserach techniques in cohort studies. Used together these techniques can open the field of investigations that would better enable us to understand behavioral dynamics in the detection and care of cancer.

ACKNOWLEDGEMENTS

The studies reported here are supported in part by contracts NO1 CP 43278 and 1-CN-35021, from the National Cancer Institute. I am grateful for the aid provided by Nancy Ampel, Ruth Roeser, and Wanda Venet in the preparation of this report.

REFERENCES

1. Shapiro, S., Strax, P., Venet, L., and Venet, W. Changes in 5-year breast cancer mortality in a breast cancer screening program. In *7th National Cancer Conference Proceedings*, pp. 663–678, J. B. Lippincott Co., Philadelphia.
2. Coburn, D., and Pope, C. R. Socioeconomic status and preventive health behaviour. *J. Health Soc. Behav.*, 15:67–78 (1974).
3. Fink, R., Shapiro, S., and Lewison, J. The reluctant participant in a breast cancer screening program. *Public Health Rep.*, 83:479–490 (1967).
4. Fink, R., Shapiro, S., and Roeser, R. Impact of efforts to increase participation in repetitive screenings for early breast cancer detection. *Am. J. Public Health*, 62:328–336 (1972).
5. Goldsen, R. K. Patient delay in seeking cancer diagnosis: Behavioral aspects. *J. Chron. Dis.*, 16:428–435 (1963).
6. Shapiro, S., Goldberg, J. D., and Hutchison, G. B. Lead time in breast cancer detection and implications for periodicity of screening. *Am. J. Epidemiol.*, 100:357–366 (1974).
7. Hochbaum, G. M. Public participation in medical screening programs: A socio-psychological study. *PHS Publ.*, 572, U.S. Govt. Print. Off., Washington, D.C. (1958).
8. Rabin, P. L., Bice, T. W., and Starfield, B. Use of health services by Baltimore Medicaid recipients. *Med. Care*, 12:561–570 (1974).
9. Sparer, G., and Okada, L. Utilization and costs of health services among OEO eligibles in prepaid medical group practice. Paper presented at *100th Annual Meeting, Am. Public Health Assoc.*, 1972.
10. Shapiro, S., Goldberg, J., Venet, L., and Strax, P. Risk factors in breast cancer—A prospective study. In *Host Environment Interactions in the Etiology of Cancer in Man*, pp. 169–182, IARC, Lyon, 1973.

Cancer: The Behavioral Dimensions, edited by J. W. Cullen, B. H. Fox, and R. N. Isom. Raven Press, New York © 1976.

Factors Related to Preventive Health Behavior

Aaron Antonovsky and Ofra Anson

Department of the Sociology of Health, Faculty of Health Sciences, Ben-Gurion University of the Negev, Beersheba, Israel

An underlying premise of this chapter is that it is helpful to study the twin problems of delay in taking action on the appearance of symptoms and of participation in detection examinations by considering them in a broader context. In previous papers (1,2), influenced by the work of Rene Dubos (3), the concept of "generalized resistance resources" was discussed (see ref. 4). It was suggested that the interaction between the resistance resources at one's disposal and the nature of the problem or threat leads to a given health behavior outcome. In using this phrase, we referred both to relatively specific variables, such as knowledge, level of anxiety, and degree of involvement with health institutions, and to more global variables, such as general value orientations and patterns of social relations. This chapter described how such resistance resources are linked to specific behavior patterns with respect to cancer control. Implicit in our argument, although not detailed here, is the idea that such resources are also related to a wide variety of health behaviors.

We found it useful [in the context of developing a model to explain visits to the doctor (5)] to use the idea of the epidemiological triangle as a way of organizing consideration of the multiple factors that influence the behavior of individuals. It may likewise be useful to do so in the present context, seeing the index case as the host, the health institution as the "agent," and the broader and immediate social and cultural relationships of the host as the environment. We suggest that the focus on only the psychological characteristics of the index case, so often found in work on preventive health behavior (including my own; e.g., ref. 6) has unnecessarily limited us. Since in the last analysis we are dealing with voluntary action on the part of the individual, the characteristics of the agent and the environment are influential only as they are filtered through the host's perception.

I think the data from the study reported here can best be analyzed and presented in terms of this approach.

STUDY DESIGN AND METHODS

In view of the limited budget at our disposal, the study was originally designed in pilot terms, aiming at the exploration of various hypotheses proposed in the literature to explain the significant degree of delay in turning to professionals after recognition of a sign, and of failure to participate in preventive and early detection screening programs (7,8).

The study was conducted in a small Israeli city in the Spring of 1972. A breast cancer detection clinic, linked to the general hospital outpatient clinics, is open several afternoons a week. Most of the women attending the clinic come in response to written invitations sent out by the Cancer Association, although some are referred by their family physicians and others come on their own initiative. The clinic has been in operation for a number of years. The response to the invitation, which is sent to women aged 35 and over, and selected randomly from the Population Registry, tends to be greater than in similar clinics elsewhere in Israel.

The "experimental" sample consisted of 58 consecutive women attending the clinic, excluding those referred for biopsy. Our intention was to select an individually matched control sample by selecting the name of the woman following the index case in the Population Registry and within the same 5-year age group. The women in the two groups were interviewed at their homes within several days after the examination. The study, however, was cut short because of budgetary reasons after only 40 of the control women had been interviewed.

Ready for data analysis, we belatedly became aware of an even more serious flaw that should have been—but was not—anticipated. Of the 40 control women, 17 had attended the clinic or had had an examination elsewhere, relatively recently, whereas 23 had not been examined for at least 4 years. In the initial data analysis, then, comparisons were made between the 40 "experimental" women for whom there were controls, the 17 controls "examined," and the 23 controls "unexamined." Given these severe limitations, the remarks based on the initial data analysis can only be regarded as suggestive, and will be limited to the major issues investigated.

INITIAL DATA ANALYSIS

Anxiety

Whether one looks at the score of generalized anxiety we obtained, or the responses to questions measuring anxiety about diseases, or anxiety which is cancer-specific (susceptibility, seriousness, salience, or image of breast cancer examinations), there is no unequivocal reason to believe that this variable can serve as a powerful predictor for participation or nonparticipation in voluntary examinations. Actually, the 23 "unexamined" women had a somewhat lower level of anxiety (as measured by a psychosomatic scale) than did the others. Quite conceivably, extremely anxious women would be so immobilized as to refrain from any action. Where anxiety measures are very low, it might be a massive denial of existent anxiety or, if genuine, it might lead to feeling no need whatsoever for action. These extremes, however, characterize few women. Given more moderate levels of anxiety, there is no reason to think that anxiety prevents women from being examined.

Knowledge of and Personal Experience with Cancer

There is no patterned difference among the groups with respect to knowledge of cancer symptoms. Actually, the great majority performed poorly on an open question about symptoms; on the series of closed questions, most correct symptoms were identified by most women, although many referred to other signs as possible cancer symptoms. Similarly, the groups did not differ on personal contact with cancer patients, optimism about the possibilities of early detection, or of a cure being found.

Image of Physician Attitudes and Preventive Examinations

In this area, too, we find no hint that would suggest why women go or do not go for examinations. Most of the women do not think that doctors either encourage or discourage participation in preventive examinations, whether generally or for cancer detection specifically. Such examinations are viewed positively by most women. Physicians, too, are generally esteemed. There is, then, no indication of any particular barrier in this area.

Norms and Supports

In contrast to the above areas, we find some indication here why women go for examinations. There is general agreement among all groups that going for a preventive examination is at least a preferred, if not a prescribed, social norm. However, the "unexamined" controls tend to perceive the woman who never goes as busy, healthy, and relaxed, rather than as lazy, foolish, tense, or irresponsible. Further, while most women believe that their friends and husbands do not object to their going for cancer examinations, and do not feel that discussing the matter with them is taboo, the "unexamined" controls less often reported that their husbands pressured them to go.

But perhaps the strongest evidence for the significance of social pressures is found in the content analysis of the responses to the series of open questions posed to the 58 women in the "experimental" sample. These questions were designed to clarify what had led them to go to the clinic. Of the 58, 40 women (69%) explicitly referred to some clear social support: they went either with a friend or relative, or at the urging of husband, doctor, or friend. That such social support is of some significance is suggested when combined with the data on anxiety in this section. Of the 39 women who gave no particular indication of anxiety, 22 (56%) reported having some social support for their participation. This contrasts sharply with the 19 women reporting anxiety: all but one of them (95%) indicated having social support. Thus, for the more anxious women, social support seems to be an important factor in going for an examination.

Involvement in the World of Illness and Medicine

Heretofore, both the methodological inadequacies of the study and the lack of clear-cut results have enabled us to do no more than tentatively point to the possible significance of the role of social supports in facilitating participation in voluntary breast cancer examinations. In the final major area covered in the questionnaire, however, the evidence seems to be much stronger. On nine of the 10 items posed in this area, the "unexamined" controls indicated substantially less involvement in the world of illness and medicine.

1. They go to the doctor less often when not really sick but suspect something
2. They were less often worried about their health in the last year
3. When worried about their health, they often delay going to the doctor
4. Fewer of them think they have any need for a special preventive examination since their doctor knows their state of health
5. Their self-estimation of health status is higher
6. They less often feel incapable of coping with their problems
7. More of them believe they see the doctor later than most other women do
8. They less often tend to define themselves as ill
9. Although a majority of all women never went for a preventive general check-up, this is even more true of the "unexamined" group

There is only one item that does not correlate. More of the "unexamined" controls than of the "examined" controls (although not of the "experimental" group) had been to a dentist for a preventive check-up.

To understand these data, it is important to consider the sociocultural context in which they were collected. Israel has the highest rate of visits to the doctor in the world (5,9). Moreover, contrary to the rest of the world, there is a clear tendency in Israel toward an inverse association between social class status and use of health services. This is particularly true of curative services. In other words, the technical, normative, and institutional barriers to the utilization of health services in Israel are relatively weak. This is not to say that this pattern extends, for most, to the use of preventive services in breast cancer detection; only a minority of women have taken advantage of the available services. But to the extent that we have been able to pinpoint differences in such utilization, it would seem that the greater involvement in the world of illness and medicine, the more likely are women to use such services, particularly when personal social supports operate in this direction.

Finally, we suggest that, given this context, which serves as a potential for most Israeli women, the most effective trigger likely to increase the use of preventive services is the active encouragement by family physicians. This is not the case today, in fact, or as perceived by most of the women interviewed. Such encouragement may not persuade women with a relatively low involvement in the world of illness and medicine, but it should be particularly effective among those with an already high involvement.

A DIFFERENT APPROACH TO THE DATA

The shortcomings of the above analysis are self-evident. Further progress, however, seemed to be promised by considering the implications of the theoretical orientation presented in the first part of this chapter. Can we formulate, we asked ourselves, a typology of orientations by studying the total set of data for each of the 98 women interviewed, irrespective of whether the woman was in the "experimental" or control group? The question then became not one of statistical comparison of groups, but rather: Under what circumstances is a woman of a given type likely to voluntarily take part in a breast cancer examination? After intensive consideration of each protocol, we were able to formulate a fourfold typology, and classify each of the women as fitting into one of the four types. We have labeled these four types the "conformist," the "rational-goal-directed," the "complacent-stoic," and the "ambivalent-anxious." It will be noted that the typology is formulated in terms of a general orientation to health behavior, and seeks to incorporate the three aspects of the epidemiological triangle.

The Conformist Woman

The crucial characteristic of this type of woman is the rote-like pattern of behavior into which she falls. The behavior does not derive from a direct, substantive connection with a specific need or cognition, but is a stereotyped response to a given situation, determined by external forces. She is characterized by a relatively high level of somaticized anxiety, which is accompanied by a fatalistic image of cancer as a dread disease. She is likely to have a low educational background, and responds to questions of a more speculative kind with reference to God and fate. Given ambiguous health symptoms, she has a strong tendency to enter the sick role. On the other hand, given a sign which is neither painful, functionally limiting, nor definitely associated with an illness, she is not likely to take action. By and large she has a positive image of the physician and full confidence in his competence. This is not a rational evaluation, but part of the rote-like, nonquestioning behavior. Her attitude toward general examinations, breast examinations, or women who go for them is neutral. It is something one does (if, indeed, one has gotten into the habit of doing so) above all because the doctor or someone else has told one that this is the right thing to do, but also because "this is what everyone does." In this sense, she is other-directed and highly sensitive to conformity to the norms of her reference groups. She is reminiscent of the women of whom Johnson et al (10) wrote in describing the lower-class American women in their Dade County study who were likely to take their children for polio prophylaxis.

The Rational Goal-Directed Woman

This is the type of woman toward whom the traditional cancer education program has been aimed. She is inner-directed, and tends to evaluate and rank alternative behavior patterns in terms of their consistency with consciously defined goals. She is likely to have a relatively high educational background. Her self-image is on the positive, satisfactory side, both in terms of her health and her general ability to cope. She ranks middling in her tendency to enter the sick role, neither denying nor exaggerating symptoms. Her anxiety level is on the low-to-moderate side. She does not particularly distinguish between cancer and other serious chronic diseases such as heart disease and mental illness. She neither denies nor exaggerates her susceptibility to them, their salience for her, or their seriousness. She is neither particularly optimistic nor pessimistic about the possi-bilities of discovering a cure for cancer or of the effectiveness of early detection. Her attitudes toward and behavior in relation to physicians, the health care system, general check-ups, and cancer examinations are molded by a notion of the goal or purpose it serves. Generally positive, the key question for her is whether or not it is worthwhile. If she is persuaded that it is, there are no particular deterrents to her going to the doctor. She may not even care for him, but the only question for her is whether a good job will be done.

The Complacent-Stoic Woman

This woman is similar to the rational-goal-directed type in that she is likely to be of high educational background, and to see herself as healthy and competent. Crucial to this type of woman, however, is that she has achieved homeostasis, at least with respect to the world of health and medicine. True, she has a positive image of the medical institution, but it is one with little personal meaning. Her manifest anxiety level is very low, as is her tendency to enter the sick role. Intellectually, and in general terms, preventive check-ups make sense. She does not see herself as less susceptible to cancer than do others. However, such cognitions are not linked, for her, with personal action; she tends to see the woman who goes for such examinations as hypochondriacal and the time as wasted. All this is not to say that there is a rigid refusal to enter the world of health care. A clear symptom, upsetting her usual ability to function, will move her to action, but it would have to be quite clear. Similarly, the death from cancer of someone close to her, or strong pressure from husband or friends, may move her.

The Ambivalent-Anxious Woman

The final type of woman we identified is most strikingly characterized by a high level of anxiety, both in general terms and with specific reference to cancer. The latter expresses itself both on the psychosomatic scale and in her refusal to answer questions linking cancer to herself, and in her negative image of cancer examina-tions and the woman who goes for them. This is part of her generally fearful picture of preventive actions. She believes they are pointless or she is afraid of what might be found. This does not mean that she avoids the medical world. Her self-image is ambivalent and shifting, as is her image of physicians and her tendency to enter the sick role. The pattern, then, is one of instability and unpredictability. There is neither a sense of mastery and stable adaptation to her world, nor a sense of submission, which can be no less stably adaptive. This type of woman is most often of a low-to-moderate educational level.

Distribution of the Four Types

The typology depicted here is made up of ideal types. We would not claim that every woman classified in a given type fits perfectly into the description. Yet by and large the protocol of each woman enabled us to classify her in one of the four types, without, we believe, significant distortion. Since the 98 women included in our study do not constitute a sample, the distribution among the four types is meaningless. We are interested, rather, in whether the use of this typology can help us predict participation in examinations in detection clinics. This time the population was divided into four groups: "regular goers", those who had been examined at least twice in the 4-year period before the study (including the study examination); "new goers," those who had been examined in the 2 years before the study, but not in the 2 years before that; "once goers," those examined 3 or 4 years before the study, but not since; and "never goers," those not examined in the 4-year period. The distribution of the four types among these four groups is shown in Table 1.

TABLE 1. *General orientation by breast examination participation*

Examination behavior	Orientation			
	Conformist (%) (N=31)	Rational-goal-directed (%) (N=27)	Complacent-stoic (%) (N=22)	Ambivalent-anxious (%) (N=18)
Regular goer	38.5	37	9	17
New goer	38.5	44	46	77
Once goer	10	4	18	—
Never goer	13	15	27	6

The data in Table 1 indicate some predictive value in the typology we have presented. More of the conformist women than of the other types are regular goers, with very few who have not gone in recent years. It should be stressed, however, that this has occurred in a very specific cultural context. Such women may, in other sociocultural contexts, very well fall into the "never goers" category. The rational-goal-directed women show a very similar distribution, but the dynamics involved are totally different. The complacent-stoic women are found at the other extreme, almost none of them being regular goers, more than twice as many of them as of any other group being never goers. The ambivalent-anxious women, as would be expected, fall in between. However, the great majority of them have indeed gone in the most recent period, although not earlier.

IMPLICATIONS

The significance of this approach, however, does not lie in the predictive capacity of the typology in a given sociohistorical context. It is more important, we believe, to conclude by taking note of its implications for action programs.

We opened our discussion by referring to the need to consider the agent and environment characteristics, objectively and as perceived by the index case, in seeking to understand the factors related to preventive health behavior. We have considered the relationship of people to the health institutions, to norms and social pressures in a given culture context, as well as the more psychological characteristics of the individuals studied. Furthermore, we suggested that the concept of resistance resources would be helpful in studying preventive health behavior. Each of the different types described controls a different type of potential resistance resource, each of which is activated in a different manner in the total gamut of health behavior. In the present context, this includes both delay and participation in detection examinations. In other words, different strategies and appeals must be made in order to induce the desired behavior.

As suggested earlier, the traditional campaigns of cancer agencies, in which rational self-interest, knowledge of symptoms and benefits, and the like are stressed, are most appropriate to the rational-goal-directed type. The conformist type, by contrast, is not likely to take independent initiative, and will respond primarily to institutionalized mechanisms and social pressures, followed by reinforcement until the behavior is ritualized. In a country like Israel, the family physician or the work group may play this role. The complacent-stoic type, it seems to us, will best respond to the stress on self-examination. Discovery of a symptom may constitute a sufficient disturbance of homeostasis to lead to action. One must, however, be skeptical and seek other ways. Increasing knowledge, however, is not likely to have any effect. But, at least, one can count on random disturbances of homeostasis. It is the ambivalent-anxious type, however, that seems to be the most difficult group. This is perhaps the one type in which a particular anxiety about cancer may play an important role and for whom locating the cancer examination within the context of general examinations may be appropriate.

Within the framework of this relatively brief presentation, we have attempted to do no more than suggest, in rough outline, an approach which seems to us to be fruitful both in advancing theoretical understanding of the health behavior of people and in suggesting implications for action programs. Clearly, much work remains to be done.

ACKNOWLEDGMENTS

The study upon which this chapter is based was supported by grants from the

Bar-Lehrmsdorf Research Fund and the Israel Cancer Association. This assistance, and the cooperation and encouragement of Mrs. Miriam Klein, secretary of the Association, and Dr. Zeev Teva, director of the clinic at which the study was conducted, are gratefully acknowledged.

REFERENCES

1. Antonovsky, A. Breakdown: A needed fourth step in the conceptual armamentarium of modern medicine. *Soc. Sci. Med.,* 6:537–544 (1972).
2. Antonovsky, A. The utility of the breakdown concept. *Soc. Sci. Med.,* 7:605–612 (1973).
3. Dubos, R. *Man Adapting,* Yale University Press, New Haven, 1965.
4. Selye, H. *The Stress of Life,* McGraw-Hill, New York, 1956.
5. Antonovsky, A. A model to explain visits to the doctor: With specific reference to the case of Israel. *J. Health Soc. Behav.,* 13:446–454 (1972).
6. Rosenstock, I.M. Health behavior: Prevention and maintenance. In Kosa, J., Antonovsky, A., and Zola, I.K. (eds.): *Poverty and Health,* Harvard University Press, Cambridge, 1969.
7. Antonovsky, A., and Hartman, H. Delay in the detection of cancer: A review of the literature. *Health Educ. Monogr.,* 2:98–128 (1974).
8. Green, L.W., and Roberts, B.J. The research literature on why women delay in seeking medical care for cancer symptoms. *Health Educ. Monogr.,* 2:129–177 (1974).
9. Shuval, J.T., Antonovsky, A., and Davies, A.M. *Social Functions of Medical Practice: Doctor-Patient Relationships in Israel,* Jossey-Bass, San Francisco, 1970.
10. Johnson, A.L., et al. Epidemiology of polio vaccine acceptance. *Florida State Board of Health Monogr.,* 3 (1962).

Cancer: The Behavioral Dimensions, edited by J. W. Cullen, B. H. Fox, and R. N. Isom. Raven Press, New York © 1976.

Site- and Sympton-Related Factors in Secondary Prevention of Cancer

Lawrence W. Green

Division of Health Education, School of Hygiene and Public Health, Johns Hopkins University, Baltimore, Maryland, 21205

A potential source of confusion in our discussion of the behavioral and communication aspects of cancer control, I predict, will be the degree to which we consider cancer as a single entity. As behavioral scientists concerned with the development of theory, we are obliged to seek generalizable probabilities about behavior across the widest possible range of neoplastic phenomena, if not all diseases. As behavioral scientists concerned with operational problems in cancer control, however, we are obliged to seek applications of behavioral concepts and theories in more specific programmatic areas. William James (p. 9, ref. 1) once characterized these two orientations as "rationalist" and "empiricist" temperaments:

...empiricist meaning your lover of facts in all their crude variety, rationalist meaning your devotee to abstract and eternal principles. No one can live an hour without both facts and principles, so it is a difference rather of emphasis, yet it breeds antipathies of the most pungent character between those who lay the emphasis differently.

In previous conferences of this kind, I have noted that the proceedings tend to lean toward the first obligation to theory and away from the latter, more frustrating concern with concrete applications in specific disease or symptom categories. Most of us here are better known for our contributions as "rationalists" than as "empiricists," so we risk playing this conference to the wrong audience, namely, ourselves and each other. As one frustrated practitioner (2) recently commented in response to a behavioral scientist's selective review of the cancer literature (3): "It is not enough for scientists to take the lid off the health care system; they must be prepared to get in among pain and death and grief and help to set things to right."

We must conceptualize, because the subject is too complex to discuss at the specific, empirical level, so we must find the proper level at which generalization does not lose touch with reality:

Properly speaking, concepts are post-mortem preparations, sufficient only for retrospective understanding; and when we use them to define the universe prospectively we ought to realize that they can give only a bare abstract outline or approximate sketch, in the filling out of which perception must be invoked (p. 99, ref. 4).

PURPOSE AND SCOPE

This chapter assesses the generalizability of perception and behavior from one kind of cancer to another, thereby determining the degree to which similar or distinct strategies should be employed in different programs. Other chapters in this volume address the question of generalizability of strategies from one population or cultural group to another (see also ref. 5). My assignment here is to focus on site- and symptom-specific variations in behavior in secondary prevention, but I attempt to place this topic in perspective for this volume by reviewing first the evidence for and against generalizing between primary and secondary preventive health behavior, and second, the degree of variability or consistency in medical care utilization behavior. Finally, the degree and possible sources of variation in delay behavior between different cancer sites and symptoms are analyzed.

APPROACH

An analysis of these questions might help to avoid certain errors of induction in theorizing about cancer behavior and certain errors of deduction in proposing strategies for specific cancer problems on the basis of oversimplified behavioral concepts or theories. The research question we must ask in order to avoid the errors of induction is whether individuals respond variably or similarly to different health threats and different health services. In secondary prevention, specifically, the question is whether the individual variations in delay between sites or symptoms exceed the variations between individuals or groups (types) of individuals. If so, then the implication for program planning is that cancer control strategies must be designed specifically for different sites and symptoms. These site- and symptom-specific programs can then be more or less standardized for different populations. If not (i.e., if the variation in delay between demographic groups exceeds the variation within groups according to sites and symptoms), then cancer control programs can be more or less standardized without regard to specific sites and symptoms but must be varied for different cultural or demographic groups. This approach characterizes the early ''Seven Warning Signs'' campaign of the American Cancer Society, and their more recent emphasis on annual check-ups (6).

The third possibility in this analysis is that interaction effects will be found in which delay varies both with site and symptom characteristics and with demographic characteristics, and the variations differ between groups on both dimensions. This finding would recommend different cancer control strategies tailored to diverse populations for each of the different site/symptom complexes. This appears to be the approach recommended by the recent Cancer Program Planning Conference (7) with its emphasis on community demonstrations.

The errors of deduction in recommending or designing specific cancer control strategies can be avoided by examining each proposition about behavioral change offered in this volume. The criterion here would be that the alleged stimulus is in fact an antecedent condition for behavioral change in relation to each of the several cancer sites or symptoms in question. The factors responsible for success in reducing delay in relation to breast lesions, for example, may not have the same relative importance in reducing delay for rectal cancer. Indeed, the relationship between an antecedent variable and reduction of delay in seeking diagnosis may be the opposite for different sites or symptoms. For example, breast cancer delay appears to have been reduced through the reduction of fear (8–13), but it may be necessary to increase the level of fear to reduce delay in response to rectal bleeding, which the patient can dismiss too easily as hemorrhoids. Thus, we must be alert to interaction effects in the interpretation of factors causing or reducing delay for different symptoms or sites.

A FRAMEWORK OF SECONDARY PREVENTION VARIABLES

The several relationships to be considered in secondary prevention for cancer control can be summarized as in Fig. 1, based on the combination of a more general model of the utilization of health services (14) and a more general model of health education planning and evaluation (15). The predisposing factors include those beliefs, attitudes, value perceptions, and social norms which are expected to influence an individual's propensity to delay or to seek care promptly in response to symptoms. Some of these factors are expected to interact with the specific cancer symptom or site in affecting delay. The same is expected of some of the variables in the general categories of enabling factors and reinforcing factors.

The classification of antecedent behavioral variables into predisposing, enabling, and reinforcing factors is convenient to identify the intervention strategies necessary to influence health behavior. An important principle of health education is that none of these three broad strategies will stand alone as a program. Public education must be supported by the mobilization and coordination of resources at the community level; both of these must be accompanied by knowledge and attitudinal and behavioral supports in the providers of care (16–20). The expectations and behavior of professionals toward patients, in turn, condition and reinforce the subsequent health behavior and the predisposition of patients (21–32). These reinforcing factors are discussed by Hayes later in this volume.

PREDISPOSING FACTORS

Primary Versus Secondary Health Behavior

The first question is whether one can generalize from data on primary preventive health behavior to infer, explain, or predict secondary preventive health behavior. Can delay or participation in cancer screening programs, for example, be understood in the same terms as immunization behavior or personal hygiene?

Kasl and Cobb (33) addressed this question and found it necessary to draw formal distinctions between health behavior, illness behavior, and sick-role behavior. Baric (34) later added "at-risk" behavior to account for the distinguishing features of behavior, which is in response to asymptomatic illness such as hyper-

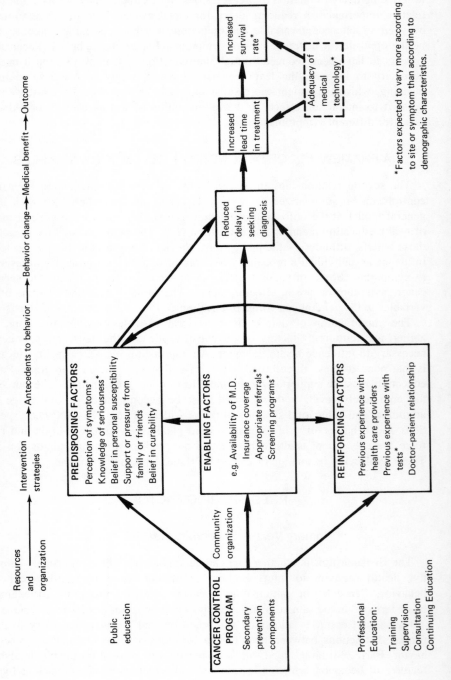

Fig. 1. Hypothesized relationships among factors in secondary prevention.

Resources
and   Intervention   Antecedents to behavior ⟶ Behavior change ⟶ Medical benefit ⟶ Outcome
organization   strategies

Public
education

Community
organization

CANCER CONTROL
PROGRAM

Secondary
prevention
components

Professional
Education:

Training
Supervision
Consultation
Continuing Education

PREDISPOSING FACTORS

Perception of symptoms*
Knowledge of seriousness*
Belief in personal susceptibility
Support or pressure from
family or friends
Belief in curability*

ENABLING FACTORS

e.g. Availability of M.D.
Insurance coverage
Appropriate referrals*
Screening programs*

REINFORCING FACTORS

Previous experience with
health care providers
Previous experience with
tests*
Doctor–patient relationship

Reduced
delay in
seeking
diagnosis

Increased
lead time
in treatment

Adequacy of
medical
technology*

Increased
survival
rate*

*Factors expected to vary more according
to site or symptom than according to
demographic characteristics.

tension or exposure to a continuous health threat. Kasl (35) has more recently examined the variations in definitions of health, at-risk, illness, and sick-role behaviors as they relate to chronic disease control. He finds little evidence even within specific categories such as "compliance" that the various forms of behavior are more than "modestly correlated with each other" and concludes that our progress may be hindered by searching for predictors of "too large a category of diverse behaviors" (p. 437, ref. 35).

Is There a General Health Predisposition?

The search for common patterns of behavior is prompted partly by the attempt to verify concepts such as "health orientation" or "general health concern," which would in turn be used to explain and predict individual variations in personal health practices (36). Although correlations between preventive health practices keep appearing, as Fink et al. (37) found between immunization and participation in the Health Insurance Plan of Greater New York (HIP) breast screening program, systematic studies of relationships among preventive health practices have generally found more unexplained variance than could be accepted in support of the concept of a single, underlying "trait" of preventive health orientation (38–43). For example, most of the common variance among a set of nine preventive health practices in a statewide sample of young mothers was attributable to socioeconomic status, and more specifically to the "maximum status identity" of the nuclear family. Thus a woman tended to behave in accordance with the preventive health norms of the highest socioeconomic stratum to which she was eligible to belong either by her own educational level, her husband's or her own occupation, or the family income. But specific health knowledge accounted for a substantial amount of variance after controlling for the status identity variable (39). These findings obviate the necessity of a "health orientation" concept to account for the moderate correlations among preventive health practices.

Secondary Preventive Actions and Illness Behavior[1]

The second question still remains, even after ruling out a general health orientation: Are there certain habits of medical care behavior that persist across a variety of symptom responses and utilization patterns for individuals? The "clinic habit" thesis formalized by Lambert and Freeman (44) applied mainly to the persistence of dental care behavior among medically indigent adolescents, but Bice (45) found correlations between anticipated use of services for sets of psychosomatic and somatic symptoms in general population surveys. His correlations between tendencies to visit a doctor for the two sets of symptoms were based on verbal reports of anticipated response to symptoms, but they were generally independent of economic or educational level.

---

[1] I am indebted to Howard Kalmer for much of the literature review for this section.

Ronald Andersen (14) concluded from his multivariate analysis of utilization behavior that beliefs and other psychological variables were relatively unimportant because he obtained weak relationships between a composite measure of these predispositions and actual use of health services. The potential misinterpretations of his conclusion are precisely what we are seeking to avoid here, namely, the inductive tendency to generalize from a specific relationship to a general rule and the deductive error of expecting a specific relationship on the basis of a general pattern of relationships. Andersen formed his composite predisposition variable from six symptoms, which formed a Guttman scale, combined with other health values and attitude measures. In view of what was shown in the foregoing review of evidence concerning the alleged general health orientation, there is little surprise that Andersen's composite yielded weak relationships with utilization. Had he correlated beliefs regarding each specific symptom with utilization of services in response to that symptom, he might have obtained more substantial coefficients.

Fischer (46), Mechanic and Volkart (47), and others have obtained such correlations between an individual's predisposition to use a health care source and actual use. Studies showing such relationships between projected and actual use have generally found that they were symptom-specific and colinear with socioeconomic status or age, or both. For example, Koos (48) found that responses to whether each of a list of symptoms required medical care were associated with social class. Shuval (49) found that older, lower SES respondents tended to see themselves more in need of medical care for mild, nonincapacitating symptoms. Similar findings were obtained in a college student population by Anderson and Bartkus (50) in their symptom sensitivity or anticipated use of a university health service.

The symptom-specificity of anticipated use has been demonstrated by Gordon (51), who found that as symptoms become more uncertain and serious, the probability increases that the projected decision will be to seek professional diagnosis or care. Hetherington and Hopkins (52) asked health insurance plan subscribers which conditions, from a list, they thought were serious enough to require a visit to a physician. "Symptom-sensitivity" (recognition of a condition as a symptom and intention to act to relieve the condition) was associated with socioeconomic, demographic, and cultural variables. The most carefully controlled study of anticipated use is probably that of Blackwell (53,54) who presented three scenarios to upper middle-class adults. Each scenario represented a symptom complex: physical (blood in stools), psychophysical (burning sensation in chest after eating for past week), and psychosocial (self-consciousness and apprehension). Projected actions of respondents were classified into seven categories ranging from "ignore" to "go to a professional immediately." The anticipated time lag between notice of symptom and the seeking of care, the type of help sought, and the alternative coping actions all differed significantly for the three types of symptoms, even though all three descriptions were eligible for immediate medical attention.

The inconsistencies in medical care behavior for individuals may be expected to increase as financial barriers are removed, extrapolating from previous studies (55–58). As the enabling factors, such as accessibility of care, are improved, the predisposing factors should take on increased importance (14). Friedman, Parker, and Lipworth (59) have found that the elimination of financial barriers to medical care by itself has not caused a reduction in delay of examination for breast symptoms, suggesting the need for health education to accompany health insurance programs. Hallauer (60) offers experimental evidence that patients do learn new utilization behavior through reinforcement from the medical care system.

Cancer Delay Versus Other Medical Care Delay

The third question is whether the usual illness behavior of individuals can be generalized to predict or explain their cancer delay behavior. Although we have seen in the foregoing section that medical care "habits" is a dubious construct, several studies suggest that established patterns of medical care behavior prevail when cancer symptoms appear (9,19,61–65). There seem to be general "delayers" and generally "prompt" persons with respect to seeking medical care. Nevertheless, the studies reviewed have used different measures of medical care practices, and most have depended on verbal reporting of past behavior. Also, what are often called prompt responses in some studies may reflect undue, even neurotic, concern about health and not necessarily rational understanding of the importance of early or regular medical attention (66).

A way of seeking care for illness may persist for an individual and prevail for cancer symptoms and for other symptoms as well. Studies (63,67,68) indicating that patients delay longer with cancer symptoms than with others suggest that emotional factors interact with habits when cancer symptoms appear, thus delaying and presumably weakening the effect of the established practices. Such findings suggest the need for multivariate analyses of the interplay between established practices of medical care and other forces affecting delay.

The striking consistency of medical care practices contrasts with the inconsistency between different preventive health practices noted above. The findings of Macdonald (69), Taylor (70), Kutner and Gordan (68), King and Leach (71), and Battistella (55) that delay was not associated with economic status provide a possible clue to this difference, because preventive health practices are almost universally and invariably associated with socioeconomic status (39). In previous, more general reviews of delay (54,72,73), it was concluded that delay was inversely associated with socioeconomic status, but our review of studies particularly focused on delay with breast cancer symptoms (13).

Delay tends to be greater with cancer symptoms than with other symptoms (63,68). Clearly, the "sick role" for cancer is significantly different from that expected with most acute illnesses (74), and adopting the sick role is only one of several decision-points along the continuum of submitting oneself to medical care (75–78). Mechanic and Volkart (47) demonstrated in a study of university students that illnesses that are relatively common, familiar, predictable, and nonthreatening are associated with a tendency to accept the sick role quite readily, whereas unfamiliar, unpredictable, and threatening symptoms lead more to stress than to action.

VARIATIONS IN CANCER DELAY AND DETECTION[2]

Nature of Symptoms

Certain departures from the normal body have come to connote cancer. The public in many countries has been alerted to cancer danger signals (79–82). The extent to which symptoms are viewed as possible cancer has therefore been investigated, as has the relationship of such interpretation to early or delayed action for care. Knowledge of cancer has also been investigated. This is discussed elsewhere in this chapter.

Simmons and Daland (83) found little association between the character of symptoms first observed (all body sites) and patient delay. In many cases, patients stated that they had delayed because they did not feel any pain. Symptoms experienced by a patient were often similar to those of nonmalignant disease, and rapidity of growth in a lesion was the chief reason for consulting a physician (93).

Smith (84), studying 95 cancer patients (six sites) admitted to a hospital in New York, reported that lack of severe symptoms and disability was the greatest delay factor. About half of the group of 41 with breast symptoms delayed because of "ignorance or procrastination" and all but two of these breast patients had seen their symptoms as mild.

Pack and Gallo (89), at about the same time, stated that reasons for delay "are probably much alike in all investigations: ignorance of the seriousness of early symptoms, fear, unwillingness to face the truth which they suspect, and perhaps financial circumstances." They studied 1,000 random cases in two hospitals (all cancer cases; several sites). They indicated that degree or severity of symptoms should have forced action earlier for some patients.

Macdonald (69) studied the first 1,000 records from 1938 in the Connecticut Cancer Record Registry and compared them with a similar group from 1946. Like Smith, she combined negligence and ignorance, which are probably quite different. These were major reasons for delay in 1938 and again in 1946.

Harms, Plaut, and Oughterson (85), studying 158 successive cancer patients in the New Haven Hospital or Turner Clinic, found more than half (all sites) failing to recognize the seriousness of symptoms, and about 7% were regarded as "ignorant" by the study observer. While fear of cancer was a cause of delay for only about 1%, only 13% had interpreted their symptoms as cancer.

---

[2]The following summary is based on the detailed reviews of Antonovsky and Hartman (72) and Green and Roberts (13). The methodological limitations of the studies mentioned here are discussed in the cited reviews.

Hackett, Cassem, and Raker (86), in a study of 563 cancer patients (all sites) at Massachusetts General, found that those who correctly labeled their condition as "cancer" were significantly earlier in seeking medical care than those who referred to their condition as a "tumor." They attribute this to socioeconomic differences in labeling illnesses.

Eardley (12) has shown that the significant reductions in delay for breast symptoms in Britian are largely attributable to the increased reassurances of curability.

Site of Symptoms

The most consistent finding regarding site is that of a greater degree of patient-caused delay with more superficial lesions than with more internal lesions. Some investigators, however, report less delay for breast symptoms (71,86,87), some report less delay with other sites (84), and some report no difference by site (61,83). Roberts, studying symptoms in the breast only, found that patients with surface manifestations (not mass type) delayed more, whereas those whose symptoms were masses were prompt in their action.

Perception of Symptoms

Several investigators report that delaying patients regarded their symptoms as not serious (8,70,88,89) or not unusual (18,62,64) more than did patients who acted promptly. Mild symptoms are specifically cited as responsible for delay by many (64,70,83,84,87,90). Some studies suggest that severity in symptoms, especially pain, ends delay by precipitating more prompt action (8,9,64,65,89).

Knowledge of Seriousness

Ignorance is referred to in a number of studies as a factor in interpreting symptoms as commonplace and not suspecting cancer (8,70,88,89). In some studies "ignorance" has been loosely classified together with "negligence" or "procrastination" (69,84), which are nothing more than descriptions of the behavior they are intended to explain (17). In some it is not clear whether the reference is to ignorance of cancer in general or failure to recognize and identify specific symptoms as related to cancer (87,90). Some studies, at the other extreme, have virtually ruled out "ignorance" as a factor in delay (85,91) and others have found no lack of knowledge regarding available treatment facilities (6,72,88).

There is some agreement in findings regarding the relationship between interpretation of possible cancer with more positive attitudes, such as belief in curability (12,70), leading to less delay. Negative attitudes, such as shame associated with cervical cancer (92) and threat to feminine roles (93), are associated with increased delay.

The action a patient takes is often attributed to the individual's manner of coping with fears and anxiety arising from the interpretations (61,64,65,89,91). Fear, variously defined, is the most commonly cited reason for delay (8,9,64,70, 89,90,92,94). Some refer to fear of cancer but some refer to other fears related to the sick role, hospitals, and so forth. Findings of several studies, especially the more recent, indicate additive and interactive relationships between knowledge and fear in determining interpretations and a decision on action to be taken (12, 18,62,70,85,86). Fear can be related to knowledge in the health belief model as knowledgeable fear about susceptibility, severity, and curability.

Methodological approaches have varied in the different types of cancer knowledge studied, making comparison of results difficult except in national opinion surveys (6,11,79–82).

Whether knowledge was measured by a recall or a recognition approach is not always clear. In some studies knowledge levels were associated only for persons voluntarily bringing cancer into discussion. Some studies have employed a retrospective question to establish knowledge levels existent at the time first action to seek care was taken; others have used a projective approach, which relates to current predispositions, but fails to distinguish action described as what would occur from what actually will occur when symptoms are perceived (53,95).

Interaction of Knowledge and Fear

Several studies make it apparent that there is no clear, one-to-one relationship between cancer knowledge and action to seek care but rather that several factors interact with knowledge. Roberts (18) and Kutner and Gordan (68) reported a clearer association between cancer knowledge and action than have others. Additional investigation is needed to analyze the interaction aspect of several factors influencing action. Study of specific types of cancer knowledge in relation to action for care is also needed. It seems quite possible that certain understandings about cancer are more salient to action than others. Some of the studies suggest knowledge areas having more relationship to action (8,18,61,64,68,70,85), especially the curability of cancer (12).

Antonovsky and Hartman (72) found no evidence in their review of the literature that knowledge of the existence of cancer detection centers or screening facilities "makes any major contribution to delay or to failure to participate in screening programs." Knowledge of the significance of symptoms, however, is almost invariably associated with reduced delay. Health educators have long recognized that this is not a simple, linear, cause-effect relationship, but rather a complex, curvilinear, multivariate relationship in which knowledge interacts with affective, personality, and sociocultural forces to influence health action in different ways under different conditions.

With anxiety or fear, for example, knowledge about the significance of cancer symptoms tends to increase delay when the fear or anxiety is intense, but reduces delay when the level of anxiety or fear is low (61,62). This finding is consistent with recent experimental studies on fear arousal in persuasive communication and health education (96).

ENABLING FACTORS

Screening Programs and Referrals

The record is more impressive for some of the specific cancer screening and testing programs than for multiphasic screening. Pap smear programs, for example, have been vigorously promoted by public and voluntary health agencies and widely accepted by women as well as by the medical profession. The evidence of reduced mortality (97) and increased survival (98) is convincing. The cost-benefit estimates vary, depending on how the earning value of housewives is calculated. Christopherson and Parker (99) suggest that screening of low income, high-risk groups reduces the program costs per detected case, but cost-benefit estimates using the tax value of survivors favor programs directed toward high-income persons living in neighborhoods of high taxation. Louis Dickinson (100) concluded from his calculations that a national health service should not expect to make a profit from cytologic screening for cervical cancer.

Breast cancer screening has been advanced by the new developments in mammography and the HIP evaluation of reduced mortality by one-third for women over 5 years of follow-up screening (31). These developments are most encouraging after decades of debate and uncertainty surrounding the efficacy of breast cancer surgery and the problems of delay in seeking diagnosis of suspicious breast symptoms (13).

One of the encouraging studies on breast screening with mammography (101) yielded a cost per examination of $26.50 (compared with $6.40 per Pap smear test). With the higher incidence of breast cancer, the cost per cancer detected was only slightly higher than that for cervical cytology, $2,223 compared to $2,212. Extrapolating from these figures and the estimated 20,000 breast cancer cases in the United States that could be saved, and the saving of $4,707 per case, which is the difference between the cost of caring for a breast cancer patient diagnosed early and one diagnosed late (101), a universal mammography screening program could yield a national monetary gain of approximately $860 million annually in earning and late treatment expenses. The costs of such a national screening program were estimated to be $622 million. Thus a net benefit of $238 million per year could be realized from mass screening for breast cancer. Using more refined biometrical arguments, Kodlin (102) also concludes that survival results from breast cancer screening "would justify the increased costs that might result from mass screening."

The major problem in launching such a program would be the paucity of mammographers and technologists. Dowdy et al. (101) therefore recommended setting up combined cervical and breast cancer screening centers throughout the country in the major medical centers. Such centers would train the necessary mammographers, technologists, and lay screeners. "These centers would serve as educational foci for both professional and lay groups." The combination of screening resources would also improve the cost-benefit ratio for cervical screening.

If cervical and breast screening are to be combined in screening centers, one would have to ask: Why not combine all cancer screening? And why should it be located in a stationary clinic that may not be accessible to some high-risk groups? These questions are answered by Lynch et al. (103) who advocate a "multiphasic mobile cancer screening unit" with as much emphasis on rectum, colon, prostate, lung, skin, lymphatic, and oral cancer detection as on breast and cervical cancer.

It is then but a small step in complexity to make the mobile screening unit a general multiphasic testing unit. Lynch et al. (103), for example, include health education services, blood pressure readings, and have incidentally identified congestive heart failure, obesity, diabetes, and chronic inflammatory disease. But they quickly disavow any interest in multiphasic health testing, and diplomatically add that any screening activity "should serve to supplement rather than to usurp the role of the practicing physicians." The usual resistance of local medical societies to such screening programs must be faced on a policy level.

The proliferation of specialized screening programs leads us into all of the same economic and dehumanizing traps that specialization and fragmentation of treatment has experienced. The arguments for comprehensive primary care might apply equally to screening. The same solutions for overcoming professional resistance to comprehensive primary care might also be applied to achieve more comprehensive screening programs. The linkage of the screening and medical care systems through referral and follow-up mechanisms is crucial to this recommendation (24,27,103,104).

Implications for Programs

My conclusions from the foregoing review of evidence follow.

1. We cannot generalize from primary preventive health behavior to secondary or illness behavior; they have some causal factors in common, but each has its own unique determinants.

2. We can generalize to a limited degree from one kind of illness behavior to another insofar as medical care utilization patterns have been colinear with socio-economic status.

3. As financial barriers to medical care access are removed, the enabling factors of accessibility will play less of a determining role and the relative importance of predisposing variables will increase the variability in personal responses to different symptoms of illness.

4. The greater delay with cancer symptoms than with noncancerous symptoms is largely attributable to predisposing factors, such as beliefs about the curability of cancer, which interact with medical care habits when cancer symptoms or

screening opportunities appear, thereby extending the delay and weakening the effect of established illness responses.

5. The combination of screening and diagnostic facilities into comprehensive, mobile testing units would improve the cost-benefit potential of cancer screening and would increase the number and range of people screened and diagnosed early.

These conclusions lead to the recommendations that public education about cancer should be specific to sites at which signs or symptoms occur and should emphasize the peace of mind that comes with knowing that nothing is wrong and the curability of cancers diagnosed early in those sites.[3]

Patient education in medical care settings should reinforce illness behavior that represents early care-seeking for other symptoms. Finally, site-specific cancer screening and detection programs should be consolidated with other, less threatening screening and risk-reduction programs in mobile units that include health education and a wide variety of testing services. The usual objections of private medical practitioners to such comprehensive screening and detection units must be overcome through careful planning of referral mechanisms and other economic reassurances. If these adjustments do not succeed in raising the early detection rates for cancer, then there will be no excuse for leaving the fragmented medical screening system intact while thousands of people suffer and die from cancers that could have been cured with earlier diagnosis and treatment. Health education must be supported by institutional arrangements conducive to the behavior expected of the public.

REFERENCES

1. James W. *Pragmatism,* Longmans, Green & Co., New York, 1914.
2. Parkes, C. M. Comment: Communication and cancer—a social psychiatrist's view. *Soc. Sci. Med.,* 8:189–190 (1974).
3. McIntosh, J. Processes of communication, information seeking and control associated with cancer: A selective review of the literature. *Soc. Sci. Med.,* 8:167–188 (1974).
4. James, W. *Some Problems of Philosophy,* Longmans, Green & Co., New York, 1911.
5. Baric, L., Stevens, R. D., Karuppaiyan, V., and Vadivelu, M. Cancer education in Kancheepuram: A case against transferring health education approaches. *Int. J. Health Educ.,* 17:32–42 (1974).
6. Lieberman Associates. *Study of Motivational, Attitudinal, and Environmental Deterrants to the Taking of Physical Examinations that Include Cancer Tests.* Vols. I and II. Lieberman Research, Inc., for the American Cancer Society, New York, 1966.
7. *Cancer Program Planning Conference: Summary Report of Working Group 8, Cancer Control.* U.S. Dept. of Health, Education and Welfare, National Cancer Institute, Bethesda, May 15, 1974.
8. Aitken-Swan, J., and Paterson, R. The cancer patient: Delay in seeking advice. *Br. Med.J.,* 1:623–627 (1955).

---

[3]Independent evidence supporting this recommendation is provided by a recent study showing that reassuring headlines about cancer got better readership and resulted in more learning than did scare headlines, especially among high anxiety subjects, smokers, and those who had a history of cancer in their families (96; see also ref. 105).

9. Aitken-Swan, J., and Paterson, R. Assessment of the results of five years of cancer education. *Br. Med. J.*, 1:708–712 (1959).

10. Balan, J. A survey of public opinion on cancer in the Argentine. *Int. J. Health Educ.*, 10:67–74 (1967).

11. Briggs, J. E., and Wakefield, J. *Public Opinion on Cancer: A Survey of Knowledge and Attitudes Among Women in Lancaster*, Regional Committee on Cancer, Christie Hospital and Holt Radium Institute, Manchester, 1967.

12. Eardley, A. Triggers to action: A study of what makes women seek advice for breast conditions. *Int. J. Health Educ.*, 17:256–265 (1974).

13. Green, L. W., and Roberts, B. J. The research literature on why women delay in seeking medical care for breast symptoms. *Health Educ. Monogr.*, 2:129–177 (1974).

14. Andersen, R. *A Behavioral Model of Families' Use of Health Services*, University of Chicago Center for Health Administration Studies, Chicago, 1968.

15. Green, L. W. Toward cost-benefit evaluations of health education: Some concepts, methods and examples. *Health Educ. Monogr.*, 2(Suppl.):34–64 (1974).

16. D'Onofrio, C. A. *Reaching our Hard-to-Reach: The Unimmunized*, California State Department of Public Health, Bureau of Health Education, Berkeley, 1966.

17. Green, L. W. Should health education abandon attitude-change strategies? Perspectives from recent research. *Health Educ. Monogr.*, 1:25–48 (1970(a)).

18. Roberts, B. J. *A Study of Selected Factors and Their Association with Action for Medical Care*. Unpublished Dr. P.H. dissertation, Harvard University School of Public Health, 1956.

19. Roberts, B. J. Factors and forces influencing decision-making related to health behavior. In *Proceedings of the Seminar on Health Education in Uterine Cancer Control*, University of Michigan School of Public Health, Ann Arbor, 1967.

20. Young, M. A. C. Review of research and studies related to health education practice (1961–1966). *Health Educ. Monogr.*, 1:23–28 (1967–1969).

21. Bernstein, L., and Dana, R. H. *Interviewing and the Health Professions*, 2d ed., Appleton-Century-Crofts, New York, 1973.

22. Caplan, E. K., and Sussman, M. B. Rank order of important variables for patient and staff satisfaction with out-patient service. *J. Health Soc. Behav.*, 7:133–137 (1966).

23. Freemon, B., Negrete, V. F., David, M., and Korsch, B. M. Gaps in doctor-patient communication: Doctor-patient interaction analysis. *Pediatr. Res.*, 5:298–311 (1971).

24. Hayes, D. M. Pathways to care for cancer patients. *Health Serv. Res.*, 89:119–127 (1974).

25. Inui, T. *Effects of Post-graduate Physician Education on the Management and Outcomes of Patients with Hypertension*, Master of Science thesis, School of Hygiene and Public Health, Johns Hopkins University, Baltimore, 1973.

26. Kalmer, H. Patient-professional congruence related to anticipated care-seeking behavior in a prepaid ambulatory setting. Mimeographed research proposal. Johns Hopkins University School of Hygiene and Public Health, Baltimore, 1974.

27. Miller, M. H. Who receives optimal medical care? *J. Health Soc. Behav.*, 14:175–182 (1973).

28. Mitchell, J. H. Compliance with medical regimens: An annotated bibliography. *Health Educ. Monogr.*, 2:75–87 (1974).

29. Rockart, J. F., and Hofman, P. B. Physician and patient behavior under different scheduling systems in a hospital out-patient department. *Med. Care*, 7:463–470 (1969).

30. Rosenzweig, S. P., and Folman, R. Patient and therapist variables affecting premature termination in group psychotherapy. *Psychother. Theory Res. Pract.*, 11:76–79 (1974).

31 Shapiro, I. S. The teaching role of health professionals in a formal organization. *Health Educ. Monogr.*, 1:40–48 (1973).

32. Waitzkin, H., and Stoeckle, J. D. The communication of information about illness. *Adv. Psychosom. Med.*, 8:180–215 (1972).

33. Kasl, S. V., and Cobb, S. Health behavior, illness behavior, and sick role behavior. *Arch. Environ. Health.*, 12:246–266 (1966); and 12:521–541 (1966).

34. Baric, L. Recognition of the "at-risk" role: A means to influence behavior. *Int. J. Health Educ.*, 12:24–34 (1969).

35. Kasl, S. V. The health belief model and behavior related to chronic illness. *Health Educ. Monogr.*, 2:433–454 (1974).

36. Becker, M. H., Drachman, R. H., and Kirscht, J. P. A new approach to explaining sick-role behavior in low-income populations. *Am. J. Public Health*, 64:205–216 (1974).

37. Fink, R., Shapiro, S., and Roester, R. Impact of efforts to increase participation in repetitive

screenings for early breast cancer detection. *Am. J. Public Health,* 62:328–336 (1972).

38. Coburn, D., and Pope, C. R. Socioeconomic status and preventive health behavior. *J. Health Soc. Behav.,* 15:67–78 (1974).
39. Green, L. W. *Status Identity and Preventive Health Behavior,* University of California, Berkeley, Pacific Health Education Reports, No. 1, (1970(b)).
40. Haefner, D. P., Kegeles, S. S., Kirscht, J., and Rosenstock, I. M. Preventive actions in dental disease, tuberculosis, and cancer. *Public Health Rep.,* 83:451–459 (1967).
41. Kirscht, J. P., Haefner, D. P., Kegeles, S. S., and Rosenstock, I. M. A national study of health beliefs. *J. Health Hum. Behav.,* 7:248–254 (1966).
42. Steele, J., and McBroom, W. H. Conceptual and empirical dimensions of health behavior. *J. Health Soc. Behav.,* 13:382–392 (1972).
43. Williams. A. F., and Wechsler, H. Interrelationship of preventive actions in health and other areas. *Health Serv. Res.,* 87:969–976 (1972).
44. Lambert. C., and Freeman, H. E. *The Clinic Habit,* College and University Press, New Haven, 1967.
45. Bice, T. W. *Medical Care for the Disadvantaged,* Johns Hopkins University School of Hygiene and Public Health, Baltimore, 1971.
46. Fischer, L. A. *The Use of Services in the Urban Scene–the Individual and the Medical Care System,* Center for Urban and Regional Studies, University of North Carolina, Chapel Hill, N.C., 1971.
47. Mechanic, D., and Volkart, E. H. Illness behavior and medical diagnosis. *J. Health Hum. Behav.,* 1:86–94 (1960).
48. Koos, E. *The Health of Regionville: What the People Thought and Did About It,* Columbia University Press, New York, 1954.
49. Shuval, J. T. The sick role in a setting of comprehensive medical care. *Med. Care.,* 10:50–59 (1972).
50. Anderson, J. G., and Bartkus, D. E. Choice of medical care: A behavioral model of health and illness behavior. *J. Health Soc. Behav.,* 14:348–362 (1973).
51. Gordon, G. *Role Theory and Illness: A Sociological Perspective,* College and University Press, New Haven, 1966.
52. Hetherington, R. W., and Hopkins, C. E. Symptom sensitivity: Its social and cultural correlates. *Health Serv. Res.,* 4:63–75 (1969).
53. Blackwell, B. L. Anticipated pre-medical care activities of upper middle-class adults and their implications for health education practice. *Health Educ. Monogr.,* 17:17–36 (1964).
54. Blackwell, B. L. The literature of delay in seeking medical care for cancer illness. *Health Educ. Monogr.,* 16:3–31 (1963).
55. Battistella, R. M. Factors associated with delay in the initiation of physicians' care among late adulthood persons. *Am. J. Public Health,* 61:1348–1361 (1971).
56. Kriesburg, L. The relationship between socio-economic rank and behavior. *Soc. Problems,* 10:334–352 (1963).
57. Ross, J. A. Social class and medical care. *J. Health Hum. Behav.,* 3:35–40 (1962).
58. Shapiro, S., and Brindle, J. Serving Medicaid eligibles. *Am. J. Public Health,* 59:635–641 (1969).
59. Friedman, B., Parker, P., and Lipworth, L. The influence of Medicaid and private health insurance on the early diagnosis of breast cancer. *Med. Care,* 11:485–590 (1973).
60. Hallauer, D. S. Illness behavior—an experimental investigation. *J. Chronic Dis.,* 25:599–610 (1972).
61. Cobb, B., Clark, R. L., MacGuire, C., and Howe, C. D. Patient responsible delay of treatment in cancer: A social psychological study. *Cancer,* 7:920–926 (1954).
62. Goldsen, R. K., Gerhardt, P. R., and Handy, V. H. Some factors related to patient delay in seeking diagnosis for cancer symptoms. *Cancer,* 10:1–7 (1957).
63. Goldsen, R. K. Patient delay in seeking cancer diagnosis: Behavioral aspects. *J. Chronic Dis.,* 16:427–436 (1963).
64. King, R. A., and Leach, J. E. Factors contributing to delay by patients in seeking medical care. *Cancer,* 3:571–579 (1950).
65. Robbins, G. F., Conte, A. J., Leach, J. E., and MacDonald, M. Delay in diagnosis and treatment of cancer. *JAMA,* 143:346–348 (1950).
66. Fischer, S. Motivation for patient delay. *Arch. Gen. Psychiatry,* 16:676–678 (1967).
67. Cobb, B. Emotional problems of adult cancer patients. *Cancer,* 7:274–285 (1969).

68. Kutner, B., and Gordan, G. Seeking care for cancer. *J. Health Hum. Behav.*, 2:171–178 (1961).
69. MacDonald, E. J. Changing reasons for cancer patient delay. *Conn. Health Bull.*, 61:91–101 (1947).
70. Taylor, H. S. Factors Associated with Culpability or Nonculpability in Delaying Medical Care for Cancer. Master's thesis, G. W. Brown School of Social Work, Washington University, 1946.
71. King, R. A., and Leach, J. E. Habits of medical care. *Cancer*, 4:221–225 (1951).
72. Antonovsky, A., and Hartman, H. Delay in the detection of cancer: A review of the literature. *Health Educ. Monogr.*, 2:98–128 (1974).
73. Makover, H. B. Patient and physician delay in cancer diagnosis: Medical aspects. *J. Chronic Dis.*, 16:419–426 (1963).
74. Callahan, E., Carroll, S., Revier, Sister Paul, Gilhooly, E., and Dunn, D. The "sick role" in chronic illness: Some reactions. *J. Chronic Dis.*, 19:883–897 (1966).
75. Kasselbaum, G., and Baumann, B. Dimensions of the sick role in chronic illness. *J. Health Hum. Behav.*, 6:16–27 (1965).
76. Roberts, B. J. A framework for consideration of forces in achieving earliness of treatment. *Health Educ. Monogr.*, 1:16–32 (1965).
77. Suchman, E. A. Stages of illness and medical care. *J. Health Soc. Behav.*, 6:114–128 (1965).
78. Sweet, R. H., and Twaddle, A. C. An exploration of delay in hospitalization. *Inquiry* 6:35–41 (1969).
79. Horn, D., and Waingrow, S. What changes are occurring in public opinions towards cancer: National public opinion survey. *Am. J. Public Health*, 54:431–440 (1964).
80. Institute for Public Opinion Research, The Czechoslovak Academy of Science: A survey of public opinion on cancer in Czechoslovakia. *Health Educ. J.*, 31:50–56 (1972).
81. Simonds, S. K. Public opinion surveys about cancer: An overview. *Health Educ. Monogr.*, 30:3–24 (1970).
82. Williams, E. M., Cruickshank, A., and Walker, W. M. *Public Opinion of Cancer in South East Wales: A Report on the Findings of a Survey of Knowledge and Opinions.* Tenovus Cancer Information Center, Cardiff, 1972.
83. Simmons, C. C., and Daland, E. M. Cancer: Factors entering into the delay and its surgical treatment. *Boston Med. Surg. J.*, 183:298–303 (1920).
84. Smith, F. M. Factors causing delay in operative therapy of carcinoma. *Surg. Gynecol. Obst.*, 60:45–53 (1935).
85. Harms, C. R., Plaut, J. A., and Oughterson, A. W. Delay in the treatment of cancer. *JAMA*, 121:335–338 (1943).
86. Hackett, T. P., Cassem, N. H., and Raker, J. W. Patient delay in cancer. *N. Engl. J. Med.*, 289:14–20 (1973).
87. Leach, J. E., and Robbins, G. Delay in the diagnosis of cancer. *JAMA*, 135:5–8 (1947).
88. Bates, F. E., and Ariel, I. M. Delay in treatment of cancer. *Ill. Med. J.*, 94:361–365 (1948).
89. Pack, G. T., and Gallo, J. S. The culpability for delay in the treatment of cancer. *Am. J. Cancer*, 33:443–462 (1938).
90. Youngman, N. V. Psychological aspects of the early diagnosis of cancer. *Med. J. Aust.*, 34:581–587 (1947).
91. Titchener, J. L., Zwerling, I., Gottschalk, L., Levine, M., Culbertson, W., Cohen, S., and Silver, H. Problem of delay in seeking surgical care. *JAMA*, 160:1187–1193 (1956).
92. Sandifer, W. G., and Pritchett, B. S. Psychologic reactions causing a delay in treatment of cancer of the cervix. *J. Obstet. Gynecol. Br. Commonw.*, 11:82–88 (1958).
93. Renneker, R., and Cutler, M. Psychological problems of adjustment to cancer of the breast. *JAMA*, 148:833–838 (1952).
94. Bard, M., and Sutherland, A. M. Psychological impact of cancer and its treatment. IV. Adaptation to radical mastectomy. *Cancer*, 8:656–672 (1955).
95. Blackwell, B. L. Upper middle class adult expectations about entering the sick role for physical and psychiatric dysfunctions. *J. Health Soc. Behav.*, 8:83–95 (1967).
96. Bishop, R. L. Anxiety and readership of health information. *Journalism*, 51:40–46 (1974).
97. Dickinson, L., Mussey, M. E. and Kurland, L. T. Evaluation of the effectiveness of cytologic screening for cervical cancer: 2. Survival parameters before and after inception of screening. *Mayo Clin. Proc.*, 47:545–549 (1972).
98. Dickinson, L., Mussey, M. E., Soule, E. H., and Kurland, L. T. Evaluation of the

effectiveness of cytologic screening for cervical cancer: 1. Incidence and mortality trends in relation to screening. *Mayo Clin. Proc.,* 47:534–544 (1972).

99.   Christopherson, W. M., and Parker, J. E. Economic considerations in the control of cervix cancer in high-risk patients. *Cancer,* 19:107–111 (1969).

100.   Dickinson, L. Evaluation of the effectiveness of cytologic screening for cervical cancer: 3. Cost-benefit analysis. *Mayo Clin. Proc.,* 47:550–555 (1972).

101.   Dowdy, A. H., Barker, W. F., Lagasse, L. D., Sperling, L., Zeldis, L. J., and Logmire, W. P., Jr. Mammography as a screening method for the examination of large populations. *Cancer,* 28:1558–1562 (1971).

102.   Kodlin, D. A note on the cost-benefit problem in screening for breast cancer. *Methods Inf. Med.,* 11:242–247 (1972).

103.   Lynch, H. T., Harlan, W., Swartz, M., Marley, J., Becker, W., Lynch, J., Kraft, C., and Krush, A. Mobile cancer screening clinic. *Cancer,* 30:774–781 (1972).

104.   Allen, W. A., MacFalls, D. E., and Mattucci, L. P. Getting the cancer message to the community. *Int. J. Health Educ.,* 16:61–68 (1973).

105.   Giesen, M., and Henrick, C. Effects of false positive and negative arousal feedback on persuasion. *J. Pers. Soc. Psychol.,* 30:449–457 (1974).

Cancer: The Behavioral Dimensions, edited by J. W. Cullen,
B. H. Fox, and R. N. Isom. Raven Press, New York © 1976.

Group Influences on Health Behavior: A Social Learning Perspective

Allen J. Enelow

Pacific Medical Center, San Francisco, California 94120

As a psychiatrist whose entry into that specialty of medicine took place nearly 30 years ago, I find it sobering to reflect on the differences in applicability between the prevalent concepts of that day and the body of behavioral science research available to the serious student of the field today. Nowhere does this become more evident than in the applications of psychiatry to general medicine, and in particular to the problems of chronic illness. The central focus of my branch of medicine has been the attempt to alter behavior, at least in this century. There have always been a number of us who are concerned with the medical patient. But the dependence on conceptual models, which attributed behavior to inner forces and unconscious conflicts and characterized the psychiatry of the 1940s, gave us little to apply to the problems of altering health behavior with respect to reducing risk factors for disease, participation in screening and illness identification programs, and compliance with therapeutic regimens. Our treatment model was that of one therapist working intensively over long periods with one patient to produce insight into the intrapsychic conflicts of the patient. Moreover, when some psychologists presented research that suggested that behavior is under external control, it was not particularly palatable; nor did it fit our experience that people behave in a relatively consistent manner. The idea that man is a passive reactor to external forces did not provide for self-determination or cognitive control of behavior. It was much too traumatic to abandon such concepts as will, motivation, and internal governing processes of behavior. In fact, however, social learning theory has provided us with a useful, and probably more complete explanation for human behavior than did the early work on learning and behavior. Further, and probably more importantly, it has given us a framework for experimental studies of behavior.

Bandura (1), for example, proposes that psychological functioning is best understood in terms of a continuous reciprocal interaction between behavior and its controlling conditions, placing special emphasis on important roles played by vicarious, symbolic, self-regulatory processes. This has not only given us a more satisfying theory dealing with cognition, affect, and behavior, but provides a starting point for research in health behavior.

Social learning theory, as developed by Rotter (2–4) and Bandura (5–8), has been applied by others (9–12) to the modification of health behavior, such as cardiovascular risk factor reduction, eating disorders, and smoking. Other research on modifying health-related behaviors includes work on chronic pain and disability after injury, on compliance with medication regimens, and on use of health facilities, to mention a few of the areas. In this chapter, I touch on a few of the relevant studies from social learning theory and social psychology in an effort to define some potential applications to cancer control, including rehabilitation. In so doing, I define some target populations toward whom programs of intervention and efforts to modify behavior might be aimed.

SOME RELEVANT PRINCIPLES OF SOCIAL LEARNING THEORY

Operant conditioning is the term for the process in which the frequency of a behavior is modified by its consequence. However, Rotter was one of the first to go beyond the study of the acquisition of new behaviors and alterations of the frequency of behaviors. Rotter concerned himself with what response from the repertoire of previously learned responses will be chosen by a given individual in a particular situation. He proposed that the subjective expectations of a person regarding the future consequences of his actions will be an important factor in predicting human behavior. The constructs developed by Rotter help us to understand why an apparent reinforcement may or may not have the expected result, and suggest that behavior can be modified by altering a person's expectations about future rewards or by changing the subjective value of anticipated rewards. This is directly relevant to altering health behavior, and suggests that patients should be exposed to supportive evidence for both the efficacy of therapeutic regimens as well as dire consequences of failing to take appropriate action. Furthermore, Rotter developed an objective index (the so-called "Internal–External Locus of Control") which measures a given subject's general expectancy that what he does is either under his own internal control or is controlled by external forces. Several studies suggest that internally as contrasted with externally oriented persons are more likely to comply with therapeutic regimens subsequent to the diagnosis of disease (13). This could be a very useful aid in the designing of behavioral strategies that differ for these two groups.

Bandura's theory was not developed directly in the field of health behavior but addresses the major problems of human learning. Bandura has compiled a great deal of evidence to support his views, which can be summarized as follows:

Man is not driven by inner forces nor is he totally controlled by environmental influences. Further, man need not learn as the product of directly experienced response consequences. In fact, practically all learning that results from direct experiences can occur on a vicarious basis through the observation of other people's behavior and its consequences for them. People can also represent external influences symbolically and later use such representations to guide their actions. People solve problems symbolically without having to enact the various alternatives; can foresee probable consequences and alter their behavior accordingly and thus are capable of both insightful and foresightful behavior. Finally, man is capable of creating self-regulated influences and different people can control their own behavior to differing degrees.

Bandura's most important conceptual contribution, in my opinion, is modeling. Modeling is based on the principle that most people learn behavior after observing others whom they wish to emulate. New behaviors can be learned through imitation. Models exemplify the cultural patterns of a given society and probably are the basis of all socialization. In Bandura's concept there are four principal components of the modeling process. These are the attentional, retentional, motoric-reproduction, and incentive-motivational processes.

Attentional processes depend on attending to or recognizing the essential features of the model's behavior. This is strongly influenced by the functional value of the behaviors displayed, the interpersonal attraction of the models, and the degree to which they are capable of holding people's attention for extended periods. For example, models presented in televised form are so effective in capturing attention that viewers learn the depicted behavior regardless of whether or not they are given extra incentives to do so.

Retention, the second factor, depends on the ability of the observer to remember, and the ability to represent, or imagine in fantasy, the processes observed. Observers who can code the modeled activities either into words or vivid imagery learn and retain the behavior better than those who simply observe without such coding or who are preoccupied with other matters while watching.

The motoric-reproduction component of modeling is concerned with those aspects of learning in which one can reproduce the behavior seen and practice it.

The reinforcement-motivational processes are those that are influenced by positive incentives to learn and practice a new behavior. In any case, having been exposed to modeling, inability to learn the new behavior could result from either failure to observe the relevant activities, inadequately representing them in memory, difficulty in retention, lack of opportunity to practice the new behavior, or lack of reinforcement of the new behavior. Attention to these processes and the provision of the necessary conditions for observation, retention, practice, and reinforcement are of greatest concern in all group efforts to influence behavior.

In social learning theory, behavior is regulated not only by directly experienced consequences from external sources but by vicarious reinforcement that encourages the individual to continue or to imitate those behaviors. Self-reinforcement is the ultimate aim of all efforts to alter behavior in a lasting way. In other words, the objective is to produce cognitive control of behavior of the individual without need for external reinforcement. Thus direct reinforcement and vicarious reinforcement help in the learning of new behaviors, whereas self-reinforcement leads to the persistence of newly learned behaviors.

Cognitive control of behavior is accomplished through imagery (the ability to fantasize or imagine consequences of behavior), symbolic coding, and thought processes. These help the individual to select appropriate courses of action by utilizing appropriate behaviors learned prior to or during the experimental or treatment-oriented behavior modification program.

Bandura's theory has been utilized by several others in the modification of eating and smoking behavior. More recently it has been utilized in group settings in the attempt to modify the major health behaviors associated with the cardio-vascular risk factors. The findings from that work appear to be relevant to cancer control and rehabilitation.

ATTITUDE THEORY AND HEALTH BEHAVIOR

In a review of research on changing health behavior through modifying atti-tudes, Leventhal (14) summarized his work in the areas of modifying smoking behavior, persuading people to take chest X-rays, take tetanus inoculations, drive carefully, and take part in systematic dental health programs. He reported that, although vivid descriptions of danger in efforts to motivate people to change their health behavior produced stronger beliefs in the danger and more behavior change, his findings suggested that it was actually the information or knowledge conveyed rather than fear-arousal that impelled the people to act. In fact, he discovered that shock material can scare an audience without persuading them. The change in attitude, in his view, did not lead to action unless a meaningful plan for action was presented. He proposes that communication attempting to alter attitudes to change health behavior must have two goals: (a) create a motive to change and (b) offer a clear-cut course of action to facilitate moving from change in attitude to change in behavior. The behavior appropriate to the changed attitude must be clearly spelled out for the individual or group whose behavior is the object of communication. He reviews other work that also gives clear guides to action in modifying health behavior. For one thing, the message must achieve a fairly wide exposure. For another, it must not be too far from the expectations of those who view or hear the message. Those who watch commercial television channels, for example, are expecting entertainment and will probably pay little heed to nonentertaining messages. On the other hand, those who watch ETV or public broadcasting networks are likely to be interested in the arts, culture, and self-improvement through education. A message would be different depending on who the potential audience might be.

Another factor is that to alter behavior one must reach the uninformed. Most of the messages that attempt to alter health behavior are heard or read by those who already are well-informed and have opinions on the issues. On the other hand, it is obvious that mass media can do a great deal in altering health behavior. McAlister (11) writes that in his work with smoking cessation considerable mod-eling occurred when Telly Savalas, star of a popular crime drama, *Kojak,* started using candy suckers on his program as an alternative to cigars and cigarettes. Clearly, if favorite television stars were to demonstrate health behavior of the type that one wishes to promote, the principles gained from social learning research and attitude research suggest that a large number of people would be influenced. This is discussed later. Leventhal's statement that interpersonal influence is a major factor shaping beliefs and behavior (14) is completely consistent with Bandura's views on modeling and vicarious reinforcement.

Janis and Hoffman (15), studying people who were trying to cut down on smoking, found that the ''buddy system'' facilitated success, suggesting the important role of personal contact and support in the maintenance of behavior changes. Byrne and Nelson (16) found strong evidence that the subjects in their experiments found another person more attractive as the similarity between the other's attitudes and those of the subject's increases. Furthermore, they found that reinforcement was more effective, in direct proportion to the degree of attraction that the subject felt for the communicator. This suggests that a patient can be more influenced to comply with a health regimen by exploring his attitudes on a number of issues and, in the process, provide cues that suggest support and agreement. Finally, in terms of applicability to the subject under consideration, a particular branch of attitude theory called "attribution theory" provides evidence that behavior changes attributed to oneself will persist or be maintained to a greater degree than behavior change attributed to an external agent, such as a drug or decision provided by someone else (17,18). This suggests that if a patient can be persuaded to make his own decision to follow a certain course of action, he is more likely to do so than if he behaves in response to an external authority's recommendations or directions.

APPLICATION: THE PATIENT, THE PHYSICIAN, AND THE HEALTH TEAM

The types of behavior of individuals, of families and small social groups, and of cancer patients and potential cancer patients that are the targets for change are: failure to come forward for screening, delay in seeing a physician upon detecting symptoms or signs that might indicate cancer, and psychological responses to treatment that are less than optimal for potential rehabilitation. Factors involved in these responses have been well summarized in Holland's review of psychological aspects of cancer (19). An important factor with which we must cope is the stigma associated with cancer in the minds of both the public and professionals. Delay in seeing the physician is often related to fear, pessimism, or fatalism, and poor or nonexistent doctor-patient relationships. A major problem is failure to take part in rehabilitation programs. A major community problem is the absence of such programs. The potential sources for altering patient attitudes include the media, the voluntary health associations, health professional organizations, health agencies, and the physician, whose attitudes, unfortunately, often must be changed.

The potential influence of the physicians in a given community, both as individuals and as a group in modifying the individual's behavior toward cancer, is far greater than they themselves realize. However, this impact is usually not maximized because of failure to use (let alone be aware of) the principles of social learning described above. The physician's relationship with a patient puts him in a position to be a powerful influencing agent. He can provide information that outlines the danger to the patient by not pursuing or treating cancer and can give him direct, clear-cut steps of action. The patient can be helped to develop independent control of his behavior, for it is quite possible to persuade him to make a decision to pursue treatment and rehabilitation where appropriate. Having done so, he can be referred to an appropriate group resource for behavior modification—either to alter risk-related behavior, or for psychosocial or physical rehabilitation with appropriate inclusion of social support and group modeling.

The group provides the greatest opportunity for facilitation of the acquisition of new health behavior. In groups there is provision for modeling, vicarious reinforcement by observing the rewards gained by others through mastery of new skills, and for the personal and public commitment of the patient to learning new health behavior consonant with the aims of that group. In fact, one study (20) indicates that if an individual can be influenced to make a public statement of intent in such a group, he is much more likely to carry out a proposed course of action. Probably the most important function that would be performed by such programs is that they would provide reference groups for the patients who would then be able to communicate and interact with others who share the common problems of cancer patients. Here, the "buddy system" previously referred to can be built in. It might be well to organize some of the groups in terms of cancer sites; thus ostomy patients might be formed into one group (many such already exist); patients with amputations of a limb or limbs into another; patients who have had mastectomies should meet together, and sometimes now do. It is important that patients compare their own situations with others in the similar situation; when dealing only with healthy others they are more likely to experience dissatisfaction and anxiety. Therefore, rehabilitation groups should facilitate the problems of adaptation to stressful life events. Also, observing the progress of fellow patients as they take steps toward independence and the resumption of social roles will strengthen their own expectations, as well as provide vicarious reinforcements that should help to strengthen new health behaviors. Finally, patients who have been anxious and fearful about the outcome of their cancer course will probably find their anxiety reduced by virtue of meeting with others under circumstances that are satisfying, pleasing, and constructive.

At the same time, special groups can be designed for those patients who represent the greatest rehabilitation problems. The patients who are chronically depressed, seriously disturbed or unduly fearful, and who fear giving up the patient role constitute special problems. The closest analogy is to the type of program designed and directed by Fordyce (21). In that program, a careful analysis is made of all environmental conditions, including family, that are reinforcing chronic pain and associated behaviors in patients who have little or no organic pathology. Patient and family are involved in a retraining program to alter the pain behavior-environmental consequence-relationships. This approach can be modified to fit a number of invalid behaviors and similar ones that are inconsistent with the actual degree of organic pathology or anatomical alteration, that is, that are greater than warranted and therefore maladaptive.

Physicians can take the lead in stimulating the formation of such groups. Physicians can be taught to pay attention to the principles of modeling (e.g., with respect to some health behaviors they propose that the patient adopt). The physician can help the patient to believe that he is not only susceptible to disease or recurrence but, more important, that preventive measures and treatment measures can be effective. By providing positive expectancies, adherence to the proposed therapeutic regimen is maximized.

This, of course, suggests two additional problems: modifying the behavior of physicians so that they will adopt the principles of social learning and become effective attitude changers and new behavior-motivators, and modifying the attitudes of the physicians and other health professionals toward working together to provide appropriate types of counseling required to motivate people to be screened, come forward when they find symptoms, and to take part in rehabilitation after treatment. This presupposes the prior provision of appropriate screening, pretreatment evaluation, treatment, and rehabilitation facilities.

It is important, too, to remember that changes in health behavior, such as taking part in screening programs, going to the physician (or, indeed, having a physician at all), compliance with therapeutic regimens, and participation in rehabilitation programs, are not the result of discrete social processes independent of the other aspects of the person's life. These behaviors are also subject to social and cultural influences, and depend on such functions as the person's level of skill in learning and executing self-changes, his perception of his own ability to control his fate, his level of alienation and disaffection from the circumstances in which he must live, and his self-image. Thus, in applying the principles that we have been discussing to the problem of health behavior in cancer patients and potential cancer patients, it is necessary that we consider the whole person and his social context (22).

The problem of making health professionals and physicians in particular, both individually and as a group, more concerned and skilled with respect to the behavioral factors in the clinician-patient relationship is a difficult one. The values and standards of the local medical community are probably the major influences in physicians' behavior with their patients. One study indicated that in every medical community there is a tendency to conform in regard to drug treatment, patterns of referral, and general treatment practices (23). One way to influence this is to identify the trend setters or innovators who are willing to try something new and persuade them to change their behavior and their public statements. If successful, this will eventually lead to diffusion and adoption by a large number of the community group. Thus the initial task is to identify in any given community the high-status physicians who are the trend setters and direct the initial attempts to influence behavior and attitudes toward them, using those professionals as the germinal centers for the diffusion of new attitudes and practices to the rest of the profession. This would include, probably, enlargement of the health team to include some individuals capable of using the necessary behavior modification principles with the patients.

Rehabilitation programs subsequent to the establishment of the diagnosis of cancer and the institution of treatment procedures probably require the greatest amount of work in bringing together groups of people whose individual skills must be applied in coordinated or integrated fashion to the needs of cancer patients. The task of modifying the behavior of the patient in rehabilitation programs must be preceded by the modification of behavior of individuals and groups of professionals. Organization of such programs requires careful structuring of informational appeals to the professional. Involvement of the concerned professionals in medicine, surgery, rehabilitation medicine, the mental health professions, nursing, social work, and others requires careful attention to all of the principles described above, because such groups do not usually work together for long periods of time in stable organized fashion outside of institutions where the hierarchies and lines of authority are clearly drawn. In the community where there are no such lines of authority, it becomes necessary to involve all of them in taking part in the organizational process, with the trend setters or opinion leaders providing the behavior to be modeled, and with careful attention to the necessity for commitment as a conscious decision of each involved professional to the goals of the program as a whole. Further, all the professionals must be persuaded to become involved in the planning process. Information campaigns should begin with such a group and include the provision of information that holds the attention. It should come from a credible source, provide clear instructions as to how to behave, and make effective use of the media. The programs themselves, whether involved with physical rehabilitation, the use of prostheses, or psychosocial rehabilitation with attention to problems of self-esteem, the resumption of family and other social roles, and coping with anxiety with respect to outcome, should include self-help groups, groups led by professionals, and groups that provide physical, vocational, and psychological programs tailored to the social and cultural characteristics of the populations to whom they are directed.

APPLICATIONS: THE COMMUNITY

The organization of community programs to provide the necessary context, as well as the resources, for cancer control programs is crucial to the success of all of the foregoing. Preventive services, screening services, and referral services to appropriate health care persons and agencies which are available, accessible, and acceptable to all segments of the population are needed. This might mean, in some communities, efforts to make a more equitable distribution of services as well as increased health education programs. A community program should also aim for an increased awareness on the part of the physician of the need for these programs and of the necessary behavioral components. Within the larger community, the professional community must be influenced to provide more continuing education to increase the behavioral science knowledge of all the health professionals as well as to include a wider range of all the health professionals within the health care system. This would lead to the development of organizations offering programs of rehabilitation counseling made up of loose networks of the appropriate health and mental health professionals. To provide these programs, a multiphasic approach is needed. This would include the constructive use of local media, including radio and television stations, information campaigns, education programs, and face-to-face discussion groups of both the providers of new services and those who would benefit from them.

A SYSTEMATIC APPROACH TO THE PROVISION OF
REHABILITATION PROGRAMS

Up to this point, I have briefly reviewed some relevant principles of social learning and the application of these principles to the modification of health behavior. I have indicated some of the areas to which change efforts should be directed and proposed some of the changes among the many that would have to be undertaken to provide the optimal program for cancer control and rehabilitation, from a behavioral perspective. In conclusion, I propose a systematic approach for the application of these principles to a given community.

For optimal effectiveness, such a program should begin at the end. In other words, the specific outcome behaviors in terms of patient outcomes should be specified first. Such a list of outcome objectives would not be applicable to every patient, and each new patient would perhaps require one or two unique objectives or highly specific ones, but the principle remains one of defining observable behaviors to be sought. These might include such objectives as finding an appropriate gainful occupation to be pursued with personal satisfaction, or an acceptable sex life, or improved communication between patient and family about their shared problems. Other outcomes representing other types of illness might include effective use of a prosthesis or reasonably acceptable pain control, or providing opportunities for the family to communicate about the impending death of the patient. But the list should be large and the specific areas needed to provide for most if not all the patient's needs should be clearly sought out at the beginning of the program.

The second step is to look at the enabling programs that would make such objectives attainable. The design of such programs should be a group effort involving all of the individuals concerned including representatives of the patient population. The resources of a given community will become an amalgam unique to each community, but one that can be organized to provide the desired outcomes. These resources might include patient self-help groups, family groups, crisis services, pain clinics, vocational retraining services, physical medicine and rehabilitation programs for prosthetic users, and others.

The third step is to identify the controlling processes by which such programs can be organized. These processes involve the use of the principles of communication, persuasion, diffusion, and adoption of innovation, and might also include education, consultation, and the mobilization of the community media and other communication channels. By such processes, community planning groups can be organized to use the media and influential citizens to persuade and educate the significant persons who would build the programs.

Finally, one can begin to identify the target groups and place a priority on when they should be recruited and what kinds of endeavors they should take part in to set in motion the necessary efforts to provide the programs from which the desired outcomes can be reached. These would undoubtedly include physicians, other health professionals, hospital administrators, community action groups, government groups, voluntary health organizations, clergy, the press, and other media.

I have covered a great deal of territory in a rather superficial way. However, if this review of a few principles of social psychology is useful, it is because it directs the attention of the behavioral science community to its role in providing the appropriate group influences to modify the health behavior of a community, the professionals, and the present and potential cancer patients to better cancer control and rehabilitation.

ACKNOWLEDGMENTS

Many of the ideas and proposals contained in this paper were developed in my work on another project, "Applying Behavioral Science to Cardiovascular Risk," supported by the American Heart Association and by a DHEW NHLI grant, Number HL16724-01 (NSS). I wish to acknowledge my special debt to the members of the American Heart Association Committee on Motivation for Risk Reduction who helped organize that project and to the behavioral scientists who reviewed the relevant literature. The list is too long to name all who contributed to that project. The proceedings of that conference are now in preparation. It was in discussion with those social scientists, and with Judith Henderson, Ph.D. and Emil Berkanovic, Ph.D., in the editing of the proceedings of the conference that the ideas contained herein were developed. The literature review was greatly facilitated by Daniel Stokols' *Research and Theory in Social Psychology Pertinent to Current Problems in Public Health,* an annotated bibliography

REFERENCES

1. Bandura, A. *Social Learning Theory,* General Learning Press, Morristown, N J., 1971
2. Rotter, J. B. *Social Learning and Clinical Psychology,* Prentice Hall, Englewood Cliffs, N.J., 1954.
3. Rotter, J. B. *Generalized Expectancies for Internal versus External Control of Reinforcement, Psychol. Monogr.,* 80 (Whole No. 609) (1966).
4. Rotter, J. B., Chance, J. E., and Phares, E. J. *Applications of a Social Learning Theory of Personality,* Holt, Rinehart and Winston, New York, 1972.
5. Bandura, A., and Walters, R. H. *Social Learning and Personality Development,* Holt Rinehart and Winston, New York, 1963.
6. Bandura, A. *Principles of Behavior Modification,* Holt, Rinehart and Winston, New York, 1969.
7. Bandura, A. Psychotherapy based upon modeling principles. In Bergin, A., and Garfield, S. (eds.): *Handbook of Psychotherapy and Behavior Change,* Wiley, New York, 1971.
8. Bandura, A., and Barab, P.G. Conditions governing nonreinforced imitation. *Dev. Psychol.,* 5:244–255 (1971).
9. Meyer, A. J., and Henderson, J.B. Multiple risk factor reduction in the prevention of cardiovascular disease. *Prev. Med.,* 3:225–236 (1974).
10. Mahoney, M. J. The behavioral treatment of obesity. Paper presented at *Conference on Applying Behavioral Science to Cardiovascular Risk,* Seattle, 1974.
11. McAlister, A. Behavioral approaches to the problem of cigarette smoking. Paper prepared for *Conference Proceedings: Applying Behavioral Science to Cardiovascular Risk,* Seattle, 1974.
12. Stunkard, A. J. Behavior modification of obesity and anorexia nervosa. *Arch. Gen. Psychiatry,* 26:391–398 (1972).
13. Lefcourt, H. M. Recent developments in the study of locus of control. In Maher, B. A. (ed): *Progress in Experimental Personality Research,* Vol. 6, Academic Press, New York, 1972.

14. Leventhal, H. Changing attitudes and habits to reduce chronic disease risk factors. *Am. J. Cardiol.*, 31:571–580 (1973).
15. Janis, I. L., and Hoffman, D. Facilitating effects of daily contact between partners who make a decision to cut down on smoking. *J. Pers. Soc. Psychol.*, 17:25–35 (1971).
16. Byrne, D., and Nelson, D. Attraction as a linear function of proportion of positive reinforcement. *J. Pers. Soc. Psychol.*, 1:659–663 (1965).
17. Davison, G. D., and Valins, S. Maintenance of self-attributed and drug-attributed behavior change. *J. Pers. Soc. Psychol.*, 11:25–33 (1969).
18. Kelley, H. Attribution theory in social psychology. *Nebraska Symposium on Motivation*, XV:192–238 (1967).
19. Holland, J. Psychologic aspects of cancer. In Holland, J. F., and Frei, E. (eds.): *Cancer Medicine*, pp. 991–1021, Lea & Febiger, Philadelphia, 1973.
20. Kothandapani, V. Validation of feeling, belief, and intention to act as three components of attitude and their contribution to prediction of contraceptive behavior. *J. Pers. Soc. Psychol.*, 19:321–333 (1971).
21. Fordyce, W. E. *A Guide to the Management of Chronic Pain by Operant Conditioning*, Department of Rehabilitation Medicine, University of Washington School of Medicine, Seattle, 1974.
22. Henderson, J., Berkanovic, E., and Enelow, A. J. Applying behavioral science to cardiovascular risk: Report of a conference. Paper presented at *Fogarty Conference on Behavioral Science in Preventive Medicine*, Washington, D.C., 1974.
23. Coleman, J. S., Katz, E., and Menzel, H. *Medical Innovation, A Diffusion Study*, Bobbs-Merrill, Indianapolis, 1966.

Cancer: The Behavioral Dimensions, edited by J. W. Cullen,
B. H. Fox, and R. N. Isom. Raven Press, New York © 1976.

Respondent

Barbara S. Hulka

Department of Epidemiology, School of Public Health, University of North Carolina,
Chapel Hill, North Carolina 27514

In order that you understand my sources of bias and areas of interest, I should say that I am an epidemiologist and also, some years ago, I was involved with the Cancer Control Program as a project director for one of their cervical cancer detection programs.

Although I realize that methodology is not the specific orientation of this volume, I think it is important; if methodology is not considered, we may come to conclusions and make generalizations that are not justified in terms of the available data in the studies. An interesting point is noted by Dr. Raymond Fink who writes of the difference in crude death rates between participants and nonparticipants in the breast cancer screening program at the Health Insurance Plan of Greater New York (HIP). This was particularly interesting taken together with the fact that when examining the differential causes of death, the nonpartic- ipants were much more likely to have died of circulatory deaths, which would presumably include the cardiovascular diseases. The possibility arises that this result could actually be due to a secondary association. Dr. Fink notes initially that the participants tended to be younger than nonparticipants. This being the case, and depending on the extent of the age differential, the observed differential death rate among nonparticipants and participants could be explained on the basis of age. In other words, if nonparticipants tended to be older, and significantly older than participants, purely on the basis of this biologic differ- ence we would expect them to have higher death rates. Also, the older one gets, the greater the likelihood that death is going to be due to a cardiovascular cause. I am therefore questioning whether the difference in death rates could be a secondary association due to age.

Dr. Antonovsky's chapter is extremely interesting and his interpretation of the findings has a great deal of intuitive appeal. However, his interpretations and conclusions were drawn from a study of 58 women in the experimental group who received breast cancer screening and 40 control women who did not. Due to the problem of unrecognized prior screening among some of his controls, he ended up with 23 matched pairs. By the usual methods of performing a matched-pairs analysis, there would have to be tremendous differences on the psychological variables of interest between the screened and the non- screened women in these 23 pairs to identify statistically significant and psychologically meaningful differences. I certainly recognize the problems that we all have in getting a sufficient number of patients into our studies, but I suggest a note of caution is making overly broad interpretations or generalizations on the basis of a very small number of patients or subjects. I would be interested in the kind of analysis that Dr. Antonovsky felt appropriate and was able to do on 23 matched pairs of cases and controls.

In Dr. Green's chapter, I became aware of an assumption that many of us accept or at least appear to accept as suggested by several of the chapters herein. This assumption concerns the nature of symptoms, particularly cancer-specific symptoms. Is there something specific or characteristic about symptoms pertaining to cancer? Dr. Green reviews data from various studies of cancer patients and the symptoms they had experienced that brought them to the doctor. Based on his review of cancer-specific symptoms, I would suggest that the literature is inadequate. Certainly, from the epidemiologic perspective, we would want to know not only what are the symptoms experienced by cancer patients but what is the distribution of these same symptoms in normal, essentially healthy persons, as well as among persons with other forms of chronic disease. Let me illustrate by using the example of hypertension. When I went to medical school, I was taught that anyone who had a history of spontaneous nose bleeds and severe headache obviously should be examined for the possibility of having high blood pressure, because these were symptoms associated with hypertension. Since then, the distribution and frequency of these symptoms were studied in a sample of essentially normal persons as well as among hypertensive patients. The results showed that there was no significant difference in the frequency of these symptoms in normals as compared with hypertensive persons. Therefore, one wonders what are the clinically pertinent symptoms of hypertension or, likewise, of cancer. This merely suggests two points. First, we cannot assume that certain symptoms are characteristic of a particular disease unless we know the frequency of those symptoms among persons without the disease. Second, if the symptoms under consideration are common occurrences in relatively normal persons, then it becomes more understandable why people delay in seeking medical advice even after the advent of those symptoms.

I would like to emphasize some issues pertaining to the health care system as it relates to screening. By screening, I mean primary or secondary prevention and early response to symptoms. I think the system of care in which screening activities take place is critically important to the effectiveness of those activities. Dr. Fink notes that participants in the breast cancer screening program were more likely to have seen a HIP physician during the prior year than were nonparticipants. He inferred from this that participants were more involved with the HIP health care system than were nonparticipants. Mammography was integrated into the HIP health care system, and women who came for screening were women who also related to that system of care. Further evidence from his study for this point of view is the finding that in the thermography program, where thermography necessarily was more distant from and in a different location from the HIP group practices, the participation rates were lower. Again, women not only had greater difficulties of accessibility but I would suggest that they had to relate to a facility that was not part of their usual source of care.

Dr. Green also refers to how best to deliver screening services, and he suggests mobile units for some locales. In his chapter he presents this topic in more detail and discusses issues pertaining to multiphasic screening versus uniphasic screening. It seems to me that whether you are dealing with multi- or uniphasic screening, it would be vastly better to have the screening activity integrated within the existing health care delivery system and preferably the patient's usual source of care. The reason for this, I believe, is that when screening is part of the existing medical care setting and organizational structure, as opposed to being separate from that structure, you are going to be much more successful in attracting patients to the screening facility. More important, the chances of getting appropriate diagnostic workup and therapy for persons with abnormalities on screening are going to be much improved. I would suggest that one of the problems with many of our screening programs has been the dichotomy between where you get screened and where you get diagnosed and treated. Certainly, there are many caveats to this statement. For example, when the technology is complex, the facilities and personnel cannot be immediately available everywhere, and undoubtedly there are areas where the existing health care system is not going to provide the service, so a separate screening facility is necessary. To give one example from my own experience, in the 1960s the Cancer Control Program had 20 cervical cancer demonstration projects. I was involved with one of them in Pittsburgh and went to a meeting of the various project directors. As we sat around the table, the program officer said: "You know, Barbara, we've learned from you how not to do cervical cancer screening"! He did not say this as a joke or as an insult. He was making a very useful point, which was the importance of learning from experience how not to do things. We were in Pittsburgh establishing separate cervical cancer screening clinics in various localities throughout the county. Administratively and economically, this proved to be a relatively unfeasible mechanism for providing services. Subsequently, the choice of screening locations and organizational settings has been within the framework of existing services where women are already coming for medical care.

Respondent

Miriam F. Kelty*

Office of Scientific Affairs, American Psychological Association, Washington, D.C. 20036

Rather than repeat Dr. Hulka's remarks or criticize methodology, which is incompletely described in the chapters, I will focus on issues that all relate in some way to health education.

After reading the chapters presented herein and the preparatory materials previously mailed to us, I am convinced that one can now find support in the literature for most theoretical orientations about the interrelationships among environmental, demographic, personality, and social factors associated with cancer and cancer-related behaviors. This is partially attributable to the complexity of health behavior and its multiple causality. However, several chapters presented here demonstrate that the contributing components of behavior can be analyzed, and that most often they are not. For example, it would be more useful to analyze behavior patterns associated with health maintenance and with illness prevention so that particular components are identifiable as such, rather than to speak in global terms as if to imply that we are dealing with unitary phenomena.

A second related point is that the chapters present multiple models of delay behavior, detection behavior, adaptation behavior, and rehabilitation behavior. These models of health behavior determinants and variables constitute useful tools for researchers and practitioners but may confuse the public. This is characteristic of the creative, developmental stage of any field that is suddenly expanding. But the public may be misled by what it perceives as conflicting messages from the scientific/medical community. This may present serious problems for health-education program planners and implementers, and may be counterproductive to fostering behavior change.

A mechanism may be needed for identifying and promoting the model that is most promising at a given time, while retaining the option of model changes as frequently as necessary to accommodate new data. Dr. Antonovsky describes psychosocial "types" that are assumed to have different resistance sources affecting their health behavior. His model, which guides his research in screening behavior of populations, predicts that different strategies for behavior change or for preventive programs will be effective for differing personality constellations. At the individual level this does not pose serious practical problems. However, at the level of wide-scale public health education it presents difficulties in predicting appropriate audiences for particular messages or programs, unless behavioral constellations of a society account for more variance between cultures than do individual differences within a culture. We were reminded of this problem by Dr. Enelow's discussion of the Children's Television Workshop experience with *Feelin' Good,* its health education program.

This entire volume focuses on the importance of health education. However, it also indicates that to a large extent we lack the knowledge on which such programs should be based. Health education has not been a high priority for our government for the last several years because of disillusionment over effectiveness and a shift to direct health care activities. In 1974, the Assistant Secretary for Health restored health education to a priority status in his 5-year Forward Plan, but curriculum, data base, and teaching methods to

*Present position: National Commission for the Protection of Human Subjects of Biomedical and Behavioral Research, DHEW, Bethesda, Maryland 20014

implement such programs on a national level have not been adequately developed and we still must demonstrate impact and cost-effectiveness.

A number of issues follow this decision to initiate a health education program. For example, to what extent should such programs increase conceptual understanding of principles based on "best knowledge" at a particular time period? To what extent should programs provide group behavior supports, or conditioning, or social role modeling? Several approaches have demonstrated areas of effectiveness. On what basis should we choose among them, or is it appropriate to employ all in a social experiment?

Ethical implications of such policies have not yet been explored herein. Should we focus on the young or on particular high-risk population subgroups? If we teach habits, and habits are difficult to change, why not focus efforts on education toward health behavior rather than on reduction of the older population? However, is it ethical to teach particular behaviors to children, particularly when knowledge is expanding so rapidly that the "facts" we teach may soon become obsolete? How do we create appropriate concern for health without teaching excessive preoccupation with illness and death? We can see the dangers of this in the preoccupation with many adults with "regularity" fostered by effective TV commercials. If we recognize that education programs have behavior modification objectives, how do we deal with the problems of producing significant and relevant behavior change to a culture that perceives behavior modification programs negatively, even if some particular behavior modification techniques have demonstrated effectiveness?

What should be the content of a public education program curriculum? Evidence to date indicates that for cancer prevention we might teach not to smoke, not to drink excessively, not to become depressed, not to live in cities, and not to engage in sexual relations with many partners at an early age—a difficult set of prohibitions to sell in our culture!

If we are to initiate public programs toward health maintenance and illness prevention it seems reasonable to implement them at the institutional level—in schools and in industry—as well as at the individual level. What are the ethical implications of initiating such programs for the individual who might be deprived of some freedom of choice? Would such deprivation of freedom be justified for the enhancement of health status at the societal level?

Finally, many of the chapters in this volume focus on secondary prevention—on diagnosis, treatment, and/or rehabilitation once disease is present. We would all agree that primary prevention is important, both to minimize individual suffering and for economic reasons. However, we also know that it is particularly difficult to modify behaviors that lead to negative consequences in the future. One large problem before us is to develop effective programs and attitudes toward behavior change in the present that will result in positive consequences for health in the future. Conceptually, this may be one of the most difficult problems we face.

Discussion

Fox: In response to Dr. Kelty's remarks about doing and not doing, it seems to me that it is quite artificial to specify that stopping a particular action should be characterized as a don't and then saying that the don'ts suffer for some reason more than the dos. There seems to be little difference in terms of actual health practice between brushing the teeth, an onerous, distasteful, disagreeable act to a 7-year-old, which is a do, and not drinking for a 16-year-old, which is a don't. Both are specific, deliberate, intentful actions that result in some change in the environment with respect to the person. This artificiality should be examined more closely. I must admit that I made the same distinction in my chapter and I'm sorry that I did, because I now disagree with myself and with Dr. Kelty.

Enelow: I would like to reply to the comment about physician bias. I don't believe that anyone working in the field of health behavior considers physician behavior to be a constant in the personality of the patient or the social factors to which the patient is subjected or is a part of as a variable at all. As a matter of fact, some of the most difficult work that we have been doing has been to alter physician behavior and attitudes with regard to prevention and with regard to utilizing what is known from behavioral science. Until we begin to do rather large-scale, quasi-controlled field intervention trials, we are not going to reach the physicians with our neatly controlled little experiments out of the social psychology laboratory. I believe that the business of altering physician bias is a very important one; it is the missing key to the whole picture and it should be in the forefront. I tried to put it there.

Kelty: One of the points I tried to make was that in the perception of the patient, physician bias is not attended to. I am not saying that the health professionals don't appreciate it, but it is the expectation of the patient that the physician or health professional is neutral and knowledgeable.

R. Fink: First, let me thank the commentators for helping to analyze the data. To answer Dr. Hulka's observation: The difference in mortality rates could in part be accounted for by the difference in age. However, I doubt very much whether that is the total story. But I think it is more important that we have characterized the nonparticipant as someone who is indifferent and unconcerned. What I am beginning to suspect from these data, which we must explore more closely, is that we have a woman who says, "My arthritis is killing me, I've got asthma, and I've recently had a heart attack, don't bother me with breast cancer, please." I think we have to be able to understand that, too. And I think I should have focused on that point a little more strongly. I thank you, too, for reminding us all that the health-care system is an important part of the whole program; that those who came were more likely to be involved in the total health-care system; and to separate a screening program from the health-care system runs the risk of losing patients, first, on their way to the screening, and second, on their way from screening into treatment. One final point I should have made is that you can involve people in a health-care system *in toto*. You can involve them in care, you can involve them in screening, and if there is any one point that perhaps I should have made, it is that I don't know whether you are changing behavior, but you can involve people.

Green: I appreciate the concerns about separate screening programs, too, and I offered that recommendation with great trepidation, recognizing past experience with separate screening programs. But it seems to me the opposition to them has usually been on the wrong grounds. I think Dr. Hulka gave the right arguments about separate screening programs. What we have to be most careful about is separating the patient into a screening program and never getting him into the medical care system. For the wrong reasons the arguments that seem to prevail when you try to set up a screening program in a community are usually more implicitly economic—the medical care system does not want competition, nor does it want to be flooded with patients for which it didn't ask.

An appropriate compromise between these two sets of arguments is to set up, where necessary, separate screening programs if the medical care system is not adequately reaching the people who need to be screened. We must be sure that adequate linkages are built to the existing medical care system so that people don't just get screened and not diagnosed, or diagnosed and not followed up with medical care.

To respond briefly to Dr. Kelty's comment, there is, in fact, some literature showing the cost-effectiveness of health education. One only needs to consider the major alternative, which is to put people in hospitals and give them surgery, and so on, and it is clear that the earlier that you can provide health education, the more cost-effective it will be; the more effectively you can do it, the more cost-effective. That is tautology, I realize, but what we have failed to do so far is invest sufficiently in health education to achieve cost-effectiveness or even the beginning of it.

L. Fink: Dr. Raymond Fink noted that there were control and noncontrol groups of women involved in and seeking breast screening. Were these prospective breast-screened women exposed to information relative to the X-ray component of mammography versus thermography and, if so, were there any data as to the effect on their behavior in seeking breast screening?

R. Fink: The mammography study screenings were started about 10 years ago. We observed the usual informed consent procedures. In the letters that went to the women we did tell them that X-rays would be taken. We do not know enough about exposure and so on to give them any more information than that. The current thermography study follows the same procedures. Women are receiving thermography and mammography both, and they are informed that X-rays will be taken.

L. Fink: Dr. Antonovsky noted that the behavior of women seeking breast screening in Israel was very seriously affected by the social norm. I question whether the social norm would be the same in our country as it is in Israel, where there is a definite cohesive nationalism that seems to be the core of behavior of all of the people in Israel.

Antonovsky: I quite agree. One has to take into account the power of the social norm in Israel, in America, in any subculture, for that matter. The contents of the social norm may vary, even from one subculture in Israel to another and certainly between Israel and America. The norm is powerful, but whether the norm pushes you in one direction or another is a different question.

Mr. Carl Symington (radiation oncologist from Ft. Worth, Texas): In looking at the Table 1 data in Dr. Fox's presentation, I find that under "personality" it is his conclusion that these conditions have been examined and found not to be precursors to the development of malignancy or to affect survival, as also are "depression" and "specific life stresses." Now, I appreciated your comments regarding the bibliography in the beginning and your specific comments regarding the difficulty in the search of the literature. My own search has been fraught with a great deal of difficulty. However, based on that search, as well as my own experience in dealing with what I have termed emotional aspects of malignancy, my conclusions are the opposite in that personality variables are indeed significant factors in certainly, survival, as shown in the work of Dr. Klopfer, Dr. West, and others. I think these matters could be clarified by coming to terms with the literature and what is acceptable, but certainly they are reported in such documents as the *Journal of the National Cancer Institute* and the *Journal of Cancer Research.* My question specifically, is where would you place the numerical rating, which you indicated was a personal judgment, on the role of personality and the other variables in both development and in cancer survival?

Fox: First of all, I did not say that personality variables were not precursors. I said it had not been proved that they are precursors, which is a very, very different matter. It is merely a statement that the studies so far have been inadequate to say anything. Now, your statement about the possibility that personality and individual characteristics can predict survival based on Klopfer's and West's data, I think, suffers from the same difficulty. I have looked over Klopfer's work very carefully and that of others who have addressed the question of survival being predicted by personality, and my conclusion is that whereas it may be true that personality could be (and I think that it has not been proved) an associated condition that goes along with greater or lesser survival, one might be able to predict on that basis, it has nothing to do with causing these greater or lesser survivals. I want to emphasize that separation between an association and a cause. You also asked my judgment as to the rating that I might give to the personality characteristics in terms of range of confidence as to their association with survival, and I have to be very careful to restrict myself to that, rather than stating something about cause. I would say that the question of personality itself is, as yet, so unsettled that whereas it is possible that there is an association, it has not been proved. There are some inklings in the literature, which I mentioned, pointing to that possibility; therefore, that is the reason I put 3-4 where 4 implies suspicion only or none at all, and 3 implies moderate-to-low confidence. I would say it is very close to the low position. Now in terms of transient or recurring states, such as mental illness, that is also in the same ball park. But because there is even less evidence in favor of there being such an association, I rated it as 4 to be on the safe side. One might, in fact, find an association with, perhaps, paranoid aspects of mental illness, which has not been thoroughly explored but is hinted at rather consistently in a number of findings.

Krant: In listening to some of the descriptions of why women go for screening and why they don't, at least three factors were not considered. One is the meaning of the breast as a sexual organ. I can't imagine that women don't pay some attention to that and it's meaning in their psychosexual sphere. What that means must have some implication as to what they will do when some threatening phenomenon, as they see it, occurs there. And I wonder why this wasn't looked into or why we didn't hear about this as a phenomenon?

Second, I would think that women would also be somewhat aware of what's to be done to them if they do, in fact, find cancer. What the outcome would be—in the form of either a standardized radical mastectomy or some other kind of technical approach to the problem—must play a role in whether they would let themselves be screened. I was wondering why this aspect was not looked at either.

And third, I would think that there has been a growing concern about decision-making and awareness of patients to be able to play a role in the way medical care is given. Namely, do I have anything to say about the way I will be operated on and what will be done to me? I am sure that must play a role, again intuitively, in how women see themselves going through any process that will leave them to be acted on by somebody else, oftentimes by a male surgeon.

Antonovsky: We did ask the question about how you feel about your body in sexual contact and so on. It is a mistake to look at this one item; that is what brought me to look at the total profile of the woman. In this specific clinical case, it may be decisive how she feels about her breast, or in that specific case, it may be decisive how she feels about her physician. But when you're trying to understand a total pattern of behavior, I think it doesn't make sense to look at the power of this or that individual item. In response to your third comment on the right of participation and what would happen to the individual, I believe you have a cultural bias here, if I may translate your comment into my typology. You are talking about one of my four types, and it makes sense for the rational goal-directed type. What you have said does not make sense for my other three types. Now what the numerical distribution of these four types is, I don't know. I doubt whether either in my country or yours or in any other country, the rational goal-directed type is most of us.

Cancer: The Behavioral Dimensions, edited by J. W. Cullen, B. H. Fox, and R. N. Isom. Raven Press, New York © 1976.

Environmental Risks Related to Cancer

Peter B. Peacock*

American Health Foundation and Cornell Medical Center, New York, New York 10019

The incidence of cancer in any population is determined by the interactions of the genome with the environment. Where genetic differences do not appear to account for geographic or subcultural variations in the incidence of cancer, we must look for environmental carcinogens that may serve as primary inducers or in an additive role. This is why geographic differences, especially among migrant populations, have always fascinated epidemiologists. A look at the various major forms of cancer reveals striking differences. Among blacks in the United States the incidence rate for cancer of the colon (excluding rectum), as recorded by the Third National Cancer Survey (1) was 24.8, which may be compared to 3.5 in Uganda (2). For cancer of the breast, age-adjusted death rates per 100,000 population in 1966–67 varied from a high of 26.45 in the Netherlands to a low of 3.99 in Japan (3). These six- or sevenfold differences can also be demonstrated for cancer of the lung, cervix uteri, stomach, and prostate. In contrast, for leukemia, where environmental factors are presumably less important, geographical differences are considerably smaller.

Perhaps more than in any other area, investigators in the cancer field have tended to jump to conclusions concerning possible environmental carcinogens with very little hard evidence. When looking at geographical or subcultural distributions and differences, it is essential that we distinguish between association and causation. An analysis of cancer figures, diet, and other factors for 37 countries (4) showed that colon cancer and breast cancer have a strong positive correlation with each other, with animal fat, with animal protein, with the number of vehicles in the community, with egg consumption, with income, and, to a lesser extent, with the number of radios and television sets and the consumption of sugar and sweets. To this list we could safely add death rates from coronary artery disease (it is the wives of our patients with coronary artery disease who get breast cancer), artificially softened water supplies, and whatever measure of industrial air pollution (e.g., sulfur oxides) suits the fancy of the investigator concerned. These variables and many others are, of course, all positively correlated with each other and with the rather artificial standard of living found in much of North America and northwestern Europe. The important question to the epidemiologist is whether we can untangle these associations.

---

*Present address: McNease Clinic, Fayette, Alabama 35555

WHAT WE BREATHE

Since 1950, when Wynder and Graham (5) and Doll and Hill (6) published their first reports, an incontrovertible body of evidence has accumulated, based on both retrospective and prospective studies, showing cigarette smokers to be at greatly increased risk of lung cancer compared with nonsmokers. The Panel on Chemicals and Health of the President's Science Advisory Committee estimated that in 1967, 17% of all deaths were directly linked to cigarette smoking (7). Possibly 40% of all male cancer deaths relate to tobacco usage.

In addition to the well-known and fully proved relationship between cigarette smoking and lung cancer, lung cancer also shows an urban excess, particularly among males (8). This urban excess has been found for smokers on both sides of the Atlantic (9) and, with relatively few exceptions, also among nonsmokers. Most investigators have reported that the urban-rural difference increases with the number of cigarettes smoked, suggesting that the two factors have a multiplicative rather than a simple additive effect. The impression that the urban factor is most probably air pollution has been based on the finding in polluted atmosphere of carcinogens (notably 3,4-benzpyrene), which produce cancer in experimental animals (10) (although not by inhalation) and which in a few studies correlate with the distribution of lung cancer (11).

The evidence linking air pollution to lung cancer is, however, far from conclusive. Some of the urban excess, and the puzzling sex difference, may be explained by the greater duration of cigarette smoking among urban dwellers and males. The remaining urban excess could be accounted for by some other variable (such as an infective or immunological state related to overcrowding and hence to urban conditions) having little or nothing to do with air pollution at the levels usually encountered. Better reporting of cases in urban areas is possible but unlikely for lung cancer. Certain arguments against the urban factor being air pollution have been summarized by Goldsmith (12) and deal with the poor correlation (for cities of each size within countries) between air pollution and lung cancer, the higher rates of lung cancer found among migrants to urban areas compared with lifetime urban residents, and the lesser impact of the urban factor on women. To these one can add the better correlation found between population density and lung cancer than between air pollution and lung cancer (13), the lack of excess cancer among garage workers and policemen exposed to heavy concentrations of motor vehicle exhaust (14), and the low death rate from lung cancer among coal miners.

The carcinogenic effects of exposure to asbestos in mining (15) (especially chrysotile), in industry (16), and in the general community (17) have been well documented. Exposure to asbestos and cigarette smoke gives a risk of mesothelioma considerably higher than that produced by either risk factor alone. Asbestos alone probably does not increase the risk of bronchial carcinoma. Industrial exposures to other minerals, such as arsenic, chromium, and nickel, have been associated with industrial respiratory cancer as have exposure to tar fumes and, more recently, to vinyl chloride (18), producing, in particular, angiosarcoma of the liver.

Although the evidence for these occupational exposures is reasonably good, the evidence relating many other so-called airborne carcinogens to human cancer is often largely nonexistent, the proponents of these calls-to-panic using the same sort of drum beating that has always been employed by antifluoridationists as a substitute for hard facts. A good example of this is the attack on many of the insecticides, which have contributed so much to human survival (19), despite good human epidemiologic work (20) showing that they have no effect on humans in doses considerably in excess of those to which the general public has been exposed. A sense of proportion is important. Compared to the risks of cigarette smoking, the effects of occupational exposures and air pollution are small.

WHAT WE EAT AND DRINK

For several major cancers there is suggestive evidence linking characteristic dietary patterns with an increased risk of cancer. Thus, in experimental animals, an increased amount of fat in the diet increases the yield of breast cancer. Animals fed high fat diets are also more liable to get breast cancer when exposed to chemical carcinogens such as 7,12-dimethylbenzanthracene. In human populations a strong positive correlation has been shown between the fat consumption of a given country (FAO figures) and the incidence of breast cancer in that country (21). For women with breast cancer there is a suggestion that cases are heavier than age-matched controls (22,23).

We have confirmed this association in older women although this difference is not as great as if found with endometrial cancer (24). A similar epidemiological correlation over several countries between cancer of the colon and fat intake can also be demonstrated (25). It is doubtful whether a single carcinogenic pathway is involved when we are dealing with a relationship such as that postulated between fat and cancer of the colon. Both adducts and proximal carcinogens are probably involved (26) and evidence suggests that the intestinal microflora participates in and is required for the activation of carcinogens by liberating the reactive intermediates from a conjugate (27). Cancers of the kidney and possibly of the prostate may follow a similar pattern, although the evidence is much more circumstantial.

Whether a lack of dietary fiber is related to large bowel cancer (28) must still be considered as unproved. Of interest is a suggestion by Hill (29) that cholestyramine used to reduce serum cholesterol levels by increasing the fecal loss of bile acids should increase the incidence of colon cancer. No evidence is yet available on this score from the trials being undertaken by the National Heart and Lung Institute. For many years an association has been suggested between stomach cancer and dietary factors and the dramatic reduction in the incidence of stomach cancer in the United States over the last 20 years has been a matter for repeated comment. One study in Japan, where the incidence is still high, suggests that the high incidence of carcinoma of the stomach in certain areas is associated with the consumption of larger amounts of salty food and smaller amounts of milk. The occurrence of 3,4-benzpyrene on and in smoked and roasted foodstuff has also attracted attention (30).

A great deal, including some excellent reviews, has been written on the subject of food additives with particular reference to possible carcinogenic effects (31,32). Carcinogens present in small amounts in food can occur naturally (e.g., senecio, cycads, chili pepper, and certain solanaceous fruits) or be the products of our modern industrialization including emulsifiers, sweeteners, preservatives, flavoring agents, dyes, pesticide residues, and hormonal contaminants. Of particular interest are the aflatoxins from certain species of *aspergillus flavus*, which have been associated with primary cancer of the liver, particularly in Africa. Strongly contrasting viewpoints can be found in the literature discussing how these possible carcinogens should be handled and whether the Delaney Amendment to the Food, Drug and Cosmetics Act can be justified. Proponents for strict control are represented by Hueper (33) and a critical look at some of the ironies introduced by the Delaney Amendment (e.g., the unnecessary banning of cyclamates) is presented by Foster (34). To test for the carcinogenicity of food additives and chemotherapeutic agents, a number of sensitive screening programs have been developed (35). It should be remembered, however, that the findings from these programs must be applied with caution to human experience, since we are dealing with doses quite unlike those found in the exposed human and we are working in an animal system that may differ widely from the human system.

The potential hazards of nitrosamines in certain foodstuffs and halogenated hydrocarbons in drinking water have received particular attention in the United States this last year. Nitrates are present in large quantities in many vegetables (36), such as spinach, eggplant, and lettuce. Nitrates are also found in small amounts as meat additives and in some water supplies. Under certain circumstances these nitrates can be reduced to nitrite, which can react with some classes of amines (e.g., trimethylamine oxide in salt-water fish) to produce nitrosamines. The nitrosamines in turn appear to behave under certain circumstances as carcinogen precursors. Examination of the New Orleans drinking water supplies and blood plasma from 21 local residents (37) demonstrated tetrachlorethylene and carbon tetrachloride in both, together with other halogenated compounds. The investigators concerned suggested that these compounds might be found accumulating in a variety of body tissues.

Three articles in the September 21, 1974, issue of *Lancet* reported a suspected association between rauwolfia therapy and breast cancer (38). In all three reported studies the use of rauwolfia appeared approximately to double the risk compared to nonusers. In the Boston study, among 150 patients with newly diagnosed breast cancer, 7.3% gave a history of taking reserpine-containing drugs compared to 2.2% among 1,200 matched surgical and medical controls. In the English study, 10 users of rauwolfia were found among 708 cancer patients and 11 among 1,430 controls with other neoplasms. In the group from Helsinki, among 438 pairs there were 68 that were discordant for reserpine use, the drug being taken by the patients in 45 pairs and by the controls in 23. The chief problems with these studies are that they cannot be regarded as independent of each other, the selection and exclusion of certain of the controls may have created some bias, and selective recall is a possibility. Nonetheless, these findings must be regarded as highly suspicious. Of considerable importance is the possible carcinogenic effect of estrogens because of their widespread use as contraceptives in addition to their use as a hormone supplement or (until recently) in agriculture. Although most recent investigators (39) have concluded that there is no evidence that the administration of female hormones, at least when given in physiological doses, is associated with the development of breast cancer, there are exceptions, and thus Black and Leis found a prior history of estrogens some three times as frequent among young nulliparas with breast cancer as in age-matched controls (40).

Another risk factor to which a large proportion of the population is exposed is alcohol. Available evidence suggests that squamous cell carcinomas of the oral cavity, pharynx, larynx, and esophagus would be uncommon in most industrialized countries without excessive exposure to tobacco and alcohol (41,42). In addition, the risk of developing a second primary cancer is significantly enhanced by more intensive combined exposures to tobacco and alcohol prior to the index cancer (43). Great gaps in our knowledge still exist regarding the relationship of vitamin intake to cancer. Thus lowering riboflavin intake may reduce the rates of growth of tumors (44) (and possibly their incidence) while at the same time there is an increased carcinogenicity of azo dyes in riboflavin-deficient animals. Similar, partly contradictory evidence has been collected for vitamin A. The role of nutrients may obviously differ for various types of cancer.

SKIN EXPOSURE

The relationship between excess exposure to ultraviolet light in sunlight and the development of skin cancer has been well documented. Of interest, because of the probable relationship between herpes virus and cancer, are recent studies demonstrating the transformation of herpes-infected cellular material by ultraviolet light. There is some concern about the use of ultraviolet light and super-vital dyes for the treatment of fever blisters about the mouth because of the possibility of producing a cancer. In addition, it has been suggested that ultraviolet light may be able to transform cholesterol into a carcinogenic metabolite.

Evidence is continuing to accumulate concerning the risk of head and neck tumors (especially involving the thyroid) among children irradiated for ringworm of the scalp (45). The risk of leukemia among children of mothers exposed to unnecessary diagnostic radiation and of bone and lung tumors among industrial workers exposed to radioactive substances such as uranium is generally well accepted today.

EXPOSURE TO INFECTION

Although no efficient human cancer-causing viruses are known, the subject of viral initiation of human cancer is receiving continued and sustained attention. Members of four different groups of viruses are known to cause cancer in animals, with all of these forming integrated viral DNA in affected cells (46). In recent years particular interest has been concentrated on suggested viral candidates related to the causation of leukemia, Hodgkin's disease (47), breast cancer (48), and, particularly, cancer of the uterine cervix. This review cannot attempt to discuss the evidence for and against a viral etiology for cancer, but it is likely that viruses have an important role in the etiology of some cancers. Other infections exerting a chronic irritative effect (e.g., schistosomiasis and bladder cancer) are also known to serve as carcinogens.

SOCIAL AND PSYCHOLOGICAL FACTORS

The literature on breast cancer includes a number of studies suggesting that breast cancer may be related to a variety of psychological states and, hence, to the social milieu. This area is worth investigating further; but at present few firm conclusions can be reached. Perhaps the most careful paper dealing with this subject, by Snell and Graham (49), failed to demonstrate any difference between breast cancer cases and controls. However, their controls contained other cancer cases, a fact that raises some question about the firmness of their conclusion. Other cancers deserve more attention. Physicians and particularly psychiatrists have noted for some years that persons with carcinoma of the pancreas often show degrees of depression quite out of proportion to any abdominal discomfort they may have. Perhaps we may be able to develop a constellation of psychological risk factors indicating an increased propensity to the development of breast cancer and other cancers that can rank along with physically established risk factors.

A simple list of environmental factors that may be related to cancer is not enough. One of the critical elements in establishing a proof of causation in human disease epidemiology is the reduction in the incidence of the disease concerned when the causal agent is controlled. Our cancer control programs must be predicated on the same need for active intervention. This intervention should be directed at those factors deserving most attention in terms of impact and our ability to modify or eliminate them. Priority attention should thus be given to those "life-style" variables that are amenable to behavior modification—tobacco usage, incorrect nutrition, and alcohol usage. Managerial control can probably exert its greatest impact on occupational exposures and exposure to radiation. We already know enough to accomplish a great deal.

REFERENCES

1. Biometry Branch, NCI. The Third National Cancer Survey advanced three-year report, 1969–1971 incidence. DHEW Publication No. (NIH) 74–637 (1974).
2. Doll, R. The geographical distribution of cancer. *Br. J. Cancer,* 23:1–8 (1969).
3. Silverberg, B., and Holleb, A. I. Cancer statistics, 1974—Worldwide epidemiology, *CA,* 24:2–21 (1974).

4. Drasar, B. S., and Irving, D. Environmental factors and cancer of the colon and breast. *Br. J. Cancer,* 27:167–172 (1973).
5. Wynder, E. L., and Graham, E. A. Tobacco smoking as a possible etiologic factor in bronchogenic carcinoma. A study of 684 proved cases. *JAMA,* 143:329–336 (1950).
6. Doll, R., and Hill, A. B. Smoking and carcinoma of the lung. Preliminary report. *Br. Med. J.,* ii:739–748 (1950).
7. *Panel on Chemicals and Health of the President's Science Advisory Committee.* Chemicals and Health, National Science Foundation, U.S. Govt. Print. Off., Washington, D.C., 1973.
8. Haenszel, W., and Tauber, K. E. Lung cancer mortality as related to residence and smoking histories. II. White females. *J. Natl. Cancer Inst,* 32:803–838 (1964).
9. Buell, P., and Dunn, J. E. Relative impact of smoking and air pollution on lung cancer. *Arch. Environ. Health,* 15:291–297 (1967).
10. Hueper, W. C., Kotin, P., Tabor, E. C., Payne, W. W., Falk, H., and Sawicki, E. Carcinogenic bioassays on air pollutants. *Arch. Pathol.,* 74:89–116 (1962).
11. Stocks, P. Recent epidemiological studies of lung cancer mortality, cigarette smoking and air pollution with discussion of a new hypothesis of causation. *Br. J. Cancer,* 20:595–623 (1966).
12. Goldsmith, J. B. Effects of air pollution on human health. In Stern (ed.): *Air Pollution,* 2nd ed., Academic Press, New York, 560 pp., 1968.
13. Ashley, J. D. B. The distribution of lung cancer and bronchitis in England and Wales. *Br. J. Cancer,* 21:243–259 (1967).
14. Lawther, P. J. Air pollution, bronchitis and lung cancer. *Postgrad. Med. J.,* 42:703–708 (1966).
15. Harrington, J. S., Roe, F. J. C., and Walters, M. Studies of the mode of action of asbestos as a carcinogen. *S. Afr. Med. J.,* 41:800–804 (1967).
16. Selikoff, I. J., Hammond, E. C., and Churg, J. Asbestos exposure, smoking and neoplasia. *JAMA,* 204:106–109 (1968).
17. Selikoff, I. J., and Hammond, E. C. Community effects of non-occupational environmental asbestos exposure. *Am. J. Public Health,* 58:1658–1666 (1968).
18. Block, J. B. Angiosarcoma of the liver following vinyl chloride exposure. *JAMA,* 229:53–54 (1974).
19. Epstein, S. S. Environmental determinants of human cancer. *Cancer Res.,* 34:2425–2435 (1974).
20. Jager, K. W. *Aldrin, Dieldrin, Endrin and Telodrin.* Elsevier, Amsterdam, 1970.
21. Carroll, K. K., Gammal, E. B., and Plunkett, E. R. Dietary fat and mammary cancer. *Can. Med. Assoc. J.,* 98:590–594 (1968).
22. De Waard, F., and Baanders-van Halewijn, E. A. A prospective study in general practice on breast-cancer risk in postmenopausal women. *Int. J. Cancer,* 14:153–160 (1974).
23. Ravnihar, B., Macmahon, B., and Lindtner, J. Epidemiologic features of breast cancer in Slovenia; 1965–1967. *Eur. J. Cancer,* 7:295–306 (1971).
24. Wynder, R. L., Escher, G. C., and Mantel, N. An epidemiological investigation of cancer of the endometrium. *Cancer,* 19:489–520 (1966).
25. Drasar, B. S., and Irving, D. Environmental factors and cancer of the colon and breast. *Br. J. Cancer,* 27:167–172 (1973).
26. Burdette, W. J. Colorectal carcinogenesis. *Cancer,* 34: (Suppl.) 872–877 (1974).
27. Weisburger, J. H. Chemical carcinogenesis in the gastrointestinal tract. In *Seventh National Cancer Conference Proceedings,* pp. 465–473. American Cancer Society, Inc., Lippincott, Philadelphia, 1973.
28. Burkitt, D. P., Walker, A. R. P., and Painter, N. S. Effect of dietary fibre on stools and transit-times, and its role in the causation of disease. *Lancet,* 2:1408–1411 (1972).
29. Hill, M. J. Bacteria and the etiology of colonic cancer. *Cancer,* 34: (Suppl.) 815–818 (1974).
30. Dickerson, J. W. T. Nutrition and the cancer patient: Food and the aetiology of cancer. *Nursing Mirror,* :33–35 (1972).
31. Philip, J. M. Toxicity and naturally occurring chemicals in food. *R. Soc. Health J.,* 90:237–42 (1970).
32. Liener, I. E. *Toxic Constituents of Animal Foodstuffs,* Academic Press, New York, 1974.
33. Hueper, W. C. Public health hazards from environmental chemical carcinogens, mutagens and teratogens. *Health Phys.,* 21:689–707 (1971).
34. Foster, E. M. Science, politics, and a safe food supply. *J. Am. Vet. Med. Assoc.,* 163:1056–1060 (1973).
35. Stoner, G. D., Shimkin, M. B., Koriazeff, A. J., Weisburger, J. H., Weisburger, E. K., and Gori, G. B. Test for carcinogenicity of food additives and chemotherapeutic agents by the

pulmonary tumor response in strain A mice. *Cancer Res.*, 33:3069–3085 (1973).

36. Wolff, I. A., and Wasserman, A. E. Nitrates, nitrites and nitrosamines. *Science*, 177:15–19 (1972).
37. Douty, B., Carlisle, D., Laseter, J. L., and Sterer, J. Halogenated hydrocarbons in New Orleans drinking water and blood plasma. *Science*, 187:75–77 (1975).
38. Editorial. Rauwolfia derivatives and cancer. *Lancet*, ii:701–702 (1974).
39. Arthes, F. G., Sartwell, P. E., and Lewison, E. F. The pill, oestrogens and the breast. *Cancer*, 28:1391–1394 (1971).
40. Black, M. M., and Leis, H. P. Mammary carcinogenesis. *NY State J. Med.*, 72:1601–1605 (1972).
41. Rothman, K., and Keller, A. The effect of joint exposure to alcohol and tobacco on risk of cancer of the mouth and pharynx. *J. Chronic Dis.*, 25:711–716 (1972).
42. Kissin, B., Kaley, M. M., Su, W. H., and Lerner, R. Head and neck cancer in alcoholics. *JAMA*, 224:1174–1175 (1973).
43. Schottenfeld, D., Gantt, R. C., and Wynder, E. L. The role of alcohol and tobacco in multiple primary cancers of the upper digestive system, larynx and lung: A prospective study. *Prev. Med.*, 3:277–293 (1974).
44. Rivlin, R. S. Riboflavin and cancer. A review. *Cancer Res.*, 33:1977–1986 (1973).
45. Modan, B., Mart, H., Baidatz, D., Steinitz, R., and Levin, S. G. Radiation-induced head and neck tumours. *Lancet*, i:277–279 (1974).
46. Temin, H. M. Introduction to virus-caused cancers. *Cancer*, 34:1347–1352 (1974).
47. Vianna, N. J. Is Hodgkin's disease infectious? *Cancer Res.*, 34:1149–1155 (1974).
48. Sarkar, N. H., and Moore, D. H. On the possibility of a human breast cancer virus. *Nature*, 236:103–106 (1972).
49. Snell, L., and Graham, S. Social trauma as related to cancer of the breast. *Br. J. Cancer*, 25:721–734 (1971).

Cancer: The Behavioral Dimensions, edited by J. W. Cullen, B. H. Fox, and R. N. Isom. Raven Press, New York © 1976.

Problems of High-Risk Populations and High-Risk Nonresponders: Smoking Behavior

Lloyd A. Shewchuck

American Health Foundation, New York, New York 10019

BACKGROUND

It was estimated that in 1975 lung cancer would claim 81,000 lives in the United States (1). This is one form of cancer in which the chief causative factor—cigarette smoking—is known. Still, cigarette sales have increased in the past 25 years. Only between the years 1965 and 1971 was there a significant trend to decreased smoking. This period is usually associated with the impact of mass media information on the dangers of smoking. It is estimated that there were approximately 29 million ex-smokers by 1971 (1). Today there are some 45 million smoking adults in the United States. Many of these want to stop smoking but have not been successful in quitting.

Recognizing the urgent need to develop procedures and programs to help people stop smoking, researchers have increasingly turned their attention to this problem (2). The solution was first seen as an educational one which led to a widespread campaign of public education about the dangers of smoking. As a result, nearly everyone, smokers and nonsmokers, now agree that smoking is harmful to health. At the same time many people also consulted their physicians, but physicians were as baffled as anyone else as to how to help people stop smoking (3). In the vacuum of proved techniques for stopping, many methods sprang up. Drug companies began producing medication to help smokers quit (4); school systems began educational programs on the danger of smoking (5,6); hypnotists began treating smokers (7,8); counseling programs were instituted (9–11); and behavior therapists began applying learning theory principles to treatment programs (12). All report varying degrees of initial success. There are intensive reviews of these intervention approaches by Schwartz and Dubitsky (13), Bernstein (14), Hunt (15), and Dunn (16).

The mass media campaign and scientific encouragement to help people to stop smoking resulted in a reaction from commercially oriented segments of society. With physicians, dentists, and scientists unable to provide the necessary service to fill the needs of people who want help in quitting, private industry has recognized the void. Quit clinics, lozenges, books, gimmicks, and other quit products for a market of about 45 million potential customers are fast becoming a $50 million industry (20). Undoubtedly, more and more ex-smokers will be produced because of this interest. But what is the dilemma facing smokers who cannot quit on their own and thus seek help? Should they turn to self-help methods, private clinics, or public clinics? All present some disadvantages. Some require the payment of a fee, most do not give sufficient information on what to expect in terms of treatment or success rate, some (especially good research programs) randomly assign smokers to treatment conditions with the possibility of assignment to a placebo or control group for some time (17). Most clinics—private or public—require the involvement of the smoker in an intensive, time-consuming, concentrated program. Help is available only in small doses or in large doses—there is no in between. Smokers seeking aid in quitting have no way of knowing what type of treatment they individually require and how extensive it must be. In fact, they are generally unaware that there are a number of approaches to smoking cessation.

LEVELS OF INTERVENTION

The American Health Foundation has involved over 2,000 persons in studies on smoking cessation in an attempt to establish a hierarchy of smoking-cessation techniques and to identify those smokers who would be most successful within each method.

So that we may identify those successful in each method, we gather information on demographic data, attitudes toward health and smoking, personality correlates, and smoking behavior. Some projects also involve blood chemistry measures.

It is clear that smoking and quitting smoking are complicated phenomena. Some smokers never quit. Of those who quit, some do so with no difficulty and others do so only with great difficulty. Some require very little help from others and some require a great deal of support and aid. Our goal is to identify the amount and type of aid needed by individual smokers.

We visualize three broad categories or levels of intervention that depend on the amount of support and aid that is given. Thus Level I, Minimal Intervention, may be applied to those who are or are not motivated to stop smoking. It provides a short message by a physician (or other health worker) in the context of the usual doctor-patient milieu. The goal in this case is to do more than simply acknowledge that cigarette smoking may be harmful to health. It is to make the patient aware that smoking is an important problem, that it has personal meaning or relevance, that there is value to be gained from stopping, and that people are indeed capable of stopping.

During one project, we found from Test 2 of the Smokers' Self-Testing Kit (18), which contains the question "What do you think the effects of smoking are?," that all persons seeking help at our clinics were aware that smoking is an important problem causing serious health risks. Furthermore, all felt that they were not exempt from the risk of serious illness as a result of smoking. However, the majority of smokers were not aware of the advantages to giving up smoking, that their related risk factors would eventually decrease to the level of a non-smoker. In addition, all believed they would have a hard time quitting. Thus, to encourage self-efforts in Level I, we reinforce the relevance and value of stopping and the smoker's ability to stop.

Level II, Intermediate Intervention, involves the utilization of audio and written material in helping the smoker to quit smoking. To date, our methods include two books and two cassette tape programs on giving up cigarettes. This level is applied to smokers who are at least sufficiently motivated to contact our smoking cessation clinic for assistance. Smokers are introduced to a step-by-step procedure which they must master on their own.

Level III, Intensive Intervention, provides a structured procedure as well as an additional support system of a therapist and/or group of persons who are also trying to quit smoking. This level is for those who are at least somewhat motivated but need a structured support system.

To make the smoking-cessation process as efficient as possible and to eliminate unnecessary extensive intervention, we ideally seek to establish proved, safe techniques at each of these three levels so that we can assign specific smokers to appropriate methods. Nonresponders may progress from one level to the next until they become ex-smokers.

Many programs experience high drop-out rates, which indicates low acceptance of the intervention method. One such method was described by Azrin and Powell (19), who reported that of 17 persons only 5 agreed to carry portable shock units containing cigarettes which they could smoke only after a shock was received. Schwartz and Dubitsky (13) discuss two factors that are necessary for any successful treatment method. First, the method must be acceptable to smokers wishing to stop; second, the method must be effective in helping them stop.

In one American Health Foundation study of 617 smokers attending group therapy sessions requiring five treatment meetings, 440 (71%) attended more than one session. Of the total, 82% attended the first session, 67% the second session, and 44% the last session. Number of sessions attended seems to be related to success in stopping. In another study with 238 group treatment smokers, the success group at end of treatment had attended an average of 4.5 out of 5 sessions, whereas failures attended only an average of 3 sessions.

Assignment on the basis of attitudes, smoking behavior, and personality characteristics to an appropriate level of intervention may counteract the rate of "drop-outs" and "no shows." We have explored three methods at Level III and are presently testing the effectiveness of four techniques at Level II and four physician messages at Level I. Thus the bulk of our experience comes from Level III work.

LEVEL III RESULTS

There is no standard method of reporting the effectiveness of a particular cessation program. The smokers in a program may drop out or continue to end of treatment. Those who drop out include failures, smokers who quit smoking seemingly without any aid, and a fluctuating group. The smokers who complete treatment similarly include failures, successes, smokers who reduce but do not stop their smoking, and fluctuators. For meaningful reporting of results, all of these categories should be considered.

In one study of 571 smokers attending American Health Foundation clinics, 26 (5%) failed to keep their appointments for treatment; another 5% dropped out after the first group session. Thus, in all, 10% of our population who were motivated enough to make an initial contact changed their minds about treatment. Some of these went on to stop on their own. Of the 51 who refused to take part in our programs, 3 (6%) quit on their own and maintained this status for a year. Seventeen of this group (34%) made no change at all in their smoking behavior throughout the entire year. The remaining 31 persons (60%) made some tempo-rary changes throughout the year by quitting or reducing their intake at various stages of the follow-up period. By comparison, of the 520 who attended treatment programs, 67 (13%) (more than double the untreated group) quit smoking and maintained this status for 1 year while another 69 (13%) continued to smoke at the same rate throughout. Thus the failure rate of the participants is about one-third that of the untreated group. One group not evident in the untreated population emerged in the treatment groups. Ten people (2%) reduced their number of cigarettes by at least 50% and maintained this status for 1 year. The bulk of the treatment group ($N = 374$; 72%) made temporary changes throughout the year by stopping for short periods or by reducing their intake. Included in this large group were 149 (29% of total 520 population) who quit at the end of treatment but who eventually returned to smoking (although not all at their original rate) at some point during the follow-up. This is the recidivist group, which many researchers have indicated should be treated separately.

We contend that the usual way of presenting treatment results of smoking programs is misleading and agree with Bernstein (17) and others (20,21), that the presentation of success rates should be standardized. Generally, success rates are based on how many end-of-treatment quitters have continued to abstain by the end of the follow-up period (20). Thus, drop-outs and failures during the initial treatment are not counted, nor are those lost to follow-up. If we applied this criterion to our own results, we would report 1-year success rates of well over 30%, but would count only 216 of the 571 registered participants. Schwartz (20) recommends that all persons registered in a program be counted and evaluated at points 1 week, 4 months, and 1 year after treatment ends. We have experienced some serious problems with such a method. First, even though every effort is made to contact people, there is always a certain percentage who cannot be found and/or do not respond. We prefer to count such "no information" as failures, although some clinics prefer to prorate their success figures to distribute the no-information data according to the distribution of the recorded responders (17). Second, we find that almost half our population fluctuates from smoking to nonsmoking status, so that if contacted at one time, they are reported as not smoking, but if contacted 1 week earlier, for example, they would have been recorded as smoking. Thus, if we report success rates at end of treatment and 1 month, 5 months, and 1 year after treatment, we report success rates of 45, 30, 24, and 20% at each of these data collection points. The question, "Are you now smoking?" should be replaced with the question, "Have you smoked more than one whole cigarette at any one time since you completed your treatment program 1, 5, or 12 months ago?" Using this criterion, we find that our 1-year success rates are 13% because all those individuals who are fluctuating from a quit to nonquit status are then excluded. This eliminates the possibility of counting temporary successes as actual ex-smokers.

In reporting results of smoking cessation activities we recommend that the following standards be utilized:

1. All individuals attending even one session must be counted and every effort made to reach all persons who began the program.
2. Those persons who cannot be reached within a reasonable time (say 1 month) or after several attempts (say 6) should be counted as failures.
3. Follow-up periods should extend to 1 year after treatment, with interim data-collection points (a) within 1 month and (b) within 6 months after treatment ends.
4. At least four basic status groups should be reported on:
   (a) those who quit by the end of treatment and maintain this status for the entire year (success group);
   (b) those who make no change by the end of treatment and make no change in their smoking status for the entire year (failure group);
   (c) those who quit by the end of treatment but fluctuate throughout the year (recidivist group);
   (d) those who do not quit by the end of treatment but who experience temporary quit periods throughout the year (fluctuation group).

In addition to these standards, it would be ideal to compare treatment groups coming from identical populations with respect to degree of motivation, smoking behavior, dosage, environmental influences, and other factors. The difficulty of meeting this criterion, however, should not dissuade us from applying more rigorous standards to the definition of effectiveness of treatment.

COMMERCIAL CLINICS

With the advent of private, profit-making, stop-smoking clinics, the question arose: Does the payment of a fee enhance the chances of success? The 149 subjects taking part in an American Health Foundation group therapy program were charged $55.00. Results after 6 months show that 36 (24%) were able to stop smoking and maintain this status for 6 months. Twenty-six (17%) did not make any changes in their smoking behavior over the 6-month period. Because the format was identical to the free services, a comparison of the two programs supports the notion that payment of a fee enhances the chance of success.

Respective rates for free clinics are 16% (success) and 15% (failure).

As part of our attempts to develop a hierarchy of techniques to help smokers to quit, the American Health Foundation is exploring the effectiveness of some of the commercial products mentioned earlier. At present, within our intermediate intervention (Level II) program, we are randomly assigning smokers to four such techniques and an appropriate control group is receiving no treatment. Our goal is to initiate a 1-week quit status and then to involve successes in a variety of maintenance programs designed to prevent recidivism. We plan to involve the failures in more intensive programs. We have not yet run enough subjects to assess these techniques. However, in trying to select appropriate products to test, we were struck by the superficial nature of some of these offerings. Some offered no more advice than to gradually cut down the number of cigarettes smoked per day so that if a smoker of 30 cigarettes smokes one less each day, then in 30 days he should not be smoking at all.

Some clinics also provide a support system which adds impetus to an individual's quit attempt. Too often this support system is withdrawn long before it does its most important work. Hunt and Matarazzo (22) demonstrated that the first 3 months after treatment is the critical time for the new ex-smoker. This is the period during which 90% of recidivism occurs. Yet many programs withdraw their support from the new ex-smokers only shortly after they give up cigarettes.

To prevent recidivism of the new ex-smoker and to further encourage the smoker to continue efforts at quitting, American Health Foundation programs instituted booster groups and a hot-line telephone service. These were available as additional service to anyone completing a program of cessation. Our experiences were discouraging; we found that very few people availed themselves of these services. When questioned, those who quit smoking invariably answered that they had quit and therefore did not need the service. Those who continued to smoke stated that they needed something more structured.

We now introduce our programs as 1-year programs concerned with two goals: getting one off cigarettes and then keeping one off cigarettes. Although our maintenance programs are new and we have not had time to assess their effectiveness, we do know that, like the initial cessation process, the maintenance process is also complex, and what suits one individual does not necessarily suit the other. We are therefore establishing a hierarchy of maintenance techniques from social reinforcements for optimal self-help procedures to total involvement in counteracting cravings for cigarettes and changing attitudes toward nonsmoking.

SUMMARY

Smokers have been encouraged to quit smoking but do not know what kind of program to go into to get help. There should be a standard measuring system to determine the success rates of various cessation programs and devices so that the variety of approaches available to the public can be objectively evaluated. A hierarchy of methods based on characteristics of the smoker would enhance the likelihood of smokers finding the right program.

ACKNOWLEDGMENTS

This research was supported in part by contract HSM-21-72-557 of the National Clearinghouse for Smoking and Health, Bureau of Health Education, Center for Disease Control, Department of Health, Education and Welfare, and in part by grant ACS MG-161 of the American Cancer Society, Inc.

REFERENCES

1. American Cancer Society, *'75 Cancer Facts and Figures*. American Cancer Society, New York, 1974.
2. U.S. Department of Health, Education, and Welfare, National Clearinghouse for Smoking and Health. *Adult Use of Tobacco–1970*. The Department, 1973.
3. Mausner, B., Mausner, J., and Rial, W. The influence of the physician on the smoking behavior of his patients. In Zagona, S. (ed.): *Studies and Issues in Smoking Behavior*, pp. 103–106, University of Arizona Press, Tucson, 1967.
4. Ejrup, B., and Wikander, P. A. Fortsatta forsok till avvanjing fran robak medelst injektions behandling. *Sven. Iakartidn*, 56:468–473 (1959).
5. Davison, R. L. An analysis of an anti-smoking research study in a college of further education. *Health Educ.*, 3:77–81 (1970).
6. Jones, J. A., Piper, G. W., and Matthews, V. L. A student-directed program in smoking education. *Can. J. Public Health*, 61:253–256 (1970).
7. Crasilneck, H. B., and Hall, J. A. The use of hypnosis in controlling cigarette smoking. *South. Med. J.*, 61:999–1002 (1968).
8. Spiegel, H. Termination of smoking by a single treatment. *Arch. Environ. Health*, 20:736–741, (1970).
9. Filbey, E. E., Reed, K. E., and Lloyd, F. T. An inpatient smoking control service. *Hosp. Manage.*,103:60–64 (1967).
10. Ross, C. A. *Smoking Withdrawal Research Clinics*, pp. 111–113. In Zagona, S. (ed.): University of Arizona Press, Tucson, 1967.
11. Lawton, M. P. A group therapeutic approach to giving up smoking. *Appl. Ther.*, 4:1025–1028 (1962).
12. Janis, I. L., and Mann, L. Effectiveness of emotional role-playing in modifying smoking habits and attitudes. *J. Exp. Res. Pers.*, 1:84–90 (1965).
13. Schwartz, J. L., and Dubitsky, M. Psycho-social factors involved in cigarette smoking and cessation. *Institute for Health Research*, Berkeley, pp. XX–554, 1968.
14. Bernstein, D. A. *The Modification of Smoking Behavior*, 174 pp., Doctoral Dissertation, Northwestern University, Evanston (1968).
15. Hunt, W. A., (ed.): *Learning Mechanisms in Smoking*, pp. VII–237, Aldine, Chicago, 1970.
16. Dunn, W. L., Jr., (ed.): *Smoking Behavior: Motive and Incentives*, pp. XII–309, Winston, Washington, D.C., 1973.
17. Bernstein, D. A. The modification of smoking behavior, a search for effective variables. *Behav. Res. Ther.*, 9:133–146 (1970).
18. U.S. Department of Health, Education, and Welfare, *Smokers' Self-Testing Kit*, DHEW Publication No. (CDC) 74–8716 (1973).
19. Azrin, N. H., and Powell, J. Behavioral engineering: The reduction of smoking behavior by a conditioning apparatus and procedure. *J. Appl. Behav. Anal.*, 1:193–200 (1968).
20. Schwartz, J. L. Recent developments in smoking cessation methods. In National Interagency Council on Smoking and Health (eds.): *National Conference on Smoking and Health*, pp. 101–113 (1970).
21. Winett, R. *Parameters of Deposit Contracts in the Modification of Smoking*, 181 pp. Doctoral dissertation, State University of New York at Stony Brook, Stony Brook, N.Y. (1971).
22. Hunt, W. A., and Matarazzo, J. D. Three years later: Recent developments in experimental modification of smoking behavior. *J. Abnorm. Psychol.*, 81:107–114 (1973).

Cancer: The Behavioral Dimensions, edited by J. W. Cullen, B. H. Fox, and R. N. Isom. Raven Press, New York © 1976.

Relationship of Sociocultural Factors to Cancer

S. Stephen Kegeles

Department of Behavioral Sciences and Community Health, University of Connecticut Health Center, Farmington, Connecticut 06032

Sociocultural variability is one of the most studied topics in the areas of health and social science. The first library search for this chapter from 1972 to 1974 produced over 500 titles, mainly from epidemiologic investigations. Articles in the *Journal of Health and Social Behavior* describing sociocultural variability are probably second in number only to those assessing the "sick-role." Of what use is such study for the control of cancer?

Organizers of the conference from which this volume is derived have taken the position that these data are important for determining "risk" for cancer. That position is accepted and risk is defined in two ways: (a) certain groups of people are more likely than others to be afflicted by or die from cancer and (b) certain groups of people do not take actions that will increase their chances of recovery from cancer.

This chapter touches on studies of subgroups in each area. For "at risk," defined as likelihood of being afflicted, questions will be raised about the yield that hypotheses derived from sociocultural study are likely to have in determining causes of cancer.

For "at risk," defined as failure to take effective actions, questions will first be raised about certain presumptions relating to the definition. Analysis of factors leading to lack of activity will then be provided. Additional questions will be raised about the potential effectiveness of strategies that might be used to obtain more frequent activity from among subgroups.

SOCIOCULTURAL STUDY TO DETERMINE CAUSES OF CANCER

Sociocultural variability in regard to cancer morbidity and mortality by site has been documented repeatedly. Studies by McMahon, Graham, Lilienfeld, and those of other investigators documented variability in subareas in the United States and among subpopulations in the world. For instance,

1. Japanese-Americans have an unusually high risk for cancer of the stomach, Japanese from Hawaii a higher risk, and Japanese from Japan an even higher risk (1,2);

2. Jews, Poles, and Russians have excess amounts of adult leukemia (3);
3. Jewish women have greater likelihood of breast cancer than Protestant or Catholic women, and women from middle- and upper-middle class groups have more breast cancer than those from lower-income groups (4);
4. An inverse relation was found between socioeconomic status and "risk" in almost all studies of cervical cancer (5).

Risks

Other than mapping sociocultural variability, epidemiologic data of this sort may provide information about why people get cancer. For instance, the environment in which they live, the food they eat, the way in which their lives are led, and the social or psychologic pressures and stresses they face may be causative factors in the excess cancer of various sites found among subgroups. Such clues may provide knowledge about how cancer works.

Hypotheses based on this line of reasoning have been tested for many years. The largest yield has come from assessment of industrial environments—from the very early discovery of scrotal cancer in chimney sweeps (6) through investigations of workers in coal and asbestos mines and plastic factories (7). Current investigations of early "life style" of women who get cervical cancer, guided by the hypothesis that the disease results from early sexual transmission of a herpes virus, are intriguing (7,8).

Studies of differential food intake based on sociocultural differentiation in gastric and colonic cancer have not yet brought results (9,10). The few studies showing a correlation between subcultural eating patterns and these cancers are not replicable. This is not surprising, since U.S. and Canadian studies of the quite firm relationship between high serum cholesterol and heart disease have yet to show any relationship between diet and heart disease [Syme, quoted in (6)]. Reliable and valid diet histories seem impossible to obtain through survey methodology.

More closely related to our interest here are formulations that link such notions as status inconsistency, alienation, anomie, relative deprivation, and sociocultural mobility to particular sociocultural groups on the one hand and to disease on the other. These have not yet been determined for cancer of any site. Psychosomatic studies that relate "repression," "denial," and "failure in emotional expressivity" to lung cancer (11–15) contain a number of research design problems and may not be replicable. Moreover, there seem to be no reasons why particular subgroups should have greater likelihood of psychologic problems of this sort.

After having studied many epidemiologic reports, I question the value of further sociocultural mapping of cancer of various sites. Study of sociocultural groups to determine causes of cancer does seem appropriate for industrial groups, but may be less relevant for testing dietary, social psychologic, or psychosomatic hypotheses about cause of cancer.

STUDY OF SOCIOCULTURAL GROUPS TO DETERMINE REASONS FOR LOW UTILIZATION

Much of the effort of the National Cancer Institute (NCI) cancer control program and of control activities of the American Cancer Society (ACS) is based on two premises:

1. Certain actions people take will reduce early mortality from cancer of various sites;
2. A great many persons from among certain subgroups fail to take these actions.

Much evidence can be marshaled to support both premises. To support the first assumption, the ACS uses data collected by the End Results Section of NCI to indicate 5-year survival rates of cancer patients whose cancers were diagnosed, respectively, as being in the "in-situ," "local," "regional," or "advanced" stage (7). ACS states that cancer diagnosed at an "in-situ" stage is mostly curable, and cancer diagnosed at an "advanced stage" is mostly incurable. They then list large percentile differences in 5-year survival rates of patients whose cancers were diagnosed at "local" and at "regional" stages. These differences are noted for such cancer sites as bladder, colon-rectum, oral cavity, breast, prostate, and uterus. ACS further states that the decreased level of cervical cancer is due mainly to increased use of cervical cytology.

However, the same End Results Section, using unpublished data gathered from a large sample of hospitals dealing with white patients but from an extremely small group of hospitals dealing with black patients, raises questions about the first premise. They show much poorer 5-year survival rates for blacks than for whites when their cancers were diagnosed at a "local" stage. This discrepancy is largest for cancer of the bladder and of the uterine corpus (16).

I am quite incapable of evaluating either these data or premises. Thus, I am willing to accept the first premise. However, as a lay-person, I have heard discussions about the differential speed of progression of cancer and read articles indicating that cervical cancer has diminished in areas where cervical cytology is not used (17). Nevertheless, examination of questions of this kind seems more appropriate for other conferences and other volumes.

Data to support the second premise derive from nationwide studies in this country (18,19) and in England (20). They show a much lower report of physical examination without symptoms, breast cancer examination, breast self-examination, and skin and proctoscopic examination for blacks than for whites, and for lower than for higher higher income and education groups. Despite the fact that the American data collected were from quite small numbers of blacks, and that such data may reveal differences in reporting ability as well as of different utilization, acceptance of the premise of lower utilization by blacks and by lower income groups is probably appropriate.

Acceptance of these two premises, albeit with some caution, leads one to raise questions about why subcultural groups fail to take appropriate actions. Two sets of answers will be examined for this purpose: those relating to these populations themselves and those relating to how these populations are dealt with by the health system. In addition, remarks will pertain primarily to action in regard to seeking cervical cytology and breast cancer examination.

SUBCULTURAL GROUP FACTORS THAT MAY LEAD TO POOR HEALTH BEHAVIOR

Although literally hundreds of studies have used sociocultural variation for analysis, unfortunately very few studies have used preventive health behavior in relation to cancer as a dependent variable. Thus, although one would expect reasons based on cultural and racial variation for the absence of preventive behavior for cancer, good data do not exist. The largest number of studies have concerned delay of breast cancer examination. For cervical cancer, many studies have been carried out by Wakefield (20) and his co-workers in England. Because of the need for brevity, these data are classified as follows.

Cognitive and Attitudinal Variables

In the relatively few studies of cervical cytology, negative predictors of action include fear of cancer (20–23), belief that cancer is incurable (20,21), belief that professional diagnosis is no better than self-diagnosis (18,24), lack of belief in the value of early diagnosis (18,20,24), and absence of felt susceptibility to cervical cancer (24).

As Dr. Raymond Fink noted these same cognitive and attitudinal statements are expressed as reasons for delay in breast cancer examination. He has provided some additional findings. These negative predictors usually vary inversely with level of education and income.

Subcultural Definitional Variables

Although not investigated directly for cervical cancer, a common finding is that racial and cultural groups each define symptomatology and its meaning differently, use different triggers for action (25), interpret the meaning of pain differently (26,27), or have different definitions of disease and cure (28,29).

Life-style Variables

Again, without data from cancer prevention activities, it is frequently asserted that different outlooks, for example, cosmopolitan-parochial (30,31), deal with health-related reactions of subcultural groups. In addition, mobility aspirations, ability to delay gratification, and high-achievement motivation, all middle-class "virtues," but supposedly absent in the lower class, have been deemed necessary for appropriate health behavior in lower income or educational groups or specific subcultural groups. In most cases, further investigation has shown these values to be expressed within most groups, though perhaps their expression is different among groups. Their direct relevance to desirable health behavior is not documented.

Familial Socialization Variables

It is often found that white, middle-class families provide frequent medical and dental visits for the children. This early training, it is said, provides a behavior retained during adulthood. Thus, a pattern of preventive behavior is passed from generation to generation. Without longitudinal study, this remains at the level of unsupported hypothesis.

This extremely limited review suggests some variables relating to subcultural groups which may limit their use of preventive cancer services. Some of these data seem quite firm, whereas other data are speculative, overinterpreted, or found in some studies and not in others. Low participation as a result of the way the health system deals with minority group members will be examined next.

HEALTH SYSTEM FACTORS THAT MAY LIMIT PARTICIPATION

In a prodigious attempt to analyze and categorize studies of utilization behavior, McKinlay (32) suggested a number of approaches used in studies. He indicates that data show the following:

1. Organizations, to maintain themselves, tend to provide services to persons who will use them most and thus avoid providing services to lower income, educational, and subgroup populations because failure of these groups to participate will make the organizations look "bad."
2. Formal settings of organizations may require skills and experiences that many members of subgroups do not possess.
3. Changes required to fit into the style demanded by preventive health behavior may have untoward effects on the social structure of subcultural groups.
4. Middle-class employees of organizations tend to provide lesser services, with greater obstacles to the acceptance of these services, to persons less like themselves than to persons who look and act like themselves, and
5. Numerous communications provided by health practitioners to clients unlike themselves seem to be misunderstood.

Many instances of each of these five points have been documented, as have a variety of other situations which potentially convey to members of subcultural groups the feeling that health establishments are run by the middle class for the middle class.

Although barely sampled by this short review, those data about characteristics of populations themselves, and those concerned with treatment of subgroups by the health establishment, suggest certain administrative and research questions about the likely success of efforts to increase frequency of cervical tests, breast examinations, and breast self-examinations. A year ago, with quite finite wisdom, I attempted to examine the utility of a number of change strategies to increase cancer screening: attitude change, public commitment, peer influence, group discussion, and mass communication (33). Many chapters in this book deal with these same strategies. Based on some of the data presented, I would like to raise certain administrative and research questions which probably have to be dealt with before these strategies will yield greater health activity among certain subcultural groups.

ATTITUDE CHANGE EFFORTS

Given the historic lack of success in translating attitudinal change to conative change, and the historic discrepancy in results between laboratory and field attempts to change attitudes:

1. Are there some new attitude change models that appear more relevant to changing utilization behavior than those used up to now?
2. Given the great fear of cancer, is it possible or even appropriate to use cognitive fear stimuli to obtain behavior?
3. With the level of distrust with which certain subgroups view the health establishment, accentuated by the recent syphilis exposé and the current failure of the health establishment to provide adequately for the "modeling" behavior created by the Ford and Rockefeller mastectomies, is the essential element of trustworthiness of the communicator sufficiently available to obtain attitudinal and/or conative change?
4. Are the cognitive elements so typically used for changing attitudes sufficient to bypass the absence of educational attainment and of differential life style of certain subcultural groups?

MASS COMMUNICATION EFFORTS

These same questions can be asked about mass communication efforts as well. In addition, however, the following questions might be asked about a mass communication strategy:

1. Given the quite recent failure to obtain differential behavior from experimental and control groups in use of seat belts (34) and contraceptives (35), what new mass communication efforts seem viable?
2. Despite the findings reported by Swinehart (36) of similar exposure to broadcast media among all subgroups, is this also true for educational television, and is there sufficient attention to and comprehension of mass media among low educational groups to produce appropriate action?
3. How does one obtain local integration of health service activities with mass communication activities to provide messages other than, "write to the National Cancer Institute"?
4. How does one provide "expertness" on a mass basis without using language and concepts beyond the level of comprehension of persons with low levels of education and still not bore persons with higher educational attainment?

PEER INFLUENCE OR DIFFUSION STRATEGIES

The diffusion of information notion, stemming from agricultural extension work and from research on physicians' acceptance of drugs coupled with the "lay referral" notion, is quite appealing as a strategy. Here too, however, I am struck with nonanswers to some questions about this strategy for urban subgroups. For instance:

1. How does one ensure that correct and appropriate information is passed from person to person?
2. Related, but somewhat separate, how is the information to be provided to the "first step" in a multistep flow of information?
3. How does one determine who the real information channels are so that they can be provided appropriate knowledge and information?
4. How does one keep from changing either the image or reality of indigenous information sources if they are incorporated into the health system?

GROUP DISCUSSION

The strategy of group discussion also has had a great deal of appeal and moderate success in the past. This strategy, too, raises a number of questions in its use among low-income and culturally divergent groups. For instance:

1. How are adult groups of lower income or minority groups to be assembled and retained for group discussion purposes?
2. How does one deal with the frequent unwillingness of lower-income and subcultural persons to verbalize within groups, especially within heterogeneous groups?
3. How does one provide "expertness" within groups without losing both trust and discussion?
4. How does verbal consensus obtained in groups of persons accustomed to providing verbal acquiescence in place of private commitment get translated into action?

In addition, it appears that such laboratory and controlled group strategies as positive reinforcement, social contract management, forced exposure, biofeedback and modeling should be translatable into community efforts. However, methods of doing so among these target populations need to be assessed very carefully and cautiously.

I wish there were time to discuss patient management, rehabilitation processes, in-hospital communication, and preparation for surgery of subpopulations. These areas present fascinating and imperative research questions. Hopefully, some of these questions will be discussed later.

SUMMARY

Analysis of data about subcultural groups was provided to deal with two definitions of risk: (1) excess morbidity and mortality for certain sites of cancer and (2) lesser utilization of preventive cancer services.

For the first definition, a few examples of the massive data available were presented. These data are potentially useful to determine causes of cancer, but most efforts have yet to yield impressive data.

Questions were raised about premises that guide the second definition. These premises were accepted with caution. Some data were presented to indicate possible causes of low utilization in cancer preventive activities, (1) those that deal with the population itself and (2) those that concern treatment of subpopulations by the health system.

Based on these data, a number of questions were raised about the use of such strategies as attitude change, mass communication, group discussion, and diffusion among urban subgroups. Certain other strategies might be translatable for community use but need careful analysis. Finally, questions about treatment of cancer patients from diverse population groups also must be answered.

REFERENCES

1. Smith, R. I. Recorded and expected mortality among the Japanese of the U.S. and Hawaii with special reference to cancer. *J. Natl. Cancer Inst.*, 17:459–473 (1956).
2. Gordon, T. Mortality experience among the Japanese in the United States, Hawaii, and Japan. *Public Health Rep.*, 72:543–553 (1957).
3. Graham, S., Gibson, R., Lilienfeld, A., Schuman, L., and Levin, M. Religion and ethnicity in leukemia. *Am. J. Public Health*, 60:266–274 (1970).
4. Silber, E. J., Trichopoulos, D., and MacMahon, B. Breast cancer in Boston, 1965–1966. *J. Natl. Cancer Inst.*, 43:1013–1021 (1969).
5. Graham, S., Levin, M. L., Lilienfeld, A. M., and Sheehe, P. Ethnic derivation as related to cancer at various sites. *Cancer*, 16:13–27 (1963).
6. Graham, S., and Reeder, L. G. Social factors in the chronic illnesses, Chapt. 3. In Freeman, H. E., Levine, S., and Reeder, L. G. (eds.): *Handbook of Medical Sociology*, 2nd ed., Prentice-Hall, Englewood Cliffs, N.J., 1972.
7. *Cancer Facts and Figures*, pp. 1–31, American Cancer Society, New York, 1974.
8. Beral, V. Cancer of the cervix: A sexually transmitted infection? *Lancet*, i:1037–1040 (1974).
9. *Conference on the Etiology of Cancer of the Gastro-intestinal Tract.* Report of the Research Committee, World Health Organization on Gastroenterology, New York, 1965. *Cancer*, 19:1561–1566 (1966).
10. Berg, J. W., Howell, M. A., and Silverman, S. J. Dietary hypotheses and diet-related research in the etiology of colon cancer. *Health Serv. Res.*, 88:915–924 (1973).
11. Kissen, D. M. Psychosocial factors, personality and lung cancer in men aged 55–64. *Br. J. Med. Psychol.*, 40:29–43 (1967).
12. Kissen, D. M., Brown, R., and Kissen, M. A. A further report on personality and psychosocial factors in lung cancer. *Ann. N.Y. Acad. Sci.*, 164:535–545 (1969).
13. LeShan, L. An emotional life-history pattern associated with neoplastic disease. *Ann. N.Y. Acad. Sci.*, 125:780–793 (1966).
14. Bahnson, C. B. Psychophysiological complementarity in malignancies: Past work and future vistas. *Ann. N.Y. Acad. Sci.*, 164:319–334 (1969).
15. Bahnson, C. B., and Bahnson, M. B. Cancer as an alternative to psychosis: A theoretical model of somatic and psychological regression. In Kissen, D. M., and LeShan, L.L. (eds.): *Psychosomatic Aspects of Neoplastic Disease*, Pitman, London, 1964.
16. Axtell, L. M., Myers, M.H., and Shambaugh, E. M. *Treatment and Survival Patterns for Black and White Patients 1955–1964.* DHEW Publication, End Results Section, National Cancer Institute, Bethesda, Md., 1974.

17. Knox, E. G. In McLachlan, J., (ed.): *Problems and Progress in Medical Care,* Oxford University Press, London, 1966.
18. Kegeles, S. S., Haefner, D. P., Kirscht, J. P., and Rosenstock, I. M. Survey of beliefs about cancer detection and taking Papanicolaou tests. *Public Health Rep.,* 80:815–823 (1965).
19. Gallup International. *The Public's Awareness and Use of Cancer Detection Tests.* Conducted for the American Cancer Society, 1970.
20. Wakefield, J. (ed.): *Seek Wisely to Prevent,* Her Majesty's Stationery Office, London, 1971.
21. Paterson, R., and Aitken-Swan, Jr. Public opinion on cancer—a survey among women in the Manchester area. *Lancet,* ii:857–861 (1954).
22. Young, Society of public health educators research committee, review of research related to health education practice. *Health Education Monogr.,* 1:70 (1963).
23. Kegeles, S. S. Attitudes and behavior of the public regarding cervical cytology: Current findings and new directions for research. *J. Chron. Dis.,* 20:911–922 (1967).
24. Kegeles, S. S. A field experimental attempt to change beliefs and behavior of women in an urban ghetto. *J. Health Soc. Behav.,* 10:115–125 (1969).
25. Zola, I.K. Culture and symptoms—an analysis of patients' presenting complaints. *Am. Sociol. Rev.,* 31:615–630 (1966).
26. Zborowski, M. (ed.): *People in Pain,* Jossey-Bass, San Francisco, 1969.
27. Weisenberg, M. Cultural and racial reactions to pain, chap. 5. In Weisenberg, M., (ed.): *The Control of Pain,* Psychological Dimensions, New York, 1975.
28. Harwood, A. The hot-cold theory of disease. *JAMA,* 216:1153–1158 (1971).
29. Paul, B. The role of beliefs and customs in sanitation programs. *Am. J. Public Health,* 48:1502–1506 (1958).
30. Suchman, E. A. Socio-medical variations among ethnic groups. *Am. J. Sociol.,* 70:319–331 (1964).
31. Suchman, E. A. Social patterns of illness and medical care. *J. Health Soc. Behav.,* 6:2–16 (1965).
32. McKinlay, J. B. Some approaches and problems in the study of the use of services—an overview. *J. Health Soc. Behav.,* 13:115–152 (1972).
33. Kegeles, S. S. Behavioral science data and approaches relevant to the development of education programs in cancer. *Health Education Monogr.,* 1: No. 36 (1974).
34. Robertson, L. S., Kelley, A. B., O'Neill, B., Wixom, C. W., Eiswirth, R. S., and Haddon, W., Jr. A controlled study of the effect of television messages on safety belt use. *Am. J. Public Health,* 64:1071–1080 (1974).
35. Udry, G. R. Can mass media advertising increase contraceptive use? *Fam. Plann. Perspect.,* 4:37–44 (1972).
36. Swinehart, J. W. Voluntary exposure to health communications. *Am J. Public Health,* 58:1265–1275 (1968).

Cancer: The Behavioral Dimensions, edited by J. W. Cullen,
B. H. Fox, and R. N. Isom. Raven Press, New York © 1976.

Respondent

Howard Leventhal

Psychology Department, University of Wisconsin, Madison Wisconsin 53706

I recently heard a radio broadcast in which an outstanding biochemist talked about his work on lipid transport and heart disease. He had developed a theory about the shape of the protein molecules that carry the lipids which eventually may cause arteriosclerosis. After validating this theory, he was going to develop a chemical to unwrap the lipids from the protein molecule so they could not be deposited in the artery wall. Although a good idea, as a psychologist I wondered why equal attention in research and public broadcasting is not given to ways of getting people to stop eating the fats that are then wrapped around those proteins. I also wondered whether the chemical to eventually be used to unwrap lipids might not have some unwanted effects, such as causing depression, that would serve as barriers to people using it, and if it might not be less expensive to keep the fats out of the system than to deal with them after they got there.

It is clear that one can attack the same problem in a variety of ways, and that biochemical and behavioral interventions may have similar end effects. It is also clear, but sometimes not foreseen, that dependence on physicochemical solutions can increase the cost of treatment and produce another set of even more complex behavioral problems than those that would be found if we attempted to intervene by encouraging preventive behaviors. Evidence for this is shown by the difficulties in securing cooperation with treatments that are unpleasant or have negative side effects. Even more important is the problem created by the development of a public attitude of passive dependency on quick, comfortable, miracle cures, an attitude that is bred by excessive emphasis on postillness chemical and surgical interventions. It is gratifying, therefore, to see the National Cancer Institute focusing attention on the full range of behavioral problems involved in all aspects of cancer from prevention and early detection, reaction to diagnosis and treatment, to reaction to success and failure in treatment with respect to work and family management.

The importance of behavioral factors and behavioral models for illness needs more emphasis. But one must not construe this need as minimizing the importance of physicochemical models in handling disease processes. Physicochemical models are important in and of themselves in understanding and treating illness, and in two major ways they are important to the proper conduct of behavioral research. First, they help us identify potential environmental antecedents and organismic conditions causally related to disease and linked to individual behavior. This knowledge allows us to move backward down the causal chain and do behavioral research in heart disease and cancer using dependent variables other than death due to either coronary or cancer. Death is a poor criterion; the rates are usually low and it is an all-or-none rather than a continuous measure. Consequently, one needs huge samples to study the impact of different amounts of behavior change on this criterion. Physicochemical models allow us to identify a more proximal risk factor as a dependent measure and use it to assess the effectiveness of particular behavior change procedures.

A second benefit of physicochemical models is the help they give us in differentiating the illness problem. A previous discussion dealt with the correlation between personality factors and cancer which needed this differentiation. Studies were reported where investigators were testing a wide range of personality traits to see if they are linked to cancer. There is no reason to do such correlational research if one knows the biological models. One should develop physicochemical models for different cancers and then link these models to behavioral factors. For example, some cancers are neuroendocrine dependent. By developing models of personality process, e.g., models describing sensitivity to environmental events and ways of defending oneself that alter neuroendocrine functioning, we can then develop hypotheses as to how these behavioral factors will influence the onset and growth rates of cancers that have a strong neuroendocrine base. If one considers everything, all cancers and all personality factors, he will see and learn nothing. Staying at a global level and working with correlational data reflect in part the absence of good physiological and behavioral models. Their absence is one reason why many psychologists avoid research in cancer and are attracted instead to research in cardiovascular disease.

I will now comment on funding: how to get the money and behavioral scientists together. The way we go after money is to compete for grants. The agency with the money competes for investigators and projects. It is not easy to put top-flight behavioral scientists, most of whom are in psychology and sociology departments, into competition for the money. First of all, most behavioral scientists do not really understand medical problems. My own experience in health research is that I can best succeed when I team up with a person who really knows the biological and clinical aspects of the problem; and the clinical side may be the more important. For example, my former student Dr. Jean Johnson and I conducted two major investigations on the preparation of patients for endoscopic examinations. Our success was greatly facilitated by her extensive experience in surgical nursing and by the astute clinical advice of Dr. John Morrissey, chief of the endoscopy clinic at the University of Wisconsin Medical Center. Together they gave the necessary familiarity and entry into the medical setting. Another example of a collaborative enterprise is our work on preparation for childbirth. I would hardly want to undertake such a venture without astute clinical advice and direct experience with both patient and physician roles! Fortunately, these are supplied in abundance by Dr. Elaine Leventhal, who experienced childbirth twice herself and has delivered numerous babies in her obstetric training.

But even the best research team can stumble when it encounters that major governmental invention and obstacle to research known as the Request for Proposal (RFP). The RFP may be government's most effective invention to prevent good behavioral research, because it can pose barriers to the investigators who are most expert in the behavioral disciplines. The RFP is a barrier to the good investigator, who is distinguished by the need and the ability to ask his own questions and the RFP often denies him that privilege. The RFP can also encourage the formation of small in-groups made up of the contractor and contractee. These in-groups develop because both parties become committed to the question posed in the contract. The group tends to be cut off from scientific scrutiny and criticism because the question, framed by the agency, will usually lack scientific meaning and the contractee is unlikely to submit the product of his research efforts to the major journals in the behavioral science disciplines. Unfortunately, the questions posed in the contract may also lack practical importance because they are usually framed with relatively limited knowledge of the practical problem and the contract can commit the participants to answering a question which probably should be discarded.

These points may seem abstract and irrelevant to the chapters I was asked to review, but I think not. The research reported and reviewed by Dr. Shewchuk and Dr. Kegeles suffers primarily, in my opinion, from a failure to address the appropriate questions. The reason for that failure may be left open at this time.

First, as to Dr. Shewchuk's chapter on the problem of smoking control: smoking research is a bag of worms because it includes everything from studies of neurotransmitters to studies of mood. At the behavioral level there are three very important problems: (a) the initiation of smoking, (b) the factors supporting or maintaining smoking, and (c) the problem posed by the process of intervention and its three subproblems: the decision to stop, the method of stopping, and ways of avoiding recidivism. One might wonder how factors in initiation, support or maintenance, and intervention are tied together. But little or no attention has been given to this in any smoking research. One reason is the absence of theory; little consideration is given to theoretical models that would allow the differentiation of variables in these different areas, and suggest ways of interconnecting them. For example, a variety of factors maintain smoking behavior, such as self-image, immediate situational factors such as social context, and the kinds of emotional rewards derived from the smoking itself. Unfortunately, when you consider the empirical work on these concepts there is really very little behavioral validation of the concepts.

Now turn to the work on intervention. There is enough experimental work on intervention to tell us that the intervention process can be treated in terms of a sequence of stages or steps going from the development of a motive for change to the structuring of the behavior that leads to change. We also know that these two steps are reasonably separate or independent; a person may be motivated to change and know or not know how to do it. But what connections exist between what is known about maintaining factors and what is known about the process of intervention?

One might suspect it to be more or less difficult to develop motivation for change depending on the factors that maintain smoking behavior; for example, it would seem relatively easy to develop a motivation to stop in the habit smoker. One would also expect that the best tactics to develop motivation for change would vary with the factors that maintain the behavior; for example, a lessening of tastiness leading to increased motivation to stop for the pleasure-taste smoker. More important, perhaps, would be the possible links between types of maintaining factors and the control of smoking cessation. Self-monitoring would appear to be more important for the habit smoker, avoidance of fear and relaxation of greater importance to the tension-reducing smoker, and the use of stimulant substitutes of greater importance to the stimulation-seeking smoker.

Unfortunately, preoccupation with the practical issue of getting people to stop smoking has directed people away from the above questions. And when considerations such as the above are ignored, one sees two quite different approaches to the entire problem of intervention. First, you see strictly empirical work; the investigators compare each known method to every other. Unfortunately, this can go on forever and in the long run it tells little and wastes the time of the investigator. Second, you see what I would call theoretical imperialism, where behavioral scientists force particular models, for example, the conditioning model, or the cognitive dissonance model, upon the intervention process whether the model does or does not fit the smoking problem.

The work that Dr. Shewchuk reported has both positive and negative features in relation to the above issues. First, he does describe what he has done to smokers and report the outcome of his intervention. He does not, however, organize his intervention procedures about any particular theoretical model. For example, he fails to consider the effects of his treatments for different types of smokers, and does not, in my opinion, give adequate consideration to the effects of the various motives for quitting, or the effect of the smokers' social relationships on success for the different treatments; at least in his report he does not mention these issues.

Another positive factor is the questions raised about how to get someone to stop smoking permanently. In discussing this interesting area, Dr. Shewchuk raises many critical questions about methods of measurement. But how do you resolve questions about measurement? Can they be resolved by devising a better measure and is the ideal measure, as suggested by Dr. Shewchuk, to ask the smoker, "Did you smoke at any time in the last year?" As a matter of fact, there is no such thing as a universal measure; the goodness of a measure is dependent on theory! The question as to whether a smoker stops and stays off for a year or forever is a practical issue for a health worker but is not a good criterion for developing a measure to evaluate an intervention program. It is insufficient because one needs separate criteria for each step of the change process; one for the motive to quit, another to see if the smokers quit for the first few days, and other measures to evaluate whether they stay off and to detect what gets smokers back to smoking. There is a sequence of steps in getting off and staying off and there are many reasons for failure. No one criterion can assess each of the different aspects of the change process, and to improve a program one must evaluate and isolate its weaknesses.

I am also surprised that no one has ever bothered to study the critical process of recidivism. Is going back to smoking externally induced or is the critical factor the rearousal of the old, internal desire to put the weed to one's lips? My conclusion, then, is that the studies reported give insufficient attention to models of process and make inadequate use of clinical experience to formulate theory and hypothesis. I also believe that theory and hypothesis should first lead to small sample studies and then be followed by larger field trials.

I now turn to Dr. Kegeles' chapter. His review raises questions about the conclusions that can be drawn when one compares two or more groups of people who differ on: (a) risk of cancer, (b) the behaviors they follow to reduce risk of cancer, and (c) the behaviors they follow to cure cancer. Does it pay to compare groups? The goal of comparing groups, I presume, is to find out about the cause of cancer and to identify ways of minimizing cancer. We all know that correlation is not causation, but when we compare groups— blacks and whites, ethnic groups, and so on, we are observing correlations between disease or preventive behavior and group membership. These correlations provide poor information because we know that the groups differ on a multitude of variables. It seems that we need to differentiate those cases where the groups compared are identified or formed on a variable that is irrelevant to the disease process from cases where the groups are identified or formed on a variable that we think is linked to the disease process. Thus it is often useful to construct groups on the basis of particular environmental factors that are suspected to cause illness, but it seems less useful to construct and compare groups identified on potentially irrelevant factors such as whether they are black or white, Italian or Jewish, or what not. I also would urge (and since I am not an epidemiologist, I can urge with impunity) that we consider studying risk factors within ethnic groups. Comparing within an ethnic group those people high on risk with those low on risk holds constant (at least to a degree) factors associated with the group and should help one tease out factors that are causally involved in increasing disease susceptibility. If the same factors can account for risk within groups and between groups, we are likely to be close to a "causal" model.

Dr. Kegeles also discusses the utilization of services. There are hundreds of studies relating social class and ethnic group to utilization of services. This knowledge helps to identify problems—for example, who is or is not getting care—but does not help much in solving them because it does not explain the "causes" of the problem. But how does one locate causes? One approach taken by health-oriented behavioral scientists (one I had something to do with when I was in the Public Health Service) was the development of the so-called health belief model. The model argues that the causes of utilization are people's belief in their susceptibility to disease, their perception of the severity of the disease, and their belief that they can take effective action at minimal cost and maximal gain. These models are supposed to account for differences within groups and differences between groups. I think this approach is an improvement over social class data, which is largely descriptive. Even so, the approach omits critical issues. First, it says nothing about where these beliefs originate. Second, it tells nothing about the process by which people respond to their bodies, to media information, and so on, and reach conclusions such as "I am susceptible to disease"; "the disease would be serious for me"; "I should, and can (or cannot) change my behavior to protect myself." There are information processing models (which now dominate cognitive and social psychology) that deal with the way an individual processes information from his environment, draws conclusions about risks, and tries to modify risks. We must use these models to answer these questions.

Finally, we must be very careful not to assume that beliefs cause behavior. Behavior might just as well be the cause of beliefs, and we need to look at more subtle links between beliefs and behavior. For example, behaviors may influence beliefs by altering social contacts and the information obtained in social interaction. For example, suppose that 20 different persons have the same physical symptom: a painful lump in the armpit. They may all do the same thing about it (talk to close friends) but may wind up with different subsequent beliefs and behaviors because their friends hold different beliefs about pain and seeking help. The health belief models do not pay close enough attention to the effect of the social context on the relationships between beliefs and behavior.

Richard I. Evans

Department of Psychology, University of Houston, Houston, Texas 77004

What bothers me about Dr. Peacock's paper is not so much its content, but rather that such information becomes disseminated in society. Findings are too often represented as more generalizable than they, in fact, truly are. What exactly are the specific behaviors we should attempt to modify, for which both an ethical and a scientific basis have been established for justifying their investigation as being definitely related to mortality/morbidity in the field? In other words, we all can agree that in oral hygiene behavior, if you brush your teeth in a certain way and use floss and a disclosant tablet, the probability of decreasing various types of periodontal disease and caries is high. Since this is well established, we moved into that view with a high degree of certainty that we could have this sort of effect, and we have demonstrated some strategies to do this.

In the area of cardiovascular disease, smoking and hypertension have been reliably linked, but you cannot point so reliably to the diet, particularly the cholesterol issue. As a matter of fact, this issue is now being tested in an intensive longitudinal study by the National Heart and Lung Institute. In the area of cancer prevention, aside from smoking and environmental considerations, what are the specific behaviors that, in terms of any probability of success in preventing cancer, would justify massive attempts to modify behavior? Breast examination may be one of the few things that Dr. Peacock didn't assault in his chapter, as he demonstrated point by point how we may be living in the era of myths concerning the validity of the relationships between various activities and cancer. I think Dr. Fox's charting, with the plusses, minuses, and question marks, is often in sharp contradiction with the kinds of skepticism in Dr. Peacock's presentation. We are asked as behavioral scientists to be of assistance in guiding and developing strategies that may be related to changing behaviors. One is concerned about whether there is enough baseline scientific support for behavioral scientists to get involved in the ethical issue that Miriam Kelty mentioned in her presentation.

Leon Festinger reported on a very interesting smoking study in his 1957 book, *A Cognitive Theory of Dissonance*. A massive campaign was undertaken to educate the people in Minnesota on the relationship between smoking and cancer. In this campaign he used two levels of careful analysis: whether people had heard about the campaign, and, if they had, whether they believed what they had heard. He found that the nonsmokers believed the most; the heavier the smoker, the less he believed what he heard. Essentially what begins to happen is that you set up the stage for a "cop-out." Festinger's results would not hold up today, because everybody believes that smoking now is related to cancer. But many other areas, such as the cyclamates or air pollution, upon which Dr. Fox and Dr. Peacock cast doubt, raise a serious question I hope this conference will consider. Dr. Fox and I have discussed listing priorities, a hierarchy. Which behaviors can you most efficiently attack? I certainly hope you don't leave the conference without seriously considering such a formulation because I think there is the capability here of dealing with this problem. I would hesitate to participate in an antiprogram, behavior modification program, even if I had the knowledge to be helpful in designing such a program, in view of many of the points Drs. Peacock and Fox, both eminent and objective scientists, have made.

The work of Janis and Feschbach at Yale some years ago, in which they used *reported* rather than *actual* toothbrushing as a criterion, created a widely accepted belief about the limitations of high fear in persuasion. In fact, their findings do not hold up if actual rather than reported behavioral measures are used. In view of this, it is unfortunate that the health clinic in which Lloyd Shewchuk and his colleagues are involved is still using essentially *reported* behavioral measures and coding these data as if they reveal *facts* about whether these people are smoking. In our present new study, we are fortunate to be working with chemist Evan Horning, author of the well-known paper on identifying nicotine in urine. Through his unique use of the mass spectrometer the technique for measuring nicotine in saliva has been developed, which we are using as a more direct measure of actual smoking. But I cannot admonish you strongly enough to keep in mind, short of the morbidity/mortality criteria Howard Leventhal discussed, that all these intervening behavioral processes that so often depend on reported behavior and verbal response can almost be ignored, because there is so much self-deception and faulty recall concerning particularly taboo behaviors. It is not a question of just using anonymous instruments; there is self-deception to such a great degree in guilt-related behavior, that I am sorry that an operation as Dr. Shewchuk's still seems to depend on reported smoking behavior, reporting such results, and using them for modifying or developing further programs. I am certain that it is not a lack of sophistication; it is simply that one is forced to use reported rather than actual behavioral measures. Much has been written about this in the social psychological, medical, and biochemical literature. I would emphasize this problem with the following. In the particular program Dr. Shewchuk has set up, although much of what he is doing is trial-and-error ingenuity in trying to shape and modify over time, the variables he seems to have ferreted out would make the data make sense. Still, with a dependent variable measure as unsure as this is, I do not even know how to interpret or even begin to react to anything he found. For example: why 1 year? There is no good evidence to show that behavior has been habituated after 6 months or a year, because there is no accurate measure of behavior. You may only be habituating reporting, maybe lying, up to a year. We know in most drug and medical areas that lying is very prevalent (except perhaps in weight modification where there is direct visible evidence). In very few areas in the health field can lying be really eliminated.

Kegeles probably had the most difficult task of all in trying to garner a case against the use of psychosocial, psychocultural, and all these correlative types of variables, because, as Dr. Leventhal stated, the question of not accounting for variances in all such studies raises tremendous questions. We must proceed from there to something more methodologically precise and more imaginative in the models that we developed. I hope Kegeles' paper helped to bury these earlier strategies.

I would like to mention some things that I think should be considered in relation to the strategies that could emerge from the fields of social and behavioral psychology. I think a real problem that many I have spoken with here have—epidemiologists, physicians, public health individuals—is a misunderstanding of what our various disciplines in the behavioral sciences, and particularly social psychology, can offer. Investigators in this field, for example, are not all behavior modifiers, and there is a peaking out of the old behavior-mod movement, as you know it now, because there is repeatedly momentary compliance, short-term compliance, and there is too often a regression to premodification behaviors.

Dr. Enelow summarized some of these points clearly. Although these points seem fruitful in this area, no one has emphasized *primary prevention* of something like smoking. I believe that the mass media are ultimately responsible for the failure to seriously modify

We are embarking on such a study, working with a huge school district, training junior high school students to cope with the pressures to begin smoking (e.g., peer, parent, media). (See Evans, R.I., Smoking in children: Developing a social psychological strategy of deterrence. *J. Prev. Med., in press.*) It would be interesting to know also how many of the other behaviors involved in either primary or secondary cancer prevention can be approached much earlier. If we develop programs to influence cancer-prone behaviors at an early age, we should specify which behaviors we think are of highest priority in cancer prevention, as Dr. Fox suggested.

As Dr. Leventhal reported, we are paying a great deal of attention to behavior modification, arranging the contingency of the environment to increase the probability that a given response will occur, but we are now also increasingly concerned about the information-processing mode. It must be remembered that to present information does not have anything to do with whether it is retained or understood, whether existing beliefs are somehow blocking this, or to what degree this, in turn, will even be converted to behavior. Even a model of a behavior should be related to an information-processing mode. Very little of what we see in this field pays attention to this process. People like William McGuire of Yale have done a fine job over the years trying to present these models, but, interestingly enough, few have seen the wisdom in recognizing that we can actually combine information processing, behavioral modification models, and communication models into an integrated system. There are possibilities for integration of these ideas around problems like cancer prevention. I hope the contributions in this volume will lead us in this direction, and that our differences of opinion as to how to attack the problem will bring forth fruitful new studies.

Discussion

Peacock: I would like to comment briefly on the objective measurement of smoking. About 3 years ago, we looked at 800 school children as part of a contract with EPA, using saliva measurements of thiocyanate. We found that about 30% of the children who said they were nonsmokers were lying and were in fact smokers. Only one of the children who said they were smokers we found was lying and was, in fact, a nonsmoker. He was presumably bragging. Interestingly enough, we found that the proportion who were giving us misleading information decreased as the age increased through 11 up to 18 and leaving school. Since then, we have been examining the same issue as part of the multiple risk factor intervention trial, for which we are the New York contractor, and we have looked at it in considerable detail among adults. Our personal belief at the moment is that between 10 and 20% of the people who say they have given up smoking are, in fact, giving us misleading information. It depends upon who asks the question, and the circumstances under which it is asked. Right now, a massive trial is going on as part of the Mr. Fit program, using serum thiocyanate as an objective measure of, in fact, whether it is true. I would like to point out one story regarding school children.

Some of you may remember the famous three-city study of a few years back using Winnipeg, Baltimore, and Edinburgh. In each of the three cities, three comparable schools were picked. One school was taught to give up smoking by the fear technique, one by saying that if you do not smoke, it will make you beautiful if you are a girl, or it will make you a great athlete if you are a boy, the so-called positive approach; and the third was the control. Of the three, the controlled school did better than either of the experimental schools, in terms of the number of kids who did not become smokers over the year of the study, which fits in exactly with the results of the drug statement that was made earlier. I would warn anybody who gets involved in school programs to be careful that you are not doing a lot more harm than good, because this has been the experience in most circumstances. I believe very strongly that kids learn by imprinting. In other words, they don't do what we say, they do what we do. This is why, if any of you visit us at the American Health Foundation and you are smoking, you will have your cigarette removed from your hand. We fire employees who smoke on the job; we fired one recently. We fired a physician because a member of the public saw him smoking on the job. We believe that you have got to practice what you preach, or else you don't work with us.

We believe what we are doing on adults—and in effect we're testing this belief—kicks back on their children. When we teach a male, for example, in dietary modification, his wife is with him, and hopefully his wife learns, hopefully both convert. In one study we found that if the wife did not convert, results in the husband were pretty lousy. This applies to both smoking and dietary modification. You've got to at least make the wife feel this is important for her husband even if she herself doesn't do it. Given wife and husband, we believe that the teenagers in that family will learn and will do it. We've just screened 7,000 students from a university in New York City, and only 18% of them are smokers today. Their average cholesterol is 220, 225; down nearly 100% from what it was just 4 years ago. This is Social Class I, males. In our adolescent populations, we find that Social Class I male adolescents are also nonsmokers. Why, because Papa and Mama teach, hopefully, that this is not a thing that a decent upperclass kid or man or woman does. It is plain bad form and dirty for them to smoke, and you don't smoke. I think that this is a pattern that is developing. I strongly believe that we are the people who have got to set the example. We don't tell the others to do it, we do it ourselves.

Leventhal: I think the modeling issue is very interesting and very important. You might look in your data not only at positive modeling, not smoking because your parents don't smoke, but the effects on a child of observing his parents trying to kick smoking and becoming aware of the problems that are involved in the longer run of that type of observation. Children often use others as negative models, not just as positive ones; that is, you don't do what he does because of the problems that it creates for him. On the behavior verbal report discrepancies, I don't share your dim view. In most settings, where in fact there is no real incentive or pressure to dissimulate, we found very high associates between reported and actual observed behavior. Obviously, the pressures to dissimulate increase if the behavior is something that is negatively valued or that you are not supposed to do, which should be the case for younger children. Obviously, you could define a situation where reported and actual behavior would be exactly the same. Unfortunately, the kinds of things with which you are dealing often involve a taboo behavior, which is a different matter.

Hulka: I think further comment on the smoking issue is pertinent because here we have that one variable that we do know, a variable that does cause cancer. We heard about Dr. Shewchuk's intervention program, which is apparently aimed at the objective of getting people to stop smoking. I suggest there might be other objectives, and the reasons for this are a couple of facts that have not been brought out in this discussion. First, nicotine as a pharmacologic agent is addicting. It is one of the most addicting agents known to man, much more so even than heroin. Those of you who are interested in this topic might take a look at a review in *Lancet* in the last half of 1974. Other information was provided, and something to consider is that the carcinogenic agent in cigarettes is not nicotine, but the tar of the cigarettes.

With that information at hand, let us consider the current interventions, which have been of the health education type, to get current smokers to stop. They have not been terribly effective, no matter what the particular intervention. Another type of intervention has been something done by the tobacco companies, and that is to try to introduce cigarettes with lowered nicotine and tar content. Well, why has this not been very effective? It has not been very effective because people just smoke more cigarettes in order to maintain the same titer of nicotine that they had before. They have to have the nicotine. This being the case, I would suggest a couple of possible recommendations. Cigarettes could be developed that would reduce the tar content but maintain the nicotine content. Therefore, current smokers would continue to smoke. We have very little experimental evidence that nicotine per se is a detrimental agent. As more experimental work is done, we may learn that nicotine does have adverse effects, not necessarily carcinogenic, but others. Currently, we do not have much evidence of that.

Second, in spite of Dr. Peacock's comments, I would think that whatever health education intervention type activity is going to be undertaken, it would have to be with the youngsters, to make every effort to prevent that first experiment in smoking.

R. Fink: With regard to Dr. Kegeles' remarks, one point has to do with the subculture. It is true that there are important differences in utilization of health services between low income and middle and upper income. In both the studies that have been reported out of Johns Hopkins, and in some of the work that we have been doing at HIP in multiphasic testing, we have found that the major part of the difference in utilization between the poverty and nonpoverty groups has to do with the use of preventive health services. When you find a health problem among poor people and nonpoor people, care for that problem is about the same for both groups. This has been observed in a number of settings. The difficulty with low-income groups has to do primarily with bringing them in for preventive health care, and I think it is important to separate the two. I am in agreement with Dr. Kegeles on the problem of replicating some of the studies that have been reported on food intake and alcohol intake. Much of the epidemilogical information I find very hard to reconcile with some of the difficulties that some of us, in survey research in particular, have had with measuring either food or alcohol intake. The ability to measure the amount of alcohol is very, very difficult. Measuring specific food intake, while difficult, is not as hard as Dr. Kegeles has indicated. We have and others have done very good nutritional studies, but it requires a kind of narrowing down and focusing on a particular topic in which you are interested. Comparing national differences in cancer as related to hypothesized differences in food intake is a very uncomfortable matter in matching.

MacCalla: I would like to comment on the failure to take effective action; namely, that we ought to consider expanding the focus of needed research in that area for the simple reason that we need to take a look at some of the social-cultural-behavioral tendencies and receptivity patterns among the consumer. In addition to making better use of clinical theory in hypotheses, we need to look at some consumer-based applied research data so that our assumption becomes not one of determining what we fail to do to promote effective action, but rather that the failure of the subcultural group is implied as it is stated now. We ought to turn that around, because it is really not the failure of the subcultural group, it is the failure of what we do. We do not have enough information to know what we do, and I am suggesting that in addition to the clinical-type research we need some applied consumer-based research. Some attempts have been made, but not in a manner that might work its way into a forum such as this one. I mentioned earlier in this conference that we should talk about the cancer-among-the-family project conducted in 1966 by the American Cancer Society in California. They recognized that they were not making contact with the Spanish-speaking population with the kind of public information material that they had, and they found that there were some very basic things that were not done properly because of faulty assumptions. They started from the other end with the materials being developed by the consumer. There you have a kind of consumer research counterpart. The laboratory is really out there and not inside. That particular model was very effective in terms of public education for special populations.

Similarly, in 1968, the ACS in California undertook (and I participated in) the development of a physiology primer, because one of the faulty assumptions was that we all know how the body works. But we all do not, and as a result we had to start from a consumer-based applied research model finding out how one is going to be able to receive the information before we start treating the problem of public education. The sociocultural variable is something that we have to look at not from the standpoint of clinical research alone, but from the receptivity to the public education that has to follow. Information alone does not treat anything, you have to do something with it. We do not know what to do with it, and that is why I think we have to expand our focus in research.

Leventhal: In talking about groups, one often tends to think in terms of problems of people understanding what you are saying, comprehension being poor in low-income groups, and so on, although I think that is generally not true. We need to distinguish between putting across conceptual information, such as defining cholesterol, versus operational information—what do you have to do in your life situation to avoid this agent. The deficit in this information may be just as high for upper and middle as for low income groups, the problem being one of not knowing how to avoid those foods that are not good. Individuals don't know enough about food. And professionals don't know enough about how to eat and live to tell them what to avoid.

McQueen: We ought to be very careful when talking about carcinogens, particularly when the information is likely to be consumed by the public. There is no question that the condensate of a cigarette does contain carcinogenic material, but beyond question the volatiles also contain carcinogens, which are yet to be defined. Perhaps one of the reasons we haven't modified the behavior of younger people is that we talk about low-tar and low-nicotine cigarettes, and I wonder if people are beginning to think that there is such a thing as a safe cigarette. I think that is an idea that we ought to try to dispel. It has been put forward quite eloquently that the only safe cigarette is the one which is not smoked, and I think that is what we ought to put across and stop talking about safe cigarettes.

Antonovsky: I have been strongly impressed in the last year by Irving Janis' work on group thinking, and because I am subject to that danger, too, I hesitated before responding. But I think there is a danger, and I would like to respond to Dr. Peacock's last remark in his chapter. I thought it was facetious when he said, all you have to do is do a simple thing like changing life styles. When he spoke now, I realized he was not being facetious, and that is because he seems to have the truth. He spoke of the anticigarette campaign with a religious fervor in which he expressed the truth. Now, I fully accept the data about cigarettes and fully share the desire to have an anticigarette campaign. But I am afraid, as a scientist and as a citizen, I must ask two questions. As a scientist, what price do you pay when you succeed in cutting out cigarettes? Is it so clear that this is the answer and that there is no boomerang in other health areas? As a citizen I must point to the dangers of knowing the truth religiously, and by God, when the revolution comes "you'll eat strawberry shortcake" whether you like it or not.

Cancer: The Behavioral Dimensions, edited by J. W. Cullen, B. H. Fox, and R. N. Isom. Raven Press, New York © 1976.

Introduction

Betty Mathews

School of Health Education, University of Washington, Seattle, Washington 98105

Our topic in this section is the health care system and its influences. By way of providing a focus, I want to point out that during recent years we have taken note of a rapid rise in the cost of medical care and, also, in the amount of malpractice litigation that has occurred. We have noted, too, that there are some research findings that suggest that from one-half to two-thirds of patients fail to comply with medically prescribed treatment. Recognition of these factors has led to policy and legislative developments in recent years, which reflects that the notion of the patient role as one of passive submissive dependence is being replaced by one of responsible independence and active involvement in decision-making about his health and medical care. This relatively new philosopy parallels the major principle of cancer control that was articulated in the 1973 program planning conference: "Cancer control is a personal responsibility." The principle implies that each individual is entitled to a full understanding of the options and the alternatives, and that based on such an understanding, one has the responsibility of choosing freely and bearing the consequences of that decision.

As I consider the points and some of the discussions we have been having, I wonder if we sometimes operate on the assumption that our task is to get persons to change their behavior, rather than to make a choice about what that behavior will be and live with those consequences. Of course, all professionals share cognitions that a patient is a whole person with needs and strivings; that care of the patient must include consideration of the social, psychological, and cultural factors that impinge upon him; and that recognition of his human dignity and his potential for assuming responsibility and productive living must be incorporated into the patient role. But the programs of activities that health professionals are swept into and are rewarded for tend to be those that support institutional regulations or the means that have been established for achieving the technical goals of health care. Frequently forgotten is the fact that many of the same activities provide a multitude of signals that impress upon consumers of health services that they have no business participating, that they are dependent on the good will of those around them, and that they are to comply in the sense of submission and cooperation. The expectations of the person who sought the health care service may have been to surrender his illness. But more often than not, he ends up surrendering himself.

We have some evidence that when people make their own decisions, they are more likely to follow through than when the decisions are imposed by external agents. The promotion of such responsible decision-making is extremely complex, because people differ greatly in their needs to be dependent or independent in their decision-making styles and skills, in their ability to process new knowledge, in their handling of anxiety, in their stage of illness, and in many other factors that we could identify.

However, the behaviors of health professionals vis-à-vis patients serve as reinforcing factors in perpetuating patient dependency or in supporting patient attempts to be responsible and independent. At the same time, the behaviors of the health professionals are a response to the influences within the health care system itself. The following chapters consider some of the characteristics of the health care system that influence behavior and the impact that such influences have on health professionals and on patients.

Cancer: The Behavioral Dimensions, edited by J. W. Cullen,
B. H. Fox, and R. N. Isom. Raven Press, New York © 1976.

System Characteristics that Influence Behaviors

William Lohr

Health Services Research Methods Branch, Bureau of Health Services Research, Department of Health, Education and Welfare, Rockville, Maryland 20852

This chapter deals with system characteristics that influence behaviors as they relate to health. We are concerned not only with the "health care system" itself but with the larger context of the social system, many aspects of which have a bearing on health. Surprisingly, not enough systematic attention has been given to this area of inquiry. However, a number of publications touch on elements of the problem in such a way that a general insight can be gained on how, and to what degree, the "system" does in fact influence behaviors. As will become clear, the system effects are both positive and negative.

Andersen and Newman dealt with some aspects of this question (1). They employed the following definition of system proposed by Barker (2):

> The general concept of system refers to a set of units or elements which are actively interrelated and that operate in some sense as a bounded unit....General systems theory is, then, primarily concerned with the problem of relationships and of interdependence than with the constant attributes of objects.

They discussed the societal determinants of utilization, itself a behavior, but what they suggested could be applied to a broader spectrum of behaviors. In their view, these societal determinants of utilization are technologies and norms. They derived their definition of technology from Taylor (3) and mean by it "a set of principles and techniques useful to bring about change toward desired ends." Specifically, by medical technology, they mean those techniques and principles providing "tools for extending the physician's power of observation and making more effective his role as therapist," as Warner suggested (4).

Their notion of norms is derived from Moore's description of "social control as representing the spectrum of modes whereby social systems induce or insure normal compliance on the part of members" (5). This definition includes "Sumner's classic distinctions of degrees of control and correlative degree of negative sanctions for violators: folkways (it is normally expected), mores (you ought to behave), and laws (you must comply)."

Technology and norms have, in Andersen and Newman's view, affected behaviors in many areas of the health care system. Technology has obviously had an enormous impact on the way that people in industrialized societies live. That these impacts have been evident in health care and medical practice is equally obvious. They cite examples, such as the decline of mortality from a range of acute, infectious diseases, as the result of antibiotic drug technology. Similarly, changes have occurred in other areas, such as altered "patterns of care for hospitalized patients in terms of case mix and length of stay."

An example of these changed patterns and the "service intensive" trends was noted by Fuchs and Kramer (6), who pointed out that from the late 1940s to 1956, technological change was "physician saving," whereas since 1956, these technologies have been "physician using." One statistic supporting this view is the average length of stay in short-term hospitals: "This statistic declined from 8.7 days in 1948 to 7.7 days in 1956. After 1956, the average length of stay leveled off and then began to rise, reaching 7.9 days in 1966." Another pattern is cited: "hospital days per capita (admissions times average length of stay) were relatively stable in the first period (before 1956) but rose appreciably in the second. The population's health did not worsen after 1956, but more cases became treatable and the average time of treatment rose. The increase in hospitalization was associated with increased utilization of physician's services because the new technology required large inputs of each."

Norms are the second factor in Andersen and Newman's view of the societal determinants of behaviors. There have been many changes in norms, reflected through "formal legislation as well as growing consensus of beliefs and homogeneity of values which pervade the society." The belief that medical care was somehow a right reached a level in the mid-1960s sufficient to see Congressional approval of legislation for Medicare and Medicaid. The steady rise in the numbers covered by health insurance plans in the past 30 years is an indication of changing norms and has produced a substratum of support, reflecting popular demand, for enactment of a National Health Insurance Plan.

The health services sytem is, in their view, structured for the "provision of formal health care goods and services in society, including physician care, hospital care, dental care, drugs, and health appliances and services by other health care practitioners...to the individual." There are two dimensions: resources and organization. Resources are the "labor and capital devoted to health care" in both their volume and geographic distribution. Organization refers to what the system does "with its resources" and describes the "manner in which medical personnel and facilities are coordinated in the process of providing medical services," and have a series of effects on access to care and the structures for delivery.

Others address themselves to these questions of systems characteristics with far more troubled spirits. The system is in "crisis" and in "chaos" and is affecting people's behavior adversely, in too many cases, by being unresponsive to individual needs. A number of publications have traced this process, often in parallel with the growth of industrialized life. The 1947 report of the New York Academy of Medicine (7) traces this history of medical care in the past 150 years. Kelman (8) follows the parallel course of the industrial and medical care world from their stages as "cottage" industries and general practitioners up through the industrial capitalism model for both. He notes that there are two almost constant characteristics found in the Western world: competition and monopoly. Competition is low in technological levels and fairly static, whereas monopoly is tied in with an ever-increasing technological level irrespective of changes in production.

When science and technology were introduced into the medical care area, a natural consequence was the greater use and importance of the hospital, the analogue of the plant in this industrial-type model, and there was understandably a decline in the role and numbers of general practitioners. This emphasis on hospital produced a need for more substantial financial bases for the delivery of care, an industrial, science-oriented delivery system, specialization, and other characteristics, which has made it difficult for the patient, now "consumer," to "shop" for care amidst all these new complexities, and has substantially increased the cost of care because of a linkage between insurance carriers and the hospital rate schedules.

The Ehrenreichs discuss this same subject in their book, in a chapter entitled "From the Family Doctor to the Medical Industrial Complex" (9). They suggest that the problem is now becoming clearer to the public:

> The proper study of the American health system is no longer medicine but medical institutions. Everyone knows that...the myth of the paternal, house-calling practitioner went out years ago. But people are only beginning to discern the outlines of a new medical establishment, based on local networks of hospitals and medical schools, backed up by a highly technological and profitable health commodities industry, and represented nationally by the corporate voices of the American Hospital Association, Blue Cross, and the American Association of Medical Schools. At the heart of the new system is no longer the free enterprise private practitioner, but the local, medical-school-centered medical empire.

Waitzkin and Waterman (10) discuss "medicine as a social institution." They see health care as set within the broad "sociopolitical structures of the societies" in which they occur. The organizational forms "which govern the treatment of the sick reflect broad normative principles within a society; the normative framework within which health workers and patients interact may be called society's *medicocivil structure.*" But these interactions are, in their view, not interactions on a one-to-one basis but manifest a stratification with the providers, both individually and collectively, assuming a dominant role. The result is a "medical imperialism" made up of "large health organizations (medical schools, hospitals, the insurance industry, companies manufacturing medical equipment and so forth...(attempting)...to expand their physical plants, services programs, patient populations or sales." Such an arrangement with its "duplication and overlap" causes health costs to rise even while distribution is poor and some facilities are underutilized.

Alford (11) argues that the system of health care in the United States is and has been in crisis for the past 40 years. He cites Rosen, an economist (12), who says that "the catalogue of problems drawn up almost forty years ago strongly resembles the latest list—inadequate services, insufficient funds, understaffed hospitals. Virtually nothing has changed." And Ginzberg (13) says, in a similar vein, that "while changes have occurred in response to emergencies, opportunities, and alternatives in the market place, the outstanding finding is the inertia of the system as a whole." This situation he describes as "dynamics without change" resulting from a "struggle between different major interest groups operating within the context of a market society—professional monopolists controlling the major health resources, corporate rationalizers challenging their power, and the community population seeking better health care."

Each of these viewpoints on the state of medical care suggests that we are in the midst of a dynamic process in which the parts or elements in the system are engaged in a continuous effort at reaching an equilibrium. The end result of that equilibrium has consequences which have an impact on behaviors. Swanson (14) discusses this process in relationship to the "politics of health" and the scope of government. He uses a figure in which the public-private sectors, contractionist, and expansionist forces are at work in health care (Fig. 1). At any given time,

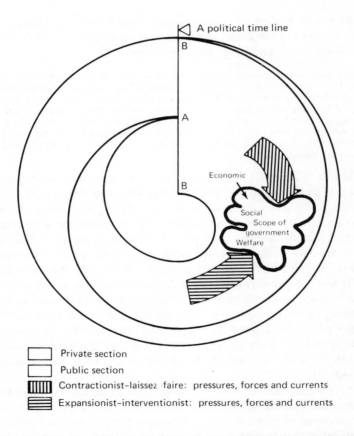

FIG. 1. Expansion-contraction continuum of the local scope of government. (Reprinted from ref. 42.)

depending on the state of the political climate, the scope of government in health care varies in degree. Swanson delineates "seven factors affecting and shaping health systems": system outputs, levels of stress, system inputs, power structures, political ideologies, political focuses, and system changes processes.

System outputs are subject to increase, decrease, or maintenance of present levels of government involvement. These efforts to increase that level may be incremental or comprehensive. *System stress* refers to the degree of "disturbances" threatening the system, ranging from invisible issues to potential and then on to routine and controversial problems. *System inputs,* both demands and supports, are a mirror of the clamor raised by public demand and the degree of political support that can be mustered for these demands. *Power structure* deals with a "key factor," and is concerned with both the distribution and exercise of power. The dimensions are the degree to which that power is "distributed broadly or narrowly throughout the citizenry and the extent to which the ideology in regard to the scope of government of the political leadership is convergent or compatible, on the one hand, or divergent and conflicting on the other." The convergent group is led by a consensual elite; the divergent by a competitive elite.

Political ideologies are the "way of perceiving and reacting to the events occurring around the individual" which help shape "the attitudes of a person's political behavior." *Political focus* deals not only with health in general, but with the "equally important aspects of decision-making structures and processes, public policies, financial resources and who shall administer the policies," and represents both a contractionist and expansionist mentality. The final factor, *system change processes,* includes the change agents "who operationalize general objectives and strategies." Increasers of the governmental role are interested in reform through "politicization" and "creative tension." Those seeking to decrease or maintain the present scope of government use the processes of "professionalization," "mediation," and "management."

Some of these forces might be mentioned as illustrative examples of these factors in health care, because each group feels that its approach to the system would beget behavioral effects. Some suggest that we let the free-market competitive processes work in the medical market place. Alford cites Harry Schwartz as a representative of this view (15). Encourage free competition between health facilities, physicians, and health insurance plans and "market pressures will drive out the incompetent, excessively high-priced or duplicated service, and the inaccessible physician, clinic, or hospital." This view would advocate "the control of the individual physician over his practice, over the hospital, and over his fees, and they simply wish to open up medical schools to meet the demand for doctors, to give patients more choice among doctors, clinics and hospitals, and to make that choice a real one by providing public subsidies for medical bills."

These "assumptions are questioned by the 'bureaucratic reformers,'"according to Alford. Because of the importance of the "hospital as the key location and organizer of health services," they wish "to put individual doctors under the control of hospital medical boards and administrators," coordinate "fragmented services, instituting planning, and extending public funding." Technological sophistication and the scientific aspects of medicine require "a complex and coordinated division of labor between ambulatory and in-hospital care, primary practitioners and specialists, and personalized care and advanced chemical and electronic treatment." The community is regarded as necessarily involved and its interests are to be represented. Dr. Roemer is, in Alford's view, a primary proponent of this approach (16).

An alternate, quasi-public utility model has been proposed by White (17). In several articles, White suggested that the "organizational prototype for the health services systems of this country...is that of the airlines. Competitive, regulated, subsidized and franchised service in which 'private' enterprise is encouraged to serve the public purposes is worth considering." An analogy could be made between health services agencies and the Federal Aviation Agency. White holds that for medicine, "the basic model of a modified public utility may be preferable to that of a welfare or social service, a 'cottage' industry or a solo storekeeper. Such a model...is in the best traditions of this country in its mix of public and private financing, participation and control: it encourages innovation and experimentation and is based on the most constructive aspects of human motivation and competition."

Waitzkin and Waterman suggested a series of characteristics of a system that would be more responsive and humanistic: (1) profits from illness must be abolished; (2) the problems of bureaucracy, often itself dehumanizing and alienating, must be surmounted; (3) there must be a national set of goals regarding health care but local control to adapt that system to specific needs; (4) a healthy "dialectic" between compulsory and voluntary systems; and (5) a modification in the medical "stratification" by insuring better and more equal distribution of resources, liberalizing and expanding medical and paramedical training, and softening the doctor-patient "stratification" patterns, now so common, so that a "more egalitarian doctor-patient relationship would be created," a development that would most certainly have a strong bearing on behaviors.

Barbara and John Ehrenreich present a series of problems with the system that seem to suggest ways it could be improved if these problems were remedied: (1) provide facilities where appropriate care would be available at reasonable cost; (2) develop ways of permitting individual patients to find their way amid the many available types of care; (3) inform people what is being done to them when they receive care; (4) develop procedures for recourse when "things don't go right"; (5) alter patterns of "racism and male chauvinism" in physicians and hospitals that are now present in the "system." It is implicit in the achievement of these objectives that more appropriate behavioral responses would result.

These critics of the "system" urge its reform and change because, in their view, it is not now sufficiently responsive to patient needs and does not benefit the population as it should. In sum, problems of availability of care and access to care, and its excessive cost, together with the lack of adequate control and power on the part of users once in the system, are not calculated to maximize the potential for improved health which this medical care system ought to have.

Some insight into the possible effects of changing the system has emerged from the English experience with the National Health Service. Has their universal entitlement policy made care more uniformly available across social classes as seen in their use of medical services? Rein (18) argued that the "availability of universal free-on-demand, comprehensive services, along with a system of medical accountability by generalists, is a crucial factor in reducing class inequalities in the use of medical services." Others, such as Titmuss (19), hold an opposite view. Titmuss states, "We have learned from 15 years of experience of the Health Service that higher income groups know how to make better use of the service; they tend to receive more specialist attention; occupy more of the beds in better equipped and staffed hospitals, receive more elective surgery, have better maternal care, and are more likely to get psychiatric help and psychotherapy than low-income groups—particularly the unskilled." Gough (20) also concludes that "inequalities in the *use* of these services persist within the National Health Service." What may account for such differences, even after the removal of such considerable barriers as payment, is discussed later in this chapter.

Some have held that the system is what it is because it represents the equilibrium of forces found in the society at any given time. Although these may change slowly over time, it is not realistic to assume that any massive restructuring of the system is possible. Odin Anderson (21), for one, in citing Crozier (22), suggests that "organizational goals stated in rational terms encounter the necessity to conform to social systems of which the organizations are a part." He does recognize that change is and has been a part of our system. In his comparison of the systems in the United States, Sweden, and Britain, he notes that each "works" because the politicians and other interest groups are responsive enough to different pressures so that each system operates with tolerable equilibrium. Within that equilibrium, however, the public is a genuine factor: "The public obviously wants health services; otherwise politicians would not enshrine access to care as a civil right." To underscore this notion, Anderson cites Charles Schultze (23), who notes that a "plan and a fistful of money will not be enough to achieve the objectives of a public program if the plan runs counter to the motivations, rewards, and penalties of the public and private institutions which must carry it out."

That the situation is not one which has easy solutions is made clear by the wealth of literature in which the effects of social class, socioeconomic status, family structure, culture, education, and many other aspects of population characteristics are described. Kasl and Cobb (24), Aday and Eichhorn (25), Andersen and Anderson (26), Lohr (27), and McKinlay (28) presented much of this literature in a systematic manner. We shall discuss only some highlights here to point out the complexities of the problem of behavioral influences on medical care on the part of users.

Bice (29) suggested that the major contribution of sociologists toward the understanding of health behaviors is a better knowledge of "(1) the social and cultural processes which influence the perception of illness; and (2) the influences of group structures on the use of professional services." R. Andersen (30) developed a model to help understand how these factors are interrelated. This model is made up of the predisposing, enabling, and need factors, influential in the decision to seek or not to seek care and under what conditions. Predisposing factors are those rooted in behaviors and attitudes inclining persons to use or not to use care or to use differentially, to perceive pain in different ways, to assume certain roles, and so on. Enabling factors are the economic and financial aspects associated with seeking care, as well as the availability of those services within the potential user's psychological and fiscal resources. Need factors are actual illnesses or threats of illness that are influential in the behavior of individuals and families.

A number of investigators have described the social dimensions of illness that accompany its biological dimensions. Freidson (31) speaks of illness as a "social deviance," which is as pertinent in society's view as the notion of "biological deviance" is to the medical practitioner's view. "In any particular empirical case," Freidson notes, "the 'sickness' may or not be biologically 'real' while the sick role is always socially 'real'." Polgar (32) put it this way: "The definition of illness involves not only the identification of signal changes in the person and the reflection on their possible causes but in his social identity as well.... To be treated as a sick person, social validation for this temporary role must be obtained." And Bloom (33) discussed the social and cultural meaning of illness: "Each illness, in theory, has a clinical entity.... But the meaning of illness, from the view of the patient, is more variable.... People perceive illness in different ways. The pattern of these perceptions and the definitions of illness vary according to culture and within culture."

Parsons (34) coined the term "sick role," which describes the way a person assumes a particular kind of behavior, fully expecting that others will behave toward him in a certain way. While in the "sick role," customary roles are not lost or dropped but simply superseded for a time.

Mechanic (35) introduced the term "illness behavior," which refers to the ways in which given symptoms may be differentially perceived, evaluated, and acted (or not acted) upon by different kinds of persons. A patient, confronted with symptoms, may choose to do one or more of the following: seek help, treat himself, or absent himself from customary duties. Each course of action includes the notion of "social deviance" from normal patterns and implies the legitimization of these "deviant" patterns by others.

Freidson (31) is even more forceful. He speaks of society, not only as the legitimizer of illness, but of a segment of society as creator of the possibility of sickness:

> Unlike Parsons, I do not argue that medicine has the power to legitimize one's acting sick by conceding that he is really sick. My argument goes further than that. I argue that by virtue of being the authority on what illness 'really' is, *medicine creates the social possibility for acting sick*. In this sense, medicine's monopoly includes the right to create illness as an *official social role*.... It is part of being a profession to be given the official power to create the shape of the problematic

segments of social behavior: the judge determines what is legal and who is guilty, the priest what is holy and who is profane, the physician what is normal and who is sick.

These kinds of considerations have genuine effects on the behaviors of the population and on subgroups within that population. The patterns of care, types of services used, use of services, and the like are very clearly dependent on many characteristics. Both Koos (36) and Ross (37) noted the differing interpretation of illness between classes. Ross found that the lower classes go to a physician (when they go at all) for a "felt complaint," whereas the upper classes devote a greater share of their visits to preventive care, "of less urgency and without the immediate goad of discomfort." Others found similar patterns. Andersen, Anderson, and Smedby (38) found that socioeconomic factors were significant in response to symptoms: the lowest income groups had a higher percentage of symptoms (67%) but a lower percentage of reporting them (69%), while the highest income group had only 49% experiencing symptoms with 75% of them seeing a physician as a result.

Ludwig and Gibson (39) studied the perception of sickness relative to socioeconomic status. Seeking care in the face of perceived poor health was influenced by the recognition and significance attached to symptoms, situational factors that make it more or less difficult to seek attention (such as income and welfare experience) and the mental set called faith in the medical care system. Low income and welfare experience were strongly "associated with failure to seek care irrespective of system orientation" and lack of faith in the medical system was more influential in the decision to seek care than the symptoms perceived. Strauss (40) and Coe and Wessen (41) suggest that lower social classes avoid care, unless pressed by extreme necessity, in part because of the perceived distance between users and providers resulting from class-induced modes of acting and behaving.

There are many other factors associated with different patterns of use, each of which has a bearing on how individuals and groups will behave and interpret their illnesses, symptoms, and complaints. These are not immutable and are influenced by changes in the system, as is evidenced by the changing patterns of physician visits since the advent of Medicaid. It would appear, in that instance, that a major deterrent to use, the financial barriers to access, was removed by that federal program.

SUMMARY

It would be wise to ask, given what is known, what ought to be done with the knowledge available in the formulation of policies. While there is much information on the patterns of behavior of groups, classes, individuals, and populations with respect to health and health care, it is not unreasonable to ask that translation of that information into policy decisions be made with judiciousness. Policies have emerged—for instance, Medicare and Medicaid—and there is no easy way to estimate their full impact. It is not known whether these two programs have really had a measurable impact on the health status of the persons they have served. We do know that the costs have been enormous and have probably contributed to the spiraling costs of care in general. They have helped to create the belief that medical care is a right—not unreasonably—and have changed and influenced the behaviors of considerable numbers of both providers and users.

With regard to health levels and behavioral change, it must be asked first and be clearly understood whether and why behavioral change or modification is a good, outweighing its opposite. If behaviors are modified, how can this be done without producing other undesirable changes? It is necessary to ask why, on what bases, and by what methods are these changes to be made? The general presumption is that scientific evidence (not always unequivocal) indicates that certain kinds of behaviors are detrimental to health and therefore ought to be changed. The clearest example of that is smoking behavior, but such clear-cut evidence is not always available. There are many ambiguities about other behavioral patterns that do not permit simple solutions. For instance, the efficacy of health services themselves is not always and in all cases a demonstrated reality, so that their use may or may not effect improvements in health levels. Should the strategy be to provide a wealth of information on the benefits of hazards of a particular set of behaviors and allow individuals to follow their own course? Or should there be specific campaigns to modify behaviors or incentives given to induce behavioral change? What is the role of evidence in making decisions about what behaviors ought to be changed and what are the limitations and tradeoffs involved?

Clearly, a good deal of consideration must be given to understanding specific dimensions of these complex problems, followed by well-articulated strategies which, when implemented, are evaluated by careful experiments. This has been done in some areas and work in other areas is under way, much of which is a tribute to serious investigators, agencies, and groups. Using this model of discovery, diffusion, and implementation, system changes have taken place and will continue to occur which will without doubt have serious effects on the behaviors of providers and users of services for better health.

REFERENCES

1. Andersen, R., and Newman, J. Societal and individual determinants of medical care utilization in the United States. *Milbank Mem. Fund Q.*, 51:95–124 (1973).
2. Barker, F. General systems theory, research and medical care. In Sheldon, A., Barker, T., and McLaughlin, C. (eds.): *Systems and Medical Care*, M.I.T. Press, Cambridge, 1970.
3. Taylor, J. *Technology and Planned Organizational Change*, University of Michigan, Ann Arbor, 1971.
4. Warner, H. Problems and priorities for health care technology in the 1980's. Presented at the *Conference on Technology & Health Care Systems in the 1980's*, sponsored by the National Center for Health Services Research & Development, San Francisco, January 21, 1972.
5. Moore, W. Social structure and behavior. In Lindzey G., and Aronson, E., (eds.): *Handbook for Social Psychology*, vol. 4, 2nd ed., Addison-Wesley, Reading, Mass., 1969.
6. Fuchs, V., and Kramer, M. *Determinants of Expenditures for Physicians' Services in the United States, 1948–1968*, DHEW, HSMHA, National Center for Health Services Research & Development, DHEW Publication HSM-73-3013, 1972.

7. *Medicine in the Changing Order,* Report of the New York Academy of Medicine, Committee on Medicine & the Changing Order, The Commonwealth Fund, New York, 1947.
8. Kelman, S. Toward the political economy of medical care. *Inquiry,* VIII, No. 3 (1971).
9. Ehrenreich, B., and Ehrenreich, J. *The American Health Empire, Power, Profits and Politics,* Random House, New York, 1971.
10. Waitzkin, H., and Waterman, B. *The Exploitation of Illness in a Capitalist Society,* Bobbs-Merrill, New York, 1974.
11. Alford, R. The political economy of health care: Dynamics without change, *Politics and Society,* 2:127–164 (1972).
12. Rosen, S. Change and resistance to change. *Soc. Policy,* 1:4 (1971).
13. Ginzberg, E., et al. *Urban Health Services,* Columbia University Press, New York, 1971.
14. Swanson, B. The politics of health. In Freeman, H., Levine, S., and Reeder, L. (eds.): *Handbook of Medical Sociology,* 2nd ed., Prentice-Hall, Englewood Cliffs, N.J., 1972.
15. Schwartz, H. Health care in America: A heretical diagnosis. *Saturday Review,* 14–17, 14 August 1971.
16. Roemer, M. Nationalized medicine for America. *Trans-Action,* 31–36, September, 1971.
17. White, K. Primary medical care for families—organization and evaluation. *N. Engl. J. Med.,* 277:847–852 (1967), and health care organization—trends and opportunities. *Am. J. Dis. Child.,* 127:549–533 (1974).
18. Rein, M. Social class and utilization of medical care services—a study of the British experience under National Health Insurance hospitals. *J. Am. Hosp. Assoc.,* 43:43–52 (1969).
19. Titmuss, R. *Commitment to Welfare,* Allen & Unwin, London, 1968.
20. Gough, I. *Inequalities in Britain,* Penguin, London, 1970.
21. Anderson, O. *Health Care: Can There be Equity?,* John Wiley & Sons, New York, 1972.
22. Crozier, M. *The Bureaucratic Phenomenon,* University of Chicago Press, Chicago, 1964.
23. Schultze, C. *Political Bargaining, Systematic Analyses and Federal Budget Decisions,* The Brookings Institution, Washington, D.C., Report No. 95, 1969.
24. Kasl, S., and Cobb, S. Health behavior, illness behavior and sick role behavior. *Arch. Environ. Health,* 12:246–266 (1966).
25. Aday, L., and Eichhorn, R. *The Utilization of Health Services: Indices and Correlates,* DHEW, HSMHA, National Center for Health Services Research (DHEW Publication HSM 73-3003), 1972.
26. Andersen, R., and Anderson, O. *A Decade of Health Services: Social Survey Trends in Use and Expenditures,* University of Chicago Press, Chicago, 1967.
27. Lohr, W. *An Historical View of the Research Done on Behavioral and Organizational Factors Related to the Utilization of Health Services.* Unpublished paper, National Center for Health Services Research, Rockville, Md., 1972.
28. McKinlay, J. Some approaches and problems in the study of the use of services—an overview. *J. Health Soc. Behav.,* 13:115–152 (1972).
29. Bice, Y. *Medical Care for the Disadvantaged,* Department of Medical Care and Hospitals. The Johns Hopkins University, Baltimore, 1971.
30. Andersen, R. *A Behavioral Model for Families' Use of Health Services,* University of Chicago, Chicago, Center for Health Administration Studies, Res. Ser. 25, 1968.
31. Freidson, E. *The Profession of Medicine: A Study of the Sociology of Applied Knowledge,* Dodd, Mead, New York, 1970. *See also* his *Professional Dominance: The Social Structure of Medical Care,* Atherton, New York, 1970, and his *Patient's Views of Medical Practice,* Russell Sage Foundation, New York, 1961.
32. Polgar, S. Health and human behavior: Areas of interest common to the social and medical sciences. *Curr. Anthropol.,* 3:159–205 (1962).
33. Bloom, S. *The Doctor and His Patient: A Sociological Interpretation,* Russell Sage Foundation, New York, 1963.
34. Parsons, T. *The Social System,* The Free Press, Glencoe, Ill., 1951. *See also* his other articles: Definitions of health and illness in the light of American values and social structure. In Jaco, E., (ed.): *Patients, Physicians and Illness,* The Free Press, Glencoe, Ill., 1958; Illness and the role of the physician: A sociological perspective. *Am. J. Orthopsychiatry,* 21:452–460 (1951).
35. Mechanic, D. The concept of illness behavior. *J. Chron. Dis.,* 15:189–194 (1962), and Mechanic, D., and Volkart, E. Illness behavior and medical diagnosis, *J. Health Soc. Behav.,* 1:86–94 (1960).
36. Koos, E. *The Health of Regionville,* Columbia University Press, New York, 1954

37. Ross, J. Social class and medical care. *J. Health Soc. Behav.*, 3:35–40 (1962).
38. Andersen, R., Anderson, O., and Smedby, B. Perceptions of and response to symptoms of illness in Sweden and the United States. *Med. Care*, 6:18–30 (1968).
39. Ludwig, E., and Gibson, G. Self-perception of sickness and seeking medical care. *J. Health Soc. Behav.*, 10:125–133 (1969).
40. Strauss, A. Medical organization, medical care and lower income groups. *Soc. Sci. Med.*, 3:143–177 (1969).
 1. Coe, R., and Wessen, A. Social-psychological factors influencing the use of community health resources. *Am. J. Public Health*, 55:1024–1031 (1965).
42. Agger, R. E., Goldrich, D., and Swanson, B. E. *The Rulers and the Ruled*, John Wiley & Sons, New York, 1964.

Cancer: The Behavioral Dimensions, edited by J. W. Cullen, B. H. Fox, and R. N. Isom. Raven Press, New York © 1976.

Impact of the System on the Patient-Practitioner Relationship

Jane Davies

School of Nursing, University of Florida, Gainesville, Florida 32611

Dr. Cullen stated that his main objective for this volume is to "determine the state of the art of behavioral principles as they relate to chronic disease, cancer in particular." It is my intent to illustrate a configuration of the system as nursing views it. The use of the word system implies to me a specific system, and this chapter outlines that system in nursing.

The general systems approach is based on the assumption that matter in all its forms, living and nonliving, can be regarded as systems, and that systems have certain discrete properties that can be studied (1). Walter Buckley defined the system as a complex of elements or components directly or indirectly related in a caused network such that each component is related to at least some others in a more or less stable way within a particular period.

According to Koesher (2), a system can simultaneously be a part and a whole. He coined the word "holon" to denote a system that is both a part of a larger suprasystem and is itself a suprasystem to other subsystems. For example, the circulatory system is made up of the heart, blood vessels, and blood. It is a whole suprasystem when related to man. It is a subsystem when related to the whole of man. Man becomes the suprasystem.

The general systems approach enables us to order our knowledge about entities with which we work. In nursing, we work with man. You and I are in the business of seeking compliance from our clients—compliance being the behavioral posture that enables the client to obtain, internalize, and apply knowledge relevant to the complexities of his illness/health continuum and, further, to modify his behavior in ways supportive of an agreed-upon therapeutic regime designed to make the patient more well, less ill. General systems approach also enables us to formulate a conceptual model of man. Since nursing practice is based on nursing knowledge, the general systems approach by our concept of humanity can also be used to develop our concept of nursing and nursing practice. We believe that man is a dynamic being who is born, lives, and dies as an individual and as a member of a group. In effect, we are saying man is both a part and a whole.

General nursing education has tended to focus primarily on either the subsystem or parts of man, or the systems, such as social systems, of which man is a part. There has been little emphasis on man as a whole.

Rogers (3) formulates a conceptual model based on the general systems theory of man as a whole—a conceptual model that provides a lens to view the relatedness of concepts that constitute the relatedness of "wholeness" of man. She indicates that certain assumptions can be made about man as a whole. From these assumptions, she evolved what we call nursing principles. I discuss the relevance that this conceptual model of man, and the ecological systems concept of health, have for nursing. The conceptualization of man's health/illness status, resulting from his interactions with his environment, led to the development of an ecological-theoretical perspective of health. According to the ecological systems approach (4), man is perceived as a system, that is, interrelated parts that mutually react to maintain themselves by exchanging energy which transacts with other systems within the environment. The health status of an individual is seen as being determined by the interaction and integration of two ecological universes: the internal environment of man himself and the external environment in which he lives and to which he relates. We are returning to the concept of holon.

Because these environments are interrelated, a change in one part of the system will necessarily produce change in other parts of the system. Therefore, all man's interactions with his environment have an effect on his health status. It is obvious then that almost any event that takes place within the life processes of man could be said to be relevant to nursing in some way. The subject matter for nursing includes the normal and pathological processes used in life in both actual and potential events. Since man and the environment continually interact and exchange energy, any phenomena with the potential to impinge on man or the environment with which he is in constant interplay could be said to constitute the subject matter of nursing. However, there are restrictions on the subject matter of nursing implied by Rogers' conceptual model.

1. The subject matter should deal with man as a living phenomenon as opposed to his postmortem state.
2. Cognizance must be taken of man as a whole as opposed to an aggregate of parts (5).

Man signifies the human being as a single system whose characteristics are identifiably those of the whole. Man is a unified whole possessing his own integrity and manifesting characteristics that are more than and different from the sum of his parts. Man is a unified whole having his own distinctive characteristics that cannot be perceived by looking at or describing the parts. The properties of man cannot be deduced from the study of biology, physics, psychology, or sociology as separate entities. This is not a denial of interactions between subsystems or between levels of organization. It emphasizes the problems arising when we as professionals fail to recognize that the properties of sodium and chlorine atoms do not enable us to foresee the properties of salt. So man is different from each of his subsystems, although it is a common practice to describe man according to one or more subsystems. A summation of these parts does not add up to man.

So what unites man's brain, mind, digestive system, circulatory system, nervous system, and so on, to create the thinking, feeling creature known as man that we are trying to deal with in pathology and in preventive areas of health? The fundamental unit of the living system is an energy field. It is this field that gives unity to the concept of wholeness. The whole and the parts cannot be perceived simultaneously nor can they successfully be directed into parts wherein nursing has a kidney, behaviorists have feeling, psychologists have tests, and so forth. The identity of man exists in his wholeness. This wholeness is central and indispensable to any science trying to observe and understand man to modify his behavior in relation to illness/health continuums.

Man is an open system—an open system characterized by constant interaction of materials and energy with his environment. *Ecosystem,* which means the interaction system comprising living things and their environment, is becoming a common word appearing often in the literature and documentaries of the ecology minded. It is becoming increasingly recognized that man not merely adapts to his environment, but rather man and environment engage in dynamic interplay in which each is continually affecting and being affected by the other. The unity of man has its counterpart in the unity of the environment. The environment possesses its own wholeness. Man-environment transactions are characterized by continuous repatterning of both man and environment. The constant interchange of matter and energy between man and environment is at the basis of man's becoming. It is the mutual changing and being changed that evolution foresees.

Changes taking place in the human field and in the environment are holistic in nature. For example, syphilis was very deadly. The germ has changed and has more long-term effects. Spirochetes were identified by man, antibiotics were developed, spirochetes became more resistant, and man starts again. General systems theory introduced the term *negentropy* to signify increasing order, complexity, and heterogeneity. In nursing, one must recognize the nurse as part of the patient's environment. She has an effect on him and he in turn affects her. This interaction should be goal directed and the nurse should be *comanaging* this interaction.

The life process evolves irreversibly and unidirectionally along the space-time continuum. It is a continuous and continuing metamorphosis—innovative in character and marking both man and his environment. Heterogeneity, diversification, and growing complexity are observable attributes of man's unfolding. The life process is a becoming. The evolution of life exhibits an invariant one-way trend. The process of change occurs in space along the time axis. The concepts of past, present, and future denote time progression. The process of life evolves through time and is concomitantly bound in space-time. At any given point in time, man is the expression of the totality of advanced present at that point in time.

The irreversible and unidirectional nature of the life process is readily perceived in the developmental process of the individual. Conception, birth, infancy, childhood, adolescence, adulthood, and old age follow one another in a predictable way with predictable attributes with each stage. The capacity of life to transcend itself, the capacity for new forms to emerge and for new levels of complexity to evolve predict the future that cannot be foretold. The question now arises as to whether life is goal seeking. Today's recognition of the negentropic, unidirectional nature of life, coupled with probability theory, suggests that, although the specific final goal may not be known, there is probabilistic purposefulness in life. Pattern and organization identify man and reflect his innovative wholeness. The existence of organization and patterning in living systems is an observable phenomenon. An energy field is the basic unit of living things. It is this field that imposes pattern and organization on the parts. It is pattern and organization that reflect man and his wholeness. Without patterning there would be chaos. Without lawful development in nature there could be no meaningful predictions. Through biorhythm research there has arisen an expanded recognition of the circadian nature of the physical phenomenon and its relationship to nature's lawfulness. For example dysrhythmia of one's circadian rhythm exemplifies the time clock out of whack. Everyone's body is regulated by a built-in time clock. (The cycle ranges from 30–20 hr and circadian means "about a day," taken from the Latin word circa—about, and dies—day.) When planes fly through time zones at jet speeds these time clocks can become temporarily disoriented. Effects on individuals vary widely.

Vaughn suggests he doesn't need a magazine called *Human Behavior* to tell him that people have alternating cycles, good and bad, physically, intellectually, and emotionally. He suggests the great aim of the social sciences is to provide us with statistical evidence with which to support our institutions. He suggests that we have a cyclical nature intellectually and wouldn't it be nice if we could say to our employer:

> Your majesty, I think it only fair to tell you that I am embarking on 16½ days of cloddishness during which I will not produce a single valuable idea and will probably make a mess of whatever routine jobs may come my way. So if Your Worship would give me that time off, the company would save a ton, plus I would have a great time since my emotional and physical cycles are on the upswing. I know the board would approve of giving me the time off—to a man who is going to sit at his desk in an emotional and physical frame of mind rather than an intellectual one. Better he should be on the golf course or fishing pond where the intellect can, so to speak, lie dormant.

He suggests that the physical cycle is a 23-day affair. Oysters move inland from their native locations and open and close while feeding according to the tide phases of the water from where they came. Why should not persons take several days to adjust biologically when they change time zones?

Patterning is a dynamic process and represents the continuous change that marks man and his environment. Covertly and overtly the patterning is expressed in the continuing of new patterns in man and environment. The patterning of life is evolutionary in nature. It is the continuous repatterning of man and environment along the life axis that characterizes the dynamic nature of the universe. Self-regulation is directed toward achieving increasing complexity or organization—not toward achieving equilibrium and stability. For example, a patient in a relatively good middle-class home who is a diabetic and is in diabetic control, will have free time to direct his energies toward doing something constructive. Conversely, the patient in a lower-class home, who is having to meet survival levels, may not have the free time to direct toward any kind of goal achievement other than surviving. He is not interested or concerned with his health status except as it affects his survival. Self-regulating mechanisms are directed toward fulfilling the needs and potentialities of life. They maintain multiple functions in the living system. Self-regulation is an expression of wholeness together with man's capacity to rearrange his environment knowingly and to exercise choices in fulfilling his potentials. Man is additionally characterized by the capacity for abstraction and imagery, language and thought, sensation and emotion.

The preceding concepts of wholeness, interaction, unidirectionality, and pattern reveal themselves in a wide range of all living systems, not just man. What is there about man that is not only different from all other living forms but places him at the forefront of the evolutionary complexity? What other living creature is aware of the past and envisions the future? Abstraction and imagery, language and thought, sensation and emotion are fundamental attitudes of man's humanness. Man's self-awareness and awareness of his world are rooted in cognizance of his own mortality. Religion, art, and philosophy all attest to man's continuing search for the meaning of life and death. How man meets death, the meaning he attaches to it, and the belief he holds relative to what comes after death reveal his gropings for cosmic understanding. Man experiences feelings as a unified being. Feelings are an expression of wholeness; they are field functions and as such encompass the totality of the individual. Biology and psychology are inadequate as independent entrepreneurs in explaining feelings on either a matter or mind principle. Behavioral sciences are focusing more and more on overt behavior and the inward experience of the individual is overlooked if not denied by behaviorists. Rogers (6) states, "The warm subjective encounter of two persons is more effective in facilitating change than is the most precise set of techniques growing out of learning theory and operant conditioning." Man's feelings are proper subjects for study.

The exploration of man's need to work through grief is an illustration of such interest. Man thinks and transmits through language. Language preserves the past and anticipates the future. Man seeks to organize his world and make sense of it. Modern scientific method is still subject to feelings that provide the basic motivation for inquiry. The joy of discovery is the motivating factor, not the rigid rules of methodology. Efforts to elevate the human predicament through scientific study and technology are rooted in social awareness, e.g., in the conquest of polio, in the effect of cancer on people, and in the stimulus to study and control it. Feelings, as well as rational thought, are positive integrating forces. Man's knowledge of his world has long been deemed to come through the five senses. Now there is growing scientific respectability to extrasensory phenomenon. Is there a trend in man's evolution to development through training to utilize this in the future? Man's capacity for experiencing himself and his world identifies his humanness. It is the ability for abstraction, thought, language, and sensation that allows man to transcend his present self. Dunn (7), in his definition of high-level wellness, summed up the dynamic interplay between man and his environment when he stated:

> High level wellness for the individual is defined as an integrated method of functioning which is oriented toward maximizing the potential of which the individual is capable. It requires that the individual maintain a continual balance and purposeful direction within the environment within which he is functioning.

Positive health measures will be directed toward determining individual differences in assisting people to develop patterns of living coordinated with environmental changes rather than in conflict with them. Man and environment change together. Man plays his role in directing change both consciously and unconsciously. Whatever goals are set, the mutuality of the process is a significant factor in the achievement.

I now return to the role of the nurse in comanaging the direction toward which the client wishes to move as a goal in health levels. From these remarks then, discussing man as holon interacting with his environment, what are the barriers in nursing and how are we trying to deal with those barriers? I present a profile of several different kinds of people. For example, What do you say after you say hello (8), because we don't know who our clients are, where they're coming from, what their value systems are, what their territorial boundaries are, who their legitimizers for advice are, what subcultures are in operation, what they are practicing by way of folklore, and what is important to them. Student and staff nurses have indicated that they are aware of these multiple stimuli operational within the client's environment. However, they did not attend to these stimuli because the process, the audit, or the punchcard did not have a space. Professionals seem to expect their patients simply to comply with medical and nursing regimes generated through the use of some tool, laboratory test, history, or process, because the process is inherently correct and the patient desires to get well. However, a regime must be tailored to the life style of the client, taking into account his or her environment, whichever, i.e., man and his environment. Otherwise the professional fails to elicit the necessary change for cooperation from the patient. The language barrier is often enormous and professionals are sometimes like the middle-class European tourist who thinks that talking more slowly and loudly in English to a Frenchman will help, even though the Frenchman does not understand English, then blaming the foreigner for not fully comprehending. You suggest (allegorically) that learning French is more effective in understanding the patient in his own environment than exclusively delivering health care messages from a medical/nursing ivory tower. Knowing the answers is usually unrelated to delivering the care.

We have become experts in understanding cause and treatment for health problems, but we are novices in effectively obtaining the client's participation in using the knowledge to increase his level of wellness. Great technical knowledge may be irrelevant without commensurate understanding of the client and who he is. Each of us brings to every stimulus of the situation that confronts us a group of assumptions, i.e., mind sets. These assumptions are predicated on prior learning wherein we have ascribed meanings and emotions to the perceived stimulus, and we apply learned behavior from our prior life experience. Each of us believes that what we individually perceive is the truth and is real. However, each individual varies greatly and uniquely in the perception of the stimuli. The more ambiguous the stimuli, the greater the distortion or variation in characterizing the stimuli. As an illustration: If a picture flashed above us of a strip of concrete approximately 3 feet wide, the concrete running in a straight line in front of houses, most of us would be willing to say that's a sidewalk. In other words, you and I, through somewhat similar life experiences, (cognitive maps), can comfortably agree that a sidewalk is not emotionally charged, and requires very little guarding of territorial imperatives. We are not placed in a defensive or protecting posture for fear our decision may be wrong.

On the other hand, let me present a profile of a client unlike us and see what our responses would be for a "proper professional approach." We are given these data: A young woman is in the lower class, and knowing what we know about that class, or what we should know, she presents a profile of fifth-grade education—and because of that fifth-grade education level has little to no ability to read or write—has an income under $3,000 per year for a family of four, and is non-skilled. She is marginally employed, if at all, and has no particular religious denomination, clearly demonstrates an inability to cope with planning beyond now—this hour, this day—and is just barely meeting survival levels (i.e., biological food and shelter needs), and is experiencing her first pregnancy. The question is: What have the behaviorists, psychologists, and our other professional colleagues told us is good professional content and should be taught to this young woman? What do we, as professionals, perceive as valuable information to give this young woman for her to behave in more healthy ways?

You and I, by our profession, are classified as either upper-middle class or upper-upper lower class. Our profiles are quite different. Most of us have one or more college degrees; many of us have two or more. We are not marginally employed, our salaries in the main are stable and well over $10,000 per year. We value material wealth. We possess many things—cars, televisions, homes in suburbia—and are capable of planning far beyond tomorrow. We have religious ties, predominately Presbyterian and Episcopalian, and communicate with ease at a rather impressive vocabulary level. In terms of hierarchy of needs, we are between the belonging and recognition levels; i.e., we belong to civic and professional groups, we have symbolic and fiscal ways of giving and receiving recognition to each other, and, finally, we are striving toward self-actualization. These values, these methods of interaction have been constant for many years. They are as much a part of our conscious behavior as brushing our teeth. Now add the dimension of my previous example: the young woman requiring specific information about a state of health. Because we are who we are, by way of our psycho-, sociocultural and cognitive map and because the patient is who she is, by way of her psycho-, sociocultural and cognitive map, our language—verbal and nonverbal—denoting a therapeutic regime in terms of value to this patient may as well be written by wind on the sand.

Is it more succinct or meaningful to us to substitute the word cancer for pregnancy? Does the practitioner/client barrier really change if we do? To many people pregnancy is as unwanted and emotionally traumatic as cancer. Don't the same parallels operate for tuberculosis and mental illness?

Would it be more appropriate to consider the professional is truly the barrier for insisting on an interaction with man as less than a holon?

REFERENCES

1. Anderson, R., and Carter, I. *Human Behavior in the Social Environment: A Social Systems Approach*. Aldine, Chicago, 1974.
2. Koesher, A. In Anderson, R., and Carter, I. *Human Behavior in the Social Environment, A Social Systems Approach,* Aldine, Chicago, 1974, p. 8.
3. Rogers, M. *An Introduction to the Theoretical Basis of Nursing,* F. A. Davis, Philadelphia, 1970.
4. Mitchell, P. *Concepts Basic to Nursing,* McGraw-Hill, New York, 1972.
5. Duffy, M., and Muhlenkamp, A. A framework for theory analysis. *Nurs. Outlook,* 22:574 (1974).
6. Rogers, C. In Rogers, M., *An Introduction to the Theoretical Basis of Nursing,* p. 69. F. A. Davis, Philadelphia, 1970.
7. Dunn, H. *High Level Wellness,* Mt. Vernon Printing Co., Virginia, 1961.
8. Berne, E. *What Do You Say After You Say Hello?* Bantam, New York, 1973.
9. Lenocher, J. Notes, discussion, unpublished lecture material, University of Florida, College of Nursing, 1974.

Cancer: The Behavioral Dimensions, edited by J. W. Cullen, B. H. Fox, and R. N. Isom. Raven Press, New York © 1976.

The Impact of the Health Care System on Physician Attitudes and Behaviors

Donald M. Hayes

Department of Community Medicine, Bowman-Gray School of Medicine, Winston-Salem, North Carolina 27103

The National Cancer Control Program Planning Conference was held in Columbia, Maryland, September 23–27, 1973. Panel Number Five of that conference identified the attitudes of providers as a real barrier to motivating consumers to use screening and detection services.

Among the themes discussed by this panel were two of particular significance to medical educators and planners: (a) Screening and detection providers must develop greater awareness of and sensitivity to the life styles, languages, needs, and beliefs of target population groups; and (b) Motivation to use screening and detection services increases with the providers' recognition that they are dealing with people who normally want to stay healthy and therefore want to be included in all phases of a screening and detection program (1).

The Panel on Consumer Motivation developed several project descriptions in detail. Among those given the highest priority was one entitled "Health Professional Attitudes Toward Cancer Patients as a Barrier to Effective Use of Cancer Care Systems" (2). The considerations of this panel and this specific proposal inspired this chapter.

The title of this chapter implies that attitudes are closely related to behaviors. In fact, educationists long ago recognized that it was attitudes that determined behavior. A group of college and university educators considering educational objectives, i.e., those things a student is expected to learn, created a threefold division: cognitive, affective, and psychomotor (3). Educational objectives in the cognitive domain are those that deal with thought processes and factual material. Those in the affective domain emphasize a feeling tone, an emotion, or a degree of acceptance or rejection. Psychomotor objectives are those that emphasize some muscular or motor skill, some manipulation of material and objects, or some act requiring neuromuscular coordination. This chapter concerns the affective domain.

If one were planning an educational program and wanted to delineate certain desirable attitudes as educational objectives, he would find himself faced with difficulties in definition and gradation. The most elementary attitude measurable is

145

that of receiving or attending. This has to do with simply being able or willing to pay attention to a stimulus of some sort. At the upper end of the hierarchy is the most complex attitude measurable—characterization. Here, the individual has not only paid attention to certain stimuli, responded to them, internalized them, and become committed to them, he has also incorporated them into his total set of beliefs to the point that they have become part of him.

It is possible for planners of educational programs to describe desirable attitudes for their students in these terms. With this assumption in mind, one can then proceed to the more specific assumption that it must also be possible to determine, measure, and impart desirable attitudes for health professionals, specifically physicians.

For purposes of this discussion, it is necessary to have a working definition of the term attitude. There is general agreement that attitudes are feelings, either for or against something. Remmers and Gage (4) defined an attitude as an "emotionalized tendency, organized through experience, to react positively or negatively toward a psychological object." Guilford's definition (15) added: "An attitude is a personal disposition common to individuals, but possessed to different degrees, which impels them to react to objects, situations, or propositions in ways that can be called favorable or unfavorable." The addition lies in the two phrases, "common to individuals" and "possessed to different degrees." The former introduces the concept that attitudes are not completely individualistic, whereas the latter suggests that there are measurable differences among attitudes.

Combining these definitions produces the following generalizations: Attitudes (a) are feelings, (b) involve a continuum of acceptance (accept-reject, favorable-unfavorable, positive-negative), (c) are held by individuals, (d) may be held in common by different individuals, (e) are held in varying degrees, (f) influence actions, (g) are changeable, and (h) are influenced by information (6).

The title of this chapter suggests, and the perceptions of the Panel on Consumer Motivation confirm, that the attitudes of physicians may be less than optimal. What are some specific items that document this perception?

Susser and Watson (7) described a study performed in the Health Insurance Program of Greater New York showing that physicians who were closer to the community which they served were more sensitive to the personal aspects of care needed by patients from that community. As an example, they pointed out that family physicians are close to the community in which they work. Although trained to act by professional criteria, they must consider the wishes and circumstances of the patient and those close to them.

Patients confront the community practitioner with problems covering the whole range of medical competence, including its social and psychological components, and exert further pressure on them to maintain their traditional responsibility for the whole person.

In contrast, the full-time hospital physician is less subject to lay pressure. The frame of reference of hospital staff comprises their colleagues and the values they share. Typically the staff consider the hospital patient with necessary if concerned detachment, as a case and an object of scientific study. Decisions about the management of the case must reflect technical competence and be justifiable to colleagues on scientific grounds. The hospital "encapsulates" patients, insulating them from their usual associations and ideas. The behavior expected from them is accepting, submissive, and dependent. Decisions about them are made with perfunctory attention to their roles in the outside world, in family, work, and leisure, and they cannot appeal to those outside for support.

These orientations among physicians have material consequences for their patients. For while the mistakes of general practice often seem to arise from technical failures, the mistakes of hospital practice often arise from failures of communication.

Peck (8) reported on 50 patients interviewed by a psychiatrist as they registered for treatment at a radiotherapy center. All patients had cancer, but only 40 (80%) correctly gave their own diagnosis. These 40 patients had not been told their diagnosis by their own physicians. Peck concluded that physicians must be in touch with their own feelings about the patient and aware of their own reactions to the disease itself, to treatment, and to their role as the physicians of patients with cancer.

If too troubled by anxiety because of working with cancer patients, a physician will be unable to learn the patients' emotional reactions to the disease. In such instances, physicians tend to defend themselves by involuntary aloofness from patients or by rigid stereotyped management of all patients with cancer. Sometimes anxiety within physicians leads them to excessive wordiness, circumlocution, omissions, and untruths when they are forced to talk with cancer patients.

Friedman (9) reported a study aimed at exploring how physicians actually work with patients suffering from fatal illnesses. Responding to a questionnaire on their methods of managing dying patients were 59 internists, 76 surgeons, 25 gynecologists, 13 general practitioners, and 5 psychiatrists. Sixty-six percent of the physicians said they sometimes informed patients of a malignancy, 25% said they always told the patient, and only 9% said they never told the patient.

The fact that very few physicians felt they could say they never informed a patient about a fatal diagnosis was in itself a modification of previous practice. However, judging from answers to other questions, the author concluded that in actual practice many physicians tend to resist informing their patients of such a diagnosis in a direct manner. Instead they are quite selective in informing only those patients described as self-reliant, independent, and able to face reality.

The public's conception of cancer is one of a horribly painful, and above all, incurable disease. McIntosh (10) stated that this belief is so deeply ingrained that for many a diagnosis of cancer is tantamount to a death sentence. There is something about cancer that causes more fear and anxiety in individuals than any other disease. All indications are that the sole responsibility for passing information to the cancer patient or his family lies with the doctor in charge. In view of this, it is doubly distressing to find that most doctors base their policies on personal conviction, with considerable emotional overtones, rather than on past experience with patients. In short, doctors are apparently not immune to the same paralyzing fear of cancer held by the rest of the public.

Another study was that of Hinton (11), who interviewed 60 patients receiving care for terminal cancer. Of these, 40 had some awareness of dying and none disapproved of open discussion of this subject. However, 21 patients reported little or no truthful conversation with the medical staff concerning their illnesses.

Certainly these studies suggest that a common difficulty experienced by patients and doctors alike is that of effective and unbiased communication concerning cancer. Physicians may be unable to handle this particular situation because of their own uncertainties and negative attitudes concerning cancer and cancer patients.

STUDIES OF ATTITUDE CHANGES IN MEDICAL EDUCATION

When one mentions attitude measurements in medical education, the study most frequently cited is that of Eron (12), who raised questions about whether the medical professions attract, or medical school admissions committees select, a higher proportion of individuals with personality maladjustments than other professions. The alternative question considered was whether the medical school curriculum itself encourages the development of personality maladjustments.

The hypothetical prediction made before the Eron study was that medical students who were most anxious would be more cynical and less humanitarian than the least anxious students. A corollary hypothesis was that the choice of specialty made by medical students would be related to the interaction of the three variables: anxiety, cynicism, and humanitarianism.

All members of the first- and fourth-year classes of an eastern medical school completed the Eron cynicism scale designed to detect anxiety, humanitarianism, and cynicism. All indicated their specialty choice at that time also. For the cynicism variable, there was a significant difference between first- and fourth-year students, with fourth-year students showing more cynicism than first-year students. On the anxiety scale, seniors were higher than freshmen, as predicted, but not to a statistically significant degree. On the humanitarianism scale, the difference was neither significant nor in the predicted direction.

The possibility that these results were merely a maturation effect was minimized by a similar study done on the first- and third-year nursing students, revealing results that were the exact opposite of those in medical students. The author pointed out that an additional important phase in the formation of attitudes is the long period of postgraduate training, during which time financial rewards are further delayed and earlier frustrations are compounded. The trend toward increasing cynicism might be worsened or improved by the physician's reaction to this phase.

A smaller but more detailed and longer-range study was that of Becker et al. (13). They pointed out that there are two ideas in medical culture and in the perspective of physicians which tell medical students in what direction they should put forth their efforts. These two ideas are medical responsibility and clinical experience.

Medical responsibility is responsibility for the patient's well-being, and the exercise of it is seen as the basic and key action of the practising physician. The physician is most a physician when he or she is exercising this responsibility. Any physicians who have patients placed in their care are responsible for seeing that the patients get well, or as much better as is possible. More important, they are responsible for seeing, if possible, that the patients do not get worse than they were before the doctor saw him. Their observation of hospital organization, and repeated mention in formal teaching and informal conversations demonstrate to them that medical responsibility is an important characteristic of the full-fledged physician.

A second major idea expressed in the organization of medical practice in the hospital, and one closely related to responsibility, is experience. This refers to clinical experience, to actual experience in dealing with patients and disease, and a major part of its meaning lies in its implied polarity to "book learning." Clinical experience, in the view implied by this term, gives doctors the knowledge they need to treat patients successfully, even though that knowledge has not yet been systematized and scientifically verified.

Students faced with the problems of medical apprenticeship ask themselves, "What should I do, in this setting, to prepare myself for medical practice?" The students studied by Becker et al. (13) took the hints furnished by the faculty and the organization of the school and developed their perspectives around the concepts of clinical experience and medical responsibility.

Becker et al. (13) found that medical student attitudes derived from three basic areas: the medical culture, the lay culture, and the student culture.

STUDENT ATTITUDES TOWARD PATIENTS DRAWN FROM MEDICAL CULTURE

Where the physician's work does not afford (at least in some symbolic way) the possibility of saving lives or restoring health through skillful practice, or losing them through ineptness, the physician is seen as lacking some of the essence of true physicianhood. This perspective, believed to be generally an important one in medical culture, furnishes a basis for classifying and evaluating patients: those patients who can be cured are "better" than those who cannot. Furthermore, those patients who cannot be cured because they are not sick in the first place are the worst of all. "Crocks," for example, are not physically ill and, although students may occasionally sympathize with them, they are not regarded as worthwhile patients because nothing can be done for them. Obese patients, too, are frequently seen as essentially incurable and not worth bothering with. Cancer patients obviously do not qualify as "not sick" in this framework but many of them do fall in the category of incurable and thus are not deemed worthy of the student's full attention.

Medical culture lies at the base of students' concern with the problem of managing interaction with patients so that patients will be pleasant and cooperative. On this view, patients can be seen as people who may possibly create embarrassing or difficult situations for the doctor, and they can be classified as to whether or not they do this or how likely they are to do this. Obviously, cancer patients possess the potential for creating the most difficult situation of all—dying.

Another set of student ideas about patients drawn from medical culture consists of variations on the theme that some patients are "bad" because they are directly responsible for their own illness. Cigarette smokers who contract lung cancer often find themselves being judged as "bad" in this context. This same attitude finds somewhat subtler expression in cases where the student has to persuade a patient to follow medical orders or to spend money on medical treatments. Students often find that without special effort on their part patients will not do these things.

STUDENT ATTITUDES TOWARD PATIENTS DRAWN FROM LAY CULTURE

Social class culture probably lies at the root of students' disgust with patients they consider immoral or immodest. Class culture also seems to furnish the basis for occasional complaints that charity patients did not act properly "poor" or submissive.

Common knowledge indicates the existence of widespread lay cultural notions about pain and death, which are systematically violated in the medical students' experience. Students are also sometimes upset by the fact of death or by what laymen would consider unpleasant and depressing sights sometimes encountered in hospitals.

STUDENT ATTITUDES TOWARD PATIENTS DRAWN FROM STUDENT CULTURE

One notion that seems to stem directly from the student culture is that patients should not take up the "valuable" time of the student without giving something worthwhile in return.

In a sort of modified "critical incident" study, Becker et al. (13) determined that about two-thirds of the student attitudes toward patients had their roots in the student culture, 20% in the medical culture, and 16% in the lay culture.

Bondy (14) pointed out that there were certain common factors in the medical education experience which led to attitude changes in medical students:

1. The student often feels a need to develop a protective carapace so that he can tolerate the unpleasant experiences of the clinic. One of his earlier tasks in the clinic is to apply dispassionate intellectual processes to studying disturbing,

painful, or even disgusting aspects of human suffering. Unless he can learn this dispassionate attitude, he will never be an effective physician. On the other hand, he must develop a balanced attitude that does not exclude a recognition of the social, behavioral, and psychiatric factors that make the patient a person rather than simply an intellectual problem in disordered physiology. The development of this balance takes time and experience. The first step usually represents an overshoot in the direction of toughness and cynicism.

2. In developing attitudes toward patients, the student will pattern himself to a considerable extent after the faculty and house officers he sees. If these people have not developed a mature attitude and are indifferent to or skeptical about the importance of social and behavioral factors, the student will tend to reinforce his tough attitude.

3. If the faculty is unaware of the adjustments the student must undergo, they are likely to be insensitive to his needs and attitudes. The faculty themselves may continue to present a facade of self-assurance that rejects the importance of factors outside the technological aspects of medicine. Commonly this attitude expresses itself in a humorous denigration of the psychosocial and behavioral aspects of medicine. Laughter is a powerful weapon which can overwhelm all but the most secure student.

Reinhardt and Gray (15) performed a follow-up study to that of Eron (12) dealing with the development of cynicism in medical students. They concluded that attitudes of cynicism are developed by medical students and retained by some physicians after they enter practice because they are functionally useful. Their findings also suggested that cynicism is less pronounced in settings where a premium is placed on affective mutual response between physician and patient (such as psychiatry and other "high interaction" specialties). This suggests that, although attitudes of cynicism appear to help the medical student now, changes in training experiences could be made so that the student would not need to develop these attitudes. As a result of such changes, medical schools could produce physicians who could meet both the medical and psychological needs of patients more effectively.

Rezler (16) recently reviewed the literature concerning attitude changes during medical school. She concluded that medical education does not seem to increase student humanism or benevolence, at best leaving these attitudes intact in those students who exhibit them to a high degree at entrance. She pointed out that a person's attitudes are strongly influenced by the groups to which he belongs. A person is rewarded by his reference group for conforming to its standards and punished for deviating from them.

Etzioni (17) maintained that solving social problems by changing people is more expensive and usually less productive than approaches which accept people as they are and seek to mend not them but the circumstances around them. The answer may lie in selecting students who possess certain important attitudes prior to entrance, rather than trying to develop such attitudes after they enter medical school.

PHYSICIAN ATTITUDES AND BEHAVIORS AS VIEWED
BY CONSUMERS OF CANCER CARE

The study described here was performed to determine what features of cancer care were most valued by the recipients of that care and, using that information, to construct a set of desirable characteristics for the cancer care program of any community (18).

The basic technique used to gather data was the "critical incident" technique as developed by Flanagan (19), and used by Sanazaro and Williamson (20) and the American Institute for Research (21). The technique was developed for defining jobs and for obtaining satisfactory criterion measures of success at those particular jobs. It was felt that by asking cancer patients and their families to recall specific instances in which something was done to or for the cancer patient, a large dossier of descriptive vignettes could be collected. These narratives, describing "incidents" that the patients regarded as "critical" to their care could then be used for defining the "job" to be done—delivery of cancer care.

The files of the Cancer Registry, North Carolina Board of Health, were reviewed for the names of patients registered at participating hospitals in 1970–71. After obtaining the approval of their physicians, patients (or surviving families) were contacted by mail asking their permission to be interviewed. Those not responding or refusing were eliminated from the list. Interviewers, furnished with a prepared interview guide, met respondents in their homes. In addition to items about demographic and clinical variables, each interview included the question: "Looking back over your illness, can you recall an instance in which something was done to you or for you which impressed you as being particularly effective (or ineffective)?" Also: "What was the event? Who was the person concerned? What was done? What might have been done that would have been less (or more) effective?"

After collection of such data from 660 interviews, the 2,741 incidents described were reviewed. Of these, 1,850 incidents were of "effective" and 891 of "ineffective" behaviors. All duplications were eliminated, leaving 258 distinctly different incidents.

An example of an "effective" incident that appeared is as follows: "Another patient of my surgeon's visited me and told me how well he got along with his colostomy and how many people live with them. He showed me how to take care of my colostomy and gave me a lot of tips."

An "ineffective" incident was: "My local family doctor fooled around for six months treating me for 'arthritis' before he found out what was wrong. He did refer me to a specialist in ——— but only after I had wasted all that time."

Analysis of the "effective" incident revealed:

Person involved: Surgeon, other patient.

What was done: Sent patient with similar problem (colostomy) to instruct and encourage patient.

What desirable behavior was depicted:

1. Surgeon should arrange for patient with recent colostomy to talk with experienced colostomy patient.

2. Patient who is well-adjusted to his own colostomy management should visit new colostomy patients to instruct in management and assist in adjustment.

Analysis of the "ineffective" incident was as follows:
Person involved: Local family practitioner.
What was done: Incorrect diagnosis was made and patient was inappropriately treated for 6 months before referral to a consultant.

What desirable behavior was depicted:

1. Diagnostic acumen
   a. Recognizing disease entities.
   b. Seeking explanation of all signs.
2. Wisdom in deciding on appropriate care
   a. Initiating correct treatment for physical sympton or disorder.
3. Referral to another physician for consultation or treatment
   a. Physician should recognize his own inability to treat a patient and refer elsewhere when appropriate.

After analysis of each incident as above, the behaviors described were restated as shown. The resultant collection of 258 desirable behaviors was arbitrarily classified in outline form. This collection represented a descriptive tabulation of the elements of an effective cancer care system as viewed by the consumer. It consisted of 140 desirable physician behaviors, 47 desirable nurse behaviors, 34 desirable behaviors of other health professionals, 18 desirable aspects of hospital care, 8 of physicial facilities, and 11 desirable elements of general support in the community (18).

Of particular note insofar as the present program is concerned is the fact that the largest number of desirable physician behaviors (25) fell under the heading "Effectiveness of Physician-Patient Relationship." This study thus attests to the concerns held by consumers for the attitudes of health professionals.

Because this paper deals with attitudes *and* behaviors, it is appropriate to cite one additional study specifically relating to the latter. Marks and Sachar (22) reported a study concerned with undertreatment of medical inpatients with narcotic analgesic drugs. Since cancer patients frequently require these drugs, and since the attitudes of their attending health professionals determine how such drugs are used in their care, we felt it appropriate to study these variables (23).

A questionnaire concerning narcotic analgesic drugs was completed by 15 Ob/Gyn, 20 Surgery, and 26 Medicine nurses in a medical center hospital. Sixty percent of the Medicine nurses said narcotics should be administered "as frequently as needed to completely relieve pain," whereas 70% of Surgery and 50%

of Ob/Gyn nurses thought "sufficient narcotics should be given to reduce pain only so it is noticeable but not distressing." Seventy-five percent of Ob/Gyn and Medicine nurses felt physicians usually order the right amount of narcotic analgesic drug for their patients, whereas only 30% of Surgery nurses agreed. Eighty percent of Ob/Gyn and Surgery nurses agreed that patients with chronic painful disorders are less responsive to narcotic analgesics, while only 54% of Medicine nurses (those who usually care for such patients) agreed. Of Surgery and Medicine nurses, 80–92% felt that an "as needed" order for meperidine (Demerol®) should be used as sparingly as possible to avoid addiction and side-effects, while only 57% of Ob/Gyn nurses agreed.

Without belaboring the specific points, it can be pointed out that these results show at least two significant things. First, there is a large percentage of nurses in all services who possess inadequate factual information concerning narcotic analgesic drugs. Secondly, those nurses in the services most likely to care for cancer patients with chronic pain are those who are least charitably disposed toward the administration of adequate doses of narcotic analgesic drugs. Again, these data point to the need for continuing education in the affective domain for those professionals concerned with the care of cancer patients.

DISCUSSION

The inescapable conclusion seems to be that physicians possess and frequently demonstrate an attitude which is suboptimal in the management of cancer patients. It is not clear whether these attitudes arise predominantly from medical culture, student culture, society in general, or from the process of medical education. There are suggestions that each of these contributes to the total attitudinal "set" of the physician.

If one accepts the evidence presented concerning the existence of unfavorable attitudes, a corollary belief must be accepted also. This is, that there must be an optimal attitudinal "set" or "profile" for physicians caring for cancer patients. If this is true, there are then two alternatives available to those charged with training cancer care physicians: (1) identifying those attributes possessed by the ideal cancer care physician and assuring that the individuals admitted to training programs possess them (17), or (2) identifying those same attributes and attempting to impart them to all individuals in such training programs.

Although Etzioni (17) favors the former approach, the latter has been the one attempted by educators to date. One study mentioned herein pointed out that there is a group of optimal attitudes identified by consumers (18). It should be possible to impart these attitudes in some way. Likewise, Haley (24) identified certain attitudes toward cancer and its care which could be imparted. Obviously, elements of all these approaches should be utilized. There is an attitudinal "set" which should be identifiable prior to admission to training and which should be sought in applicants for medical school. Likewise, given a group of medical students possessing this attitudinal profile, it should be possible to enhance the desirable traits by appropriate reinforcement in the educational process.

One of the first steps in accomplishing this would be the broadening of admissions policies to medical schools. Haynes (25) wrote of the potential value of admitting students of a wide social background to medical school. As he pointed out, medicine has advanced much during the past 50 years, but there has been little real advancement in medical education. A totally white, middle-class institution consisting only of students with a grade point average of 3.5 or above and an average MCAT (Medical College Admissions Test) of 600 plus is a culturally deprived institution in desperate need of help. The health of the American people cannot be entrusted to the graduates of such an institution for they will not have learned some of the basic issues of health education.

Every subculture has different characteristics and approaches to life. The generally literate white can learn much about communication from the generally oral, albeit less-literate black. There is much the generally aggressive non-Indian can learn from the generally nonaggressive Indian. All such subcultures approach differently the problems of illness, specifically cancer, and all that it implies.

Finally, several recommendations made by Bondy (14) are appropriate to consider here. These suggestions were made with the general aim of fostering favorable attitudes in medical students. However, the need for these same attitudes in those charged with the care of cancer patients is even greater than in physicians generally. The following measures were suggested to encourage and protect these desirable attitudes:

1. Recognizing as part of the medical school admission policy that exposure in depth to college courses in the behavioral sciences is desirable along with exposure to the "hard" sciences.
2. Organizing the curriculum in such a way that students may take courses in the behavioral sciences in the university while enrolled in medical school, and encouraging them to do so.
3. Exposing students early in the first year of medical school to contact patients and emphasizing, during this contact, the behavioral or social aspects of the patients' problems, as well as the physical and medical considerations.
4. Encouraging the participation of faculty members in study and research in the behavioral aspects of medicine.
5. Introducing into the clinical curriculum a constant awareness of the importance of these factors.
6. Helping students to understand their own reactions toward patients.
7. Providing an opportunity to learn about the methods of delivering medical care, in which context the relations between the physician and the patient might be explored fruitfully.
8. Exploring, within the medical center, many factors of interest to behavioral scientists that affect the interrelations of students, faculty, patients, and administrators.

It is certain that any medical school which successfully implemented the recommendations above would produce a brand of physician who would demonstrate many of the attributes of an "ideal" cancer care physician.

SUMMARY

The attitudes of health care providers have been identified as one of the barriers to effective use of the cancer care system by patients. Since attitudes frequently determine behaviors, a review of physician attitudes and behaviors relating to cancer patients was undertaken. After establishing a working definition of attitudes, several studies from the medical literature were reviewed. In general, these studies confirmed the perception that cancer patients and their doctors experience great difficulty in achieving effective and unbiased communication.

On examining the literature of medical education, several studies were found concerning the impact of the process of medical education on the formation of physician attitudes. Medical student attitudes seem to arise from at least three sources: the medical culture, the lay culture, and the student culture. The most recent review of the literature concerning attitude formation in medical students concluded that medical education does not seem to increase student humanism or benevolence, at best leaving these attitudes intact in those students who exhibit them to a high degree at entrance to medical school.

Two original studies were presented. One demonstrated that consumers of cancer care place a high premium on effectiveness of the physician-patient relationship. The second study showed that negative attitudes toward pain and narcotics among health professionals were associated with an inability or unwillingness to administer narcotic drugs to cancer patients in the most effective fashion.

It was concluded that the most effective means for producing cancer care physicians possessing optimal attitudinal profiles were broadening medical school admissions policies and instituting instructional programs aimed at influencing attitudes positively. Such efforts are unlikely to succeed if either of these measures is introduced in the absence of the other.

REFERENCES

1. *National Cancer Institute, Report of Panel 5, Consumer. (People) Motivation,* National Cancer Control Program Planning Conference, September 23–27, 1973, U.S. Department of Health, Education, and Welfare, Bethesda, Md.
2. Hayes D. M. Health Professional Attitudes Toward Cancer Patients as a *Barrier to Effective Use of the Cancer Care System.* In *Report of Panel 5, Consumer (People) Motivation,* National Cancer Control Program Planning Conference, September 23–27, 1973. U.S. Department of Health, Education, and Welfare, Bethesda, Md.
3. Krathwohl, D. R., Bloom, B.S., and Masia, B.B. *Taxonomy of Educational Objectives, Handbook II: Affective Domain,* David McKay, New York, 1956.
4. Remmers, H. H., and Gage, N. L. *Educational Measurement and Evaluation,* Harper & Row, New York, 1955.
5. Guilford, J. P. *Psychometric Methods,* McGraw-Hill, New York, 1954.
6. Miller, G. E., (ed.): *Teaching and Learning in Medical School,* Harvard University Press, Cambridge, 1961.
7. Susser, M. W., and Watson, W. *Sociology in Medicine,* 2nd ed., Oxford University Press, New York, 1971.

8. Peck, A. Emotional reactions to having cancer. *Am. J. Roentgenol. Radium. Ther. Nucl. Med.,* 114:591–599 (1972).
9. Friedman, H. J. Physican management of dying patients. *Psychiatry Med.,* 1:295–305 (1970).
10. McIntosh, J. Processes of communication, information seeking and control associated with cancer. *Soc. Sci. Med.,* 8:167–187 (1974).
11. Hinton, J. Talking with people about to die. *Br. Med. J.,* ii:25–27 (1974).
12. Eron, L. D. Effect of medical education on medical students' attitudes. *J. Med. Educ.,* 30:559–566 (1966).
13. Becker, H. S., Geer, B., Hughes, E. C., and Strauss, A. L. *Boys in White,* University of Chicago Press, Chicago, 1961.
14. Bondy, P. K. Evolution of students' attitudes during medical school. In: Cope, O., *Man, Mind and Medicine,* J. B. Lippincott, Philadelphia, 1968.
15. Reinhardt, A. M., and Gray, R. M. A social psychological study of attitude change in physicians. *J. Med. Educ.,* 47:112–117 (1972).
16. Rezler, A. Attitude changes during medical school: A review of the literature. *J. Med. Educ.,* 49:1023–1039 (1974).
17. Etzioni, A. Human beings are not very easy to change after all. *Saturday Review,* pp. 45–47, June 3, 1972.
18. Hayes, D. M. Desirable characteristics of an effective cancer care program. Appendix A in *Report of Panel 5: Consumer (People) Motivation,* National Cancer Control Program Planning Conference, September 23–27, 1973, U.S. Department of Health, Education and Welfare, Bethesda, Md.
19. Flanagan, J. C. Critical requirements: A new approach to employee evaluation. *Personnel Psychol.,* 2:419–425 (1949).
20. Sanazaro, P. J., and Williamson, J. Physician performance and its effects on patients: A classification based on reports by internists, surgeons, pediatricians, and obstetricians. *Med. Care,* 8:299–308 (1970).
21. American Institute for Research. *Rationales for Clinical Skill Areas Intern and Resident Performance.* Pittsburgh (AIR-C2 1-6/60-IR) June 17, 1960.
22. Marks, R. M., and Sachar, E. J. Undertreatment of medical inpatients with narcotic analgesics. *Ann. Intern. Med.,* 78:173–181 (1973).
23. Hayes, D. M., Kosinski, E., and Edwards, J. Nurse attitudes toward narcotic analgesic drugs as determinants of their clinical use in cancer patients. *Proc. Am. Soc. Clin. Oncol.* (1974).
24. Haley, H., Juan, I. R., and Gagan, J. F. Factor-analytic approach to attitude scale construction. *J. Med. Educ.,* 43:331–336 (1968).
25. Haynes, M. Influence of social background in medical education. *J. Med. Educ.,* 48:45–48 (1973).

Cancer: The Behavioral Dimensions, edited by J. W. Cullen, B. H. Fox, and R. N. Isom. Raven Press, New York © 1976.

Respondent

Harold B. Haley

School of Medicine, University of Virginia, Roanoke, Virginia 24016

There are three parts to this presentation: first, a discussion of the definitions of "system," second, my responses to the foregoing chapters by Lohr, Davies, and Hayes (most of these responses demonstrate how care of individual patients is affected by different components of the various "systems;" specific suggestions for future work are made), and third, some data and ideas of mine relevant to the subject.

THE SYSTEM

In this section we are considering effects of "system" on its constituents. The two levels of "systems" can be called "macrosystem" and "microsystem." The components of the macrosystem are institutional, organizational, may cover wide geographic areas, and are the object of planning legislation and big thinking. Microsystem refers to the firing line where one patient does or does not seek and receive care from other individuals.

A large unit of the macrosystem is the Cancer Control Program of the National Cancer Institute. An example of the problems the National Cancer Program is attempting to solve is whether the cancer patients of this nation will receive the best care in high technology tertiary-care centers or in upgraded local secondary-care centers. Some administrators at the National Institutes of Health feel that cancer care quality is lower in secondary-care centers than in tertiary centers. This needs objective study by people not precommitted to tertiary care, the human side of which has many defects.

Cancer care is being affected by microsystem problems. For instance, the frequency of proctosigmoidoscopic examinations in hospitalized patients is affected by the procedural ease or difficulty of performing it. If the doctor can see a patient, order the procedure, have an immediate preparatory enema given to the patient, a proctoscopic set brought quickly to the floor from central supply, and do the procedure in a treatment room on the patient's floor, it is not too much trouble. But if it has to be scheduled a day in advance and performed in the operating room or a special treatment room, it is just too much trouble. Sometimes it is more efficient to bring the mountain to Mohammed.

A second microsystem example problem is in sequencing patient follow-up procedures. Successfully treated colon cancer patients should have yearly sigmoidoscopic and barium enema examinations. If I see a follow-up patient today, how do I arrange these studies for 1 year from now? Do I have the patient come back in 1 year for an office visit to schedule these procedures? Or in a year can a secretary, clerk, or nurse telephone or write the patient, ascertain the patient's status at that time, schedule the procto and barium enema, and have the reports ready when I see the patient? If I see the patient first, do the procto, find everything to be satisfactory, and order the barium enema, how do we make certain that I get to read the X-ray report rather than having it attached, unread, in the patient's chart? This kind of nit-picking is a factor in the success of screening and early diagnosis. It is surprisingly difficult to establish effective microsystems in large institutions.

These examples emphasize that we are doing macro-thinking about things that affect cancer patients at micro-levels.

To point this up again—in your hospital how many patients have Pap smears? Too few do in reality, no matter what the plan and the individual rule.

Persons do things for and to other persons. Our problem is to establish systems—macro and micro—that make it desirable, easy, and consistent for cancer patients to receive ideal care.

RESPONSES

In discussion of relationships between various units of systems, Lohr mentions that the system creates behavioral patterns. For instance, in medicine the patient most often enters the system through a professional. Therefore, he concludes that the professional controls the patient and the patient's behavior in the system. Examples can be given that agree and/or disagree with this position. There has always been a degree of negotiation between the patient and the physician in the private practice setting. In institutional settings where the patient was in a dependent position, the patient had fewer options and less negotiation. In this age of consumerism, there is increasing negotiation between patient and professional and, correspondingly, less dominance by the professional. On the other hand, I well remember being disturbed by a scheduling pattern for hernia repair in children in Chicago. Large numbers of hernias had to be repaired in the Cook County Hospital. When it appeared that there would be room on the surgical schedule for such patients to receive immediate care, they would be called from a waiting list to enter the hospital. The necessary variability in emergency load in the hospital from day to day made precise scheduling impossible. As a result, children often waited in the hospital many days before having their elective surgery. I once naively suggested that these children could not afford to miss this much school. When the suggestion was made that such surgery should be concentrated in vacation times, it was quickly pointed out that the volume of work was such that it had to go on all year and could not be concentrated in vacation periods. This was probably true, yet I was always dissatisfied because these borderline children were losing important school time.

Lohr suggests that the presence of technology has major effects on how the system operates. For example, he mentions that patients could be kept alive by machines in nursing homes at very low cost and that the primary beneficiary was the nursing home continuing to receive fees for the patient care. I disagree. Very few patients with this degree of illness are in nursing homes and maintenance of life for any extended time by life support machines requires not only expensive equipment but also round-the-clock expensive personnel and tends to be a high cost operation.

Davies explores general systems theory in relationship to nursing. My comments expand some of her concepts.

In discussion of the nurse response to the system, clinical experience with nurse patients suggests that the nurse's views of other people with cancer are conditioned by her own beliefs and experiences with cancer and, particularly, her own thoughts about the disease and its meaning if she had cancer. The nurse who, in her training, has seen only two kinds of patients—those who have big operations and those who come to the hospital to die of advanced cancer—will have a different perspective from the office or clinic nurse who has gotten to know many "cured" patients through long follow up.

Davies states: "One must recognize the nurse as part of the patient's environment. She has an effect on him and he, in turn, affects her." In 1971 I coined the word "aerogenic." Iatrogenic means the things in patients caused by doctors; "aerogenic" is the opposite. Things in nurses or doctors caused by patients may be subtle and unrecognized, but gravely affect their behaviors. We are all part of the patient's environment, affecting and being affected by the patient.

"The patient in a lower-class home who is having to meet survival levels does not have the free time to direct toward any kind of goal achievement other than surviving." An application of this is the adjustment of patients to colostomies. During my surgical residency, I remember the chief resident saying that a colostomy was an IQ test. My experience of 7 years in the Tumor Follow-Up Clinic of Chicago's Cook County Hospital led to a different thesis. Every Wednesday afternoon I saw about three patients with colostomies. Some did well, but many had their lives dominated by their colostomies. My conclusion was that patients with limited incomes, limited education, and a low stimulus environment had little else to think about so the colostomy became the dominating factor in their lives.

Davies emphasizes well the problems in communication and viewpoint resulting from background and other differences between nurses (also doctors) and their clients. For example, professional and patient may be using the same words but neither recognizes that the other understands a different meaning. A common example is the description and meaning of pain.

In exploring patient compliance it is important to suggest that doctors and nurses must comply with good care of cancer patients. Sometimes we do not. Is this due to lack of knowledge, lack of appropriate motivation, or barriers in the system?

Lastly, Davies raises the critical importance of self-actualization. This is a major control and stimulus of behavior. I am a cancer doctor, a dean, an educator, a researcher, an anthropologist, a speed-boat driver, citizen, and husband-father, because in my value systems these are things that make life—life. My actualization is different from yours. How can each of us have a self-actualization of rewards to ourselves from doing good work for ourselves and others in all of living as well as cancer?

I agree with Ms. Davies that differences between professionals and patients do occur, but I believe effective intercommunication can and does occur by effort and understanding by both. Different cognitive maps may exist, but they should not build separative fences.

In discussing the impersonalization of relationship between tertiary-care physicians and patients, Hayes shows how this depersonalization is situational. However, it is probably also psychological. Some problems may result from inappropriate coping mechanisms of physicians resulting from threatening diseases or threatening interpersonal contacts. Work is needed in the area of helping medical students and physicians develop coping systems that are nondestructive for both patient and doctor.

Review of Hayes' analysis of the Peck study suggests application of some grains of salt. Patient self-histories are not completely reliable. Forgetfulness and denial are only two of the reasons patients commonly report not being told things that they have been told. Physician-patients are the same as other patients in this.

Hayes states: "Doctors are apparently not immune to the same paralyzing fear of cancer held by the rest of the public." Years ago, after interviewing parents of leukemic children 6 months after the child's death, Dr. Joseph Simone was impressed by the frequency with which parents said, "If the doctor could look death in the eye, so could we." Apparently, some of us cannot.

Since Hayes has outlined Eron's work on cynicism and humanitarianism, I would like to call attention to a 1974 *Journal of Medical Education* paper entitled "Social Concern in Medical Students: A Reconsideration of the Eron Assumption." Dr. Philip J. Perricone strongly challenges the Eron concept.

In light of the results of this study, it would appear that many workers in the area of medical education have been attributing more to the meaning of Eron's humanitarian and cynicism scales than was warranted. These data strongly suggest that humanitarianism and cynicism are but small parts of the Social Concern and Authoritarian orientations, respectively. The results also lend support to Becker and others who claim that the medical student does not permanently lose his social concern, but that he simply is responding to the demands of his student role. His response is temporary and specific and does not seem to extend to his general social concern. The results seem more consistent with the obvious trend within the medical student subculture toward increasing involvement in the problems of delivering needed medical services to population groups generally considered medically indigent and deprived. In fact, it appears that many medical school faculties have been "humanized" by their students—i.e., they have begun to offer courses in the social and behavioral sciences which meet this new demand for a more relevant and committed approach to the problems of health care delivery. This does not imply, of course, that medical faculties have not always been concerned with 'humanizing their students, only that they have recently been moved to formalize their concern in the form of more socially relevant courses.' In light of these recent social trends in medical education the data and method of this analysis makes the original Eron thesis extremely questionable.

Dr. Hayes discusses the effects of clinical experience in the development of the physician's perspective. The randomness of clinical experience is such that results may be "good" or "bad." A specific aspect is student exposure to inappropriate role models. Role modeling deserves considerable exploration in studying professional socialization of physicians. "Bad" clinical experience plus threatening experience may result in inappropriate coping by the doctor.

To quote Dr. Hayes: "Patients can be seen as people who may possibly create embarrassing or difficult situations for the doctor, and they can be classified as to whether or not they do this or how likely they are to do this." This is particularly true when the patient has body odor. Odor has an aegrogenic effect.

Hayes reviews Agnes Rezler's conclusion that: "Medical education does not seem to increase student humanism or benevolence." Drs. Paiva, Juan, Huynh, and I have a manuscript in preparation which reports freshman, sophomore, and senior scores of 545 medical students on the Cancer Attitude Survey. In this instrument, Factor I measures attitudes toward the psychic resources of patients to carry the burden of cancer. From freshman to senior year, the mean score on this factor increased with twice as many showing increased scores as compared to those with decreased scores. Apparently, clinical experience increases the student's respect for the psychic resources of cancer patients. This could be a part of humanism.

Hayes' critical incident study is important and should be useful. One question: Could Dr. Hayes develop a critical incident evaluation microsystem that could be used in evaluation of clinical performance of individual students, residents, or physicians? This could include either positive or negative incidents.

Hayes gives two alternatives to trainers of physicians: either admit students with proper attitudes or impart such attitudes while in training. I agree. The core of the problem is how to do either. This may be the toughest question of this entire volume.

The issue of medical school admissions policies is so broad that I cannot even touch on it here. An all-out admissions program could change the mix of medical students somewhat, but our ability to predict performance outcomes is so limited that much hope should not be placed on this.

Hayes' recommendations on how to encourage and protect desirable attitudes are cogent. I will comment on several.

1. Almost all medical students now admitted have had more than one behavioral science course in college. Twenty-five years ago only a small minority had any. The medical schools want students to have more behavioral courses but premedical students and advisors have difficulty in accepting this.

2. Many medical students are so preoccupied with immersion in clinical medicine that simultaneous behavioral science courses are looked on as "soft" or not "real medicine." For such courses to be effective, they will have to be perceived by medical students as concrete, pragmatic ways to become a better doctor.

3. Early exposure of students to patients and behavioral aspects of care is being done in many schools. A few, including some distinguished schools, have not introduced this approach. In at least one school where this was not being done, the students organized meaningful experience on their own.

4. Encouraging faculty members to study and do research in the behavioral aspects of medicine is important and difficult.

In my experience, basic medical scientists do not accept behavioral work as science. Clinicians are more open to behavioral work, but since medical research is based on tangible quantitative measurements to the fourth decimal place, behavioral research has little credibility in medical schools, few avenues of publication, and little financial support.

The behavioral area is important and in relation to cancer has a very limited data base. The small data base suggests that the possibility of short-term, immediately applied behavioral techniques and demonstrations is not very good. It may very well be more important for the Cancer Control Division to recognize the need for basic solid research and shift more emphasis to grants. If they don't support in-depth behavioral research in cancer, who else will?

HYPOTHESES AND SPECULATIONS ABOUT BEHAVIORAL ASPECTS OF CANCER CONTROL

Different attitudes have different bases. "Attitudes" is a global (and unusable) term. Specific attitudes must be clearly defined. Our study of cross-cultural aspects of attitudes toward cancer shows that attitudes toward psychic resources of the patient to carry the burden of cancer relate to general cultural influences that vary from country to country. Our present studies of attitude change in medical students also show that this particular set of attitudes changes while in medical school, with students in general placing a higher value on the psychic resources of patients to handle cancer at the end of medical school than they did at the time of admission. The cross-cultural study also shows that attitude toward personal immortality and acceptance and preparation for death are deeply related to religious beliefs. For example, a marked difference is seen between attitudes in this area of Israeli doctors in comparison with non-Jewish American doctors, with Jewish-American doctors scoring somewhere between the other two. On the other hand, attitudes toward the value of early diagnosis and aggressive treatment of cancer appears to be related neither to religion nor to general culture. Our studies of students show that attitudes in this area, particularly toward the value of aggressive treatment, change while in medical school, apparently resulting from education and experience.

Table 1 presents bases for some specific attitudes of physicians. Comparison of items 1 and 2 shows that almost all physicians queried agree with aggressive treatment of cancer having high cure rates, while only three-quarters are certain about the value of aggressive treatment in low cure rate cancers.

Item 3 in the table speaks for itself.

Our studies suggest that there may be a time component in attitude change. Medical students studied at 1½- to 2-year intervals showed changes in attitudes. Residents studied at 3- to 12-month intervals showed no changes in attitudes. The differences could be due to a different level of education as well as to the difference in interval between measurements.

It is hard to define "good" attitudes, behaviors, or physicians because there are many ways of being "good." It should be easier to define "bad" attitudes and behaviors and then try to change or negate them.

In studying attitudes and behavior of patients and cancer professionals, we should explore how life experiences and coping mechanisms affect the function of persons.

Is a particular physician primarily oriented toward people or disease? Does this affect career choices and which patients or diseases are cared for? In the same individual can this

TABLE 1.

Statement	No. of Doctors	Percent answering:		
		Agree	Uncertain	Disagree
1. Cancers in which a high percentage of 5-year survivals are seen (e.g., breast, cervix, colon) should be aggressively treated.	161	99	1	0
2. Patients with cancers of low 5-year survivals (e.g., esophagus, lung, stomach, pancreas) are not improved by aggressive treatment.	255	19	8	73
3. Doctors' attitudes are influenced more by personal experience with a few cases than by statistics and generalizations.	96	72	5	23

orientation change with time and experience? Is the person who leaves general practice to become a subspecialist (including a cancer specialist) shifting from a person to a disease orientation?

The research of ourselves and others has shown that the intellectual challenge of clinical problem-solving is one of the most characteristic traits of doctors and a motivating factor attracting specific kinds of people into medicine. From some viewpoints, cancer is often an insoluble problem. If doctors are problem-solving organisms, will they tend to avoid problems that they cannot solve?

Our studies of trainees and staff at the Memorial Hospital for Cancer and Allied Diseases show that cancer doctors are special people and have special attitudes. Entering trainees and staff doctors hold the same attitudes, which are different from the attitudes of other groups we have studied.

An almost totally untapped area of research is the study of what happens in residency education. Careful review of the book published some years ago entitled *The Intern* shows close correlation between house staff experience and development of physicians' attitudes. Throughout this book, the author refers to cancer as the "Bad Disease." The average young physician spends 4 years after medical school in residency training, many spending more time than this. This is the time when the undifferentiated physician concentrates into an area of specialty. It would seem logical that this is a time when clinical attitudes are defined and formed. There is almost no study of this long and important part of medical education.

TABLE 2. *Data from a questionnaire obtained in 1972–73 from 325 interns in 24 hospitals from 89 medical schools.*[a]

Did instruction in psychological or psychosocial problems of the cancer patient in your medical school include:

specific lectures	22[b]	other	8
seminars	13	none	38
both	19		

When was this given?

first 2 years	21	all four years	19
second 2 years	26	none at all	33

By whom was this given?

Psychiatry	38	Pediatrics	3
Surgery	5	Others or	
Internal Medicine	14	combinations	40

Answer yes (a) or no (b) if you, as a student, had occasion to participate in or observe a situation in which the following occurred:

	Percent answering "Yes"
A patient was told that he had cancer, but that it was probably curable.	76
A patient was told that he had disseminated or incurable disease.	65
A patient was told that death was imminent.	33
A patient was told that a colostomy was necessary.	74
A patient's impending death was discussed with his family.	80

What is the longest time you personally followed an individual cancer patient—including in- and outpatient care, etc.?

1–4 weeks	55	3–6 months	9
5–10 weeks	30	More than 6 months	4

---

[a]The questionnaire was distributed by a curriculum committee of the American Association for Cancer Education (Susan Mellette, M.D., Chairman; V. Vaitkevicius, M.D., and H. Haley, M.D., members).

[b]Answers are given as percentages of "yes" answers.

Discussion

Lohr: I must correct Dr. Haley's belief that I am an economist. I am not. With respect to the 30¢ that will be out of pocket for the nursing home, actually the rest of the money will be paid out of Medicare or Medicaid. It doesn't cost the nursing home anything. There are other hard data from a research project on this point but I may not divulge them yet.

Hayes: I can't disagree with most of the things Dr. Haley said, and I don't sense disagreement with me in what he said. I sense amplification. I think that with regard to his point about medical faculty members doing research in and more teaching of behavioral sciences that unless they are masochistic, they will not pursue such research. On the other hand, for behavioral sciences teaching to be effective for medical students, the only people to whom they listen effectively are those who wear the long white coats. Therefore, if a physician does not teach the behavioral sciences to medical students, they will not perceive it as having much value or being beneficial. I think it is up to the physicians to do it.

Goldstein: My major interest is the area of behavioral control, of both infrahuman and human organisms. I have heard a lot of convictions expressed here but very little data. As a matter of fact, I counted the number of convictions people have about behavior control, and there were 18. There have been very little data, although there have been some citations of leading behaviorists such as Al Bandura, and I was very interested in the comments. Dr. Enelow's early reference to Bandura in some ways is highly appropriate. What concerns me is that out of the selection of people from Ferster to Bandura and all of the work of human interval control (there are over 100 references in recent reviews), the proximity of the consequence to the behavior seems to have a serious and profound effect on the future and fate of that behavior. One of the things that this group is concerned about is early detection and another is the control of some behaviors that seem to be self-destructive. In cancer, most of the consequences are delayed—in smoking, in eating, and in other aspects of behavior control. So serious is the delay that it is extremely difficult to demonstrate to young human organisms that the effects of smoking, no matter what you say, eventuate in lung cancer. It is hard to demonstrate to the entire population, as a matter of fact. What we have learned from behavior control is that vicarious experiences and Bandura's real data rest on immediate consequences, to the best of my knowledge, delivered to children observing things happening 20 years later, even in the movie, but in highly unique circumstances. It is hard for me to see the relevance of Bandura to the demonstration or to the origination of projects that might come to control behavior in successful ways. It is easier for me to see the relevance of human interval control studies, operant control studies, as in fixed and variable intervals, which is what we are talking about here. One of the things that everybody seems to have agreed on is that people return consistently at fixed interval times to centers, that these will be a source of primary and early detection. There is ample evidence in the literature that you can generate human behavior in fixed interval patterns; no one has commented on it. The license bureau knows how, although they may apply sanctions that we can not, but they are successful in getting people to come once a year to renew driving licenses, and we are under control, no matter whether we feel we are or not. That is one very broad illustration of offering rewards to people to bring them under control. The work of Jack Turner in Huntsville shows how a bus stationed outside of a facility can work, if you give green stamps when people enter it. And they will come in and do things for green stamps; that is very interesting work. None of these suggestions was offered. As a matter of fact, the talk was 99% about antecedents and very little about consequences and included a lot of putdowns of behavioral modification. I am wondering how these things about the people who are concerned with behavior control interact with what they see as the future of using these principles in a really sophisticated applied technique of bringing some of the behaviors of concern under control.

Brown: Mr. Lohr suggested perhaps that physicians should be a public utility. Dr. Kelty said that we should look at physicians' bias as they inform patients to obtain their consent. Dr. Enelow said his work in modification of physicians' behavior was very difficult. Dr. Hayes did imply some optimism, however, that we might be able to change some behavior if we work with some very concrete small types of experiences that patients report are helpful. In that respect I am encouraged.

When Dr. Antonovsky divided patients into four groups, he implied that maybe two of those groups—the rational goal-directed and the complacent stoic—might be most of us here. In taking care of patients, I would have been more comfortable if the patients fit that mold. Ralph Nader, I understand, is compiling directories of physicians and what they charge, what their qualifications are, what their competence is. Perhaps he could expand that to something that would include a rundown on physicians in terms of their attitudes toward the kind of a scale that Dr. Antonovsky has given us; in other words, our value systems. In selecting a physician or in selecting a place to plug into the health-care system, if the patient would get in where his values are similar to values of the system that he got into, he might fare a lot better. In other words, there may be situations where we cannot change behavior, but perhaps we can get people together who behave in a similar fashion.

William Zwartjes, Pediatric Oncologist, Denver, Colorado: I am a Pediatric Oncologist. I would like to draw together what has been said here. We started talking about delay in treatment and the factors that affected it; later, we started talking about how the physician approaches his patients and the fact that most physicians who graduate from medical school are in no way capable of dealing with the patient with cancer or dying or chronically ill patients. The obvious conclusion is that until we can get any type of system started toward improving patient care in regard to delay of diagnosis and having the patient interested, we have got to work on the doctors, and there is no doubt that the doctors' attitudes right now are not conducive to the type of treatment we want to give. Furthermore, we should consider a comment that the only way to get things off the ground is going to be a unification of the behavioralist and the oncologist. It is my feeling that we should point in this direction for our goals in the future.

Enelow: I would like to respond to Dr. Goldstein. I had no intent of putting down behavioral modification; I was merely attempting to show some applications of social learning as characterized in some other work of Rotter, Bandura and other people in attitude and communication therapy. By having left out the area of operant conditioning in the behavioral modification sense, I think the only putdown, if it was such, was the statement I made very early that when the first data appeared about the shaping of behavior by external responses, it was very threatening to those of us in psychiatry and we had great difficulty in accepting that it was useful. For a long time, it was quite fashionable to put down behavioral modification. I think that day is over in psychiatry as it is in physiology. In regard to the difficulty in changing physician behavior, I said our results were not spectacular. I will go further and say that our results were spectacularly poor. We never really had much alteration of behavior. We found that we were able to alter the behavior of those physicians who came to us already in agreement with us; those who did not left us without having modified their behavior. Festinger notwithstanding, we were able to alter their attitudes without in any respect altering their behavior; furthermore, when we taught them behaviors and had them perform under supervision, the attitudes did not follow. They reverted to their usual more comfortable office behavior after they left us. Finally, I do want to make one point about teaching behavioral science in medical school as suggested by Dr. Hayes. I was involved in a noble experiment to attempt that for about 5 years; it was a terrible failure. Medical students do not take to behavioral science. In fact, if they had behavioral science in undergraduate school, they were even more negative about it when they got into medical school, and they could be quite angry and difficult. We found, on the other hand, that if we put a white coat on our behavioral scientist and took him along with us when we made rounds in the clinic, and had him show us specific practical applications of behavioral science knowledge to the clinical problem at hand, that he was listened to and very much appreciated. So behavioral sciences in medical school—yes—but not behavioral science courses.

Pearson: I am a psychologist temporarily teaching in a medical school at the University of Nevada. I have two general comments. First, just as we have talked about our failures in trying to change the behavior of adults and are beginning to shift more toward the younger age levels, I feel the same way about reaching medical students in their freshman and sophomore years, prior to their clinical experiences. We have our behavioral sciences program begin the first week of the freshman year in terms of an interviewing course, which goes on for the entire semester. In the sophomore year, we have students who are taking part in placements at nursing homes with patients who have chronic disease and who are dying. These students are learning how to talk, and relate to dying people in their sophomore year before they begin their clinical experiences. They do not seem to be as hostile or as opposed to the whole concept of behavioral science when it becomes part of their basic program.

The other comment has to do with behavior modification, which I do not think has been put down enough at this conference. I think it offers a false hope in a simplistic manner in dealing with multicausal behavior, I want to quote Israel Goldiamond, one of the pioneers in behavioral modification, who said its only significant contributions have been in teaching pigeons how to play ping pong and teaching humans to deal with teaching machines. Beyond that, he does not feel that there has been much progress. But I think the real concern is that we have talked about false reports and deception on the part of subjects. Most behavior modification programs that I am familiar with have built into them such a fear of failure, such a concern about meeting the contract that we are encouraging our subjects to lie and deceive in order to not see failures.

Stein: We talk a lot about attitudes, and we spend a lot of money looking at attitudes. I think there is a great deal of merit in that, but we need to have more about outcome. What is the cost effectiveness of what we are doing, how is it helping to rehabilitate the patient, where is he in his life status as a useful productive citizen of our community? I think that in trying to answer these questions, there are new technologies that are now evolving, which my colleague, Dr. Goldstein, has referred to, namely, applied behavioral analysis. This is an area that I never heard of in medical school and which I think holds a great deal of promise for the future. Regarding the comments concerning medical students having more exposure to behavioral sciences, from what I have heard today, I think that would be a waste. I do not think there is much to be offered in that realm, or to put it a little differently, much more development will be needed in the behavioral sciences before doctors need to be concerned with this area. I am one who is wearing the hair shirt of trying to do behavioral research. I suffer enormously among my colleagues and the reason for that is, up to this time, behavioral sciences for physicians has lacked solid empirical data. The newer technologies that I have alluded to, I think, will successfully resolve this issue.

Kegeles: In regard to the teaching of behavioral science in medical schools, we at the University of Connecticut have for the past 5 years offered an extremely extensive program in behavioral science to medical students and dental students simultaneously. Let me describe it and talk about our evaluative mechanisms, which are pretty poor. The course is provided during the first 6 weeks of the medical and dental students' curriculum. It is the first subject committee that these students get before the remainder of the basic science faculty, and later the clinical faculty, has had time to turn them off some of their interests from undergraduate school. The students we have had at Connecticut are not terribly different from those who come to most places. We pride ourselves that we are better than most schools as, I am sure, does every medical school. We have had evaluation by students, blind evaluations originally done by our group, but done in the last 3 years by the Department of Educational Research, which evaluates all of the basic science subject committees over the first 2 years in the same fashion. We have turned out to be higher in student rating than any basic science subject committee in the whole curriculum over the first 2 years. We have some problems with the medical students in retaining their interest in the field, because we see them for the first 6 weeks, and we see them again at the end of the second year in the 8-week growth and development curriculum. However, only 2 1/2 weeks have to do with biobehavioral kinds of things, and although some of our same faculty teach, there has been some slippage in the 2-year period. We lose the students almost completely when they enter the clinical program, when medicine becomes the laying on of hands.

To tell you what kinds of things we do and to indicate some of the problems with behavioral science programs in other medical schools, we do not have a single behavioral scientist teaching an entire curriculum. We have a very extensive group of people in our medical and dental schools, joint program at the health center, and we have within the subject committee a number of physicians, primarily from the department of pediatrics, but from the department of psychiatry as well, who are teaching with us. It is quite clear, however, to the students that the behavioral scientists are the economists who are teaching basic economics as well as health-care economics; the sociologists who are teaching medical sociology; the anthropologists who are providing both physical anthropology and cultural anthropology; and the social psychologists, of whom there are four at the moment, who are providing a whole variety of things on social psychological variables in health care. We have managed to convince the remainder of the basic science faculty, because we got there as early as they did and have sat on important committees with them, that we, too, can judge scientific endeavor. We sit on promotions committees, on councils, medical school councils, and dental school councils. So far, we are way ahead, and I am very concerned about the generalization, which seems to be occurring here, that behavioral science should not be taught in medical schools, and if taught, should be taught primarily by physicians or behavioral scientists masquerading in white coats.

Haley: The point of the behavioral person being in the white coat is not masquerading, it is moving into a situation to make it relevant. The teaching to medical students of behavioral work has to have surface validity, and an aspect of it is the area of teaching from a concerned pediatrician, internist, or surgeon, because their patients die. Many medical schools fall into the trap of having death and dying taught by psychiatrists, and the student does not buy because he does not see it as reality. I think if you put the behavioral scientist out where the patient is, he can show you how you can care for the patient better. This is real, and it is not masquerading. Most of the time, I think it is effective.

Bahnson: I agree that it is very important to relate the behavioral sciences directly to the clinical, medical problems we are encountering. My own experience, having taught this area for some 15 years at Pennsylvania Hospital in Jefferson Medical College, has been that when you start with the psychosomatic and the sociosomatic areas rather than with some abstract behavioral sciences that hark back to undergraduate levels, then you can really capture the interest and the cooperation of the medical students and of the medical residents. What has happened in our settings is that the medical students have wanted to do research with us, and have become some of the most ardent supporters of the more global or holistic approach to disease, if we start with a clinical setting. In terms of Dr. Enelow's discussion on Rotter's internal/external control, he said that there were no real publications in this area related to cancer.

Enelow: What I said was, nobody has studied the relationship of the internal/external differentiation to the efforts to apply attribution theory to the influencing of health behavior because of the fear that attribution theory undoubtedly would be more valid for those who have internal locus of control as differentiated by the internal/external system of Rotter. I did not say that there were no publications on internal/external control at all.

Bahnson: I still maintain that this is relevant, because several studies now have uncovered that, including our own, cancer patients compared to normal control and random control patients or to any other group, feel that they are operating on internal rather than external control. And this is very, very important when we consider entrances to change in behavior or change in perception.

Cancer: The Behavioral Dimensions, edited by J. W. Cullen, B. H. Fox, and R. N. Isom. Raven Press, New York © 1976.

Focus and Introduction

Godfrey M. Hochbaum

School of Public Health, University of North Carolina, Chapel Hill, North Carolina 27514

The fact that nearly one-fourth of this volume is devoted to the topic of communication attests to the unquestioned importance ascribed to communication processes in the fight against cancer. A number of experts discuss various issues involved in making our communication efforts more effective.

In introducing this section, I observe the role of communication within the larger perspective of cancer control.

There are two major dimensions to be considered: (a) communication to or with lay population, whether it addresses itself to individuals, groups, or the entire public; and (b) communication to, with, and among scientists and professionals engaged in cancer-related activities. I will discuss the former first.

Unquestionably, human behavior plays a decisive role in the causation, prevention, treatment, and recovery from cancer. People's actions can increase or decrease the risk of some types of cancer, as is most evident in relation to smoking and lung cancer; early detection and seeking prompt medical help are human behaviors, as is cooperation in the course of medical treatment. Unless people act intelligently and conscientiously, all the efforts of the health professions, all the advances in medical know-how, and all the economic, physical, and medical resources invested in the fight against cancer will be wasted.

Therefore, this fight of ours has always focused on three goals:

1. Intervention to reduce carcinogens in the environment.
2. Medical intervention, that is, continuous development and application of more effective methods and tools to deal with biological factors.
3. Behavioral intervention, that is, continuous development and application of more effective methods and tools to influence people's behavior.

One of the most powerful tools to influence people's behavior is communication—from person to person and to large audiences through use of the mass media. I said "one of the most powerful tools" because it is neither the only, nor necessarily always the most powerful.

By definition, communication affects only intrapersonal processes and conditions. By "intrapersonal processes and conditions" I mean that through communication we may increase people's knowledge, change their attitudes, generate or increase motivations, and so forth.

Adequate knowledge, proper attitudes, and sufficient motivation are certainly critical elements for the emergence of the desired behaviors. For this reason alone, we must be concerned with them. And, as the expected large-scale behavioral changes in our public fail to materialize, our educational and communication efforts are blamed for being ineffective.

The frequently voiced disappointment in and cynicism toward the actual value of health education, especially through the mass media, are due largely to mistaken beliefs as to what education through communication can achieve. These expectations are based on a belief that people's behavior is solely or predominantly determined by those factors that are responsive to communication input, factors such as knowledge, attitudes, and motivation. If this were so, we would be far advanced in terms of getting people to engage in the kinds of behaviors we recommend. This is because cancer education has actually been highly successful in creating a knowledgeable public and in improving cancer-relevant attitudes and motivations even though it has not been as successful as we all wish. More people are better informed today about cancer than have ever been about any disease. More people (including smokers) know about the hazards of cigarettes than know what the first amendment to our Constitution is. The number of people whose attitudes and motivations in regard to cancer are as we would like them to be has steadily increased in recent years.

Thus, measured against what we can reasonably expect educational programs through the mass media to accomplish, they have been rather effective; albeit there is considerable room for improvement. But we are bound to be disappointed if we expect—quite unreasonably—that such programs will assure, by themselves, profound behavior changes in our society.

Such an expectation is unreasonable because human actions are determined or at least influenced by a host of factors, events, and conditions, many of which are neither directly responsive to educational instructions nor always under complete control of the individual. These factors may be found in the individual's social and physical environments, in his style of life, in the social, economic, and political systems—even the health-care system itself—of which he is a part, and in the complex technology that shapes much of our daily lives.

Both the preventive and much of the treatment and rehabilitive actions that we urge people to seek must be taken where people live and work and pursue their leisure-time pleasures. It is here that people, even those who have fully absorbed the requisite knowledge and are deeply motivated to follow our advice, may encounter all kinds of obstacles to taking these actions. Some of these obstacles may merely make adherence more inconvenient or difficult; others may render it impossible.

For example, the recent ex-smoker may be constantly tempted to return to cigarettes by the sight of other smokers or by the easy availability of cigarettes, and this may cause him to yield to his as yet only partially conquered urge to smoke. Inconvenience and other problems may counteract the interests of women to go to a clinic for a Pap smear. The desire not to contribute to the health hazards of polluted air by the burning of leaves and trash may be obviated when no other means of disposal are readily available.

On a larger scale, health insurance policies do not usually provide for coverage of preventive health services such as routine medical checkups. This creates not only a financial barrier to seeking such services but may also reduce their importance in the eyes of people who have been influenced by what they have learned through the media about benefits from prevention.

Similarly, we may have successfully convinced a group of women that they should have periodic Pap smears. But some of them may not have a physician to whom they go regularly and may hesitate to go to one whom they hardly know, merely to request a Pap smear. Others in the group may encounter hesitation on the part of the physician to perform or even recommend the procedure for any one of several reasons, and this apparent indifference may destroy the motivation induced by the educational program.

The point of all this is that in each of these examples the health messages have been effectively communicated but have not produced the intended behavior because of factors that are not directly responsive to influences through communication alone.

If we are concerned, as we surely are, with behavioral change, we must view communication as only one of the tools available to us, a tool that, despite its power and no matter how effectively it is used, can affect only some of the factors crucial to behavioral change.

Communication technology and our skills and sophistication in its use for health purposes have grown tremendously in the last few decades. Further improvements are certainly yet to come. But I believe we have reached something of a plateau of effectiveness in terms of its impact on the health behavior of the American people and for that matter, on cancer patients. Any further investment of ingenuity and resources will probably be beneficial but will bring diminishing returns. We can rise beyond this plateau only if we place communication in the larger context of behavioral change.

It is not enough to provide knowledge, to modify attitudes, and to motivate people to protect themselves against cancer. We must, with equal zeal and with the investment of equal resources, attempt to remove barriers to desirable behavior as much and as widely as possible. In other words, in addition to making people want to do the right things, we must try to enable them to do so.

I believe strongly, for example, that coverage of preventive medical services by insurance companies may do more to attain greater utilization of such services than further education; and may do even more if educational attempts to make people value these services were linked to simultaneous attempts to assure financial coverage for them.

Similarly, I doubt that further extension and intensification of our media-carried antismoking endeavors will bring much corresponding gain. I have been impressed with the quality and probable effectiveness of television spots stressing the importance and urgency of smoking cessation. Yet, I do not recall any such messages on television that offer helpful advice to smokers who wish to stop but are unable to cope with internally and externally imposed difficulties in doing so.

On the positive side, the antismoking movement is doing exactly what I would advocate. It will probably emerge as the single most effective health education movement ever, because it has fused communication with intervention into concrete political, economic, administrative, and other affairs through affecting legislation, regulation of smoking in many situations, and through other similar measures. This movement should serve as a model of multidimensional, comprehensive attacks on hazardous practices in which the media contribute to the effectiveness of other dimensions, just as these contribute to the effectiveness of the media.

To give one other positive illustration: There has been a substantial increase in the number of women who practice breast self-examination and seek medical checkups for breast cancer, even for cervical cancer, in the aftermath of Mrs. Betty Ford's mastectomy. This educational success has been due mainly, I believe, to three factors. One was the exhaustive and generally commendable and instructive coverage of the event in the media which utilized the fact that the public was, first, intensely interested in events affecting the First Lady and other prominent women who underwent such surgery. The second was the prevailing tenor of most of the coverage. It contributed greatly to reducing the stigma surrounding breast and other cancers, opening it to freer discussion, and also reducing the blind fear that has surrounded cancer, by stressing that prompt cancer treatment may save one's life and does not necessarily render a victim unattractive or incapable of still enjoying life fully. The third factor was that at the same time these educational activities were addressed to the public, the medical professions and medical resources were mobilized to meet the increased demand for help. I do not know how many potential barriers which in the past may have prevented women from coping with their fear of cancer were thereby removed, and thus facilitated the appropriate actions. But there is no question that this played a significant role.

I have dwelt at length on this interplay between the roles of communication and the role of other means to effect behavioral change, although it may seem self-evident once it is stated explicitly. Those who work directly with individuals who are at risk of, or already victimized by, cancer are probably well aware of it and have integrated it in their work. But those whose interests are primarily in the communication field (whether they are researchers and theorists, or are writers, producers, public health educators, or other professionals) tend at times to view communication and particularly the media as *the* key to producing broad behavioral changes in the public, thereby neglecting the fact that these are only part of a dynamic and interdependent complex of influences on people's actions, and even the fact that the effectiveness of communication processes is often determined by conditions outside the communication system.

In the following chapters several prominent experts will discuss various theories pertaining to communication and to the diffusion and adoption of new ideas and practices. These theories, based on extensive research, have helped tremendously to sharpen our understanding of communication processes and have furnished us with means for utilizing these more effectively. But the *full* practical benefits that could be harvested from these theories, and from the methods and techniques deriving from them, are often limited by this relatively frequent neglect of how they fit in with the realities in people's lives.

Another problem which I do not believe will be dealt with in any of the chapters, but which must be of considerable interest to us, concerns one of the critical elements of effective communication—the confidence that an audience has in the content and source of a message. A problem arises when several presumably trustworthy sources transmit different and even mutually contradictory messages, or when messages transmitted by a source contradict previous messages from the same source. This has occurred with increasing frequency in recent years.

For example, in the aftermath of Mrs. Ford's mastectomy, the media gave wide coverage to the medical controversy concerning the nature and extent of surgical procedures recommended for breast cancer with equally renowned surgeons on both sides of the controversy. The possible effect on the psychological state of patients and on their willingness to undergo surgery is easy to guess.

Another example is provided by the frequent withdrawal of drugs from the market by the Food and Drug Administration (FDA) as potentially carcinogenic—the same drugs that have been heretofore prescribed by physicians for one or another disease with the approval of the FDA—perhaps followed after some time by reapproval.

A third example is the almost steady flow of news in the media concerning discoveries (often dubious or actually unjustified) of more and more substances suspected of increasing the risk of cancer, substances that have been ingested or otherwise used by millions of people and have become almost an irreplaceable part of our daily life. The accumulation of such news may well lead to a loss of hope that one can protect himself against such an avalanche of threats, and therefore to a weakening of the will to defend himself against *any* of the threats with which the public is bombarded.

Conflicting messages from various sources, repeated shifts in approval and disapproval of drugs, and precipitous public announcements of new and still unverified scientific findings are bound to confuse people, weaken their confidence in our messages, and make them less responsive to our educational programs.

At present, there is no agency, organization, or other official body in a position and with the power to effect at least some moderate change in this situation. Perhaps the new Bureau of Health Education in the Department of Health, Education, and Welfare and/or the soon-to-be-established National Center for Health Education in the private sector will in time be able to do so. Some of our efforts might be directed at educating the public to understand *why* such disagreements and changes in judgment are unavoidable, and how people may still be able to reach sound decisions even when it is not yet clear in the fluid state of scientific progress where the truth lies. Virtually nothing of this nature is currently done. Instead, the proponents of one side of a controversial scientific issue try to proselytize the lay public to their point of view by pitting their communication skills against those of their opponents, much as two producers of the same kind of commercial product compete for the consumer's dollar by making their own messages more impressive than the competitor's.

More generally, our educational efforts might be more profitably directed at helping people to make decisions and choices rather than at getting them to do what we want them to do. Behavior that occurs merely in response to persuasive communication is less likely to be carried out completely and conscientiously and is less likely to persist than behavior that stems from a decision which the person has reached on his own. To help people reach *such* decisions, our communication must be attuned to beliefs, motives, needs, and problems, as people experience them. But many, perhaps most, of our communications are generated by skillful, capable, creative professionals on the basis of what *they* believe will affect their audiences. Often they are right, but as often they are wrong. The people whose thoughts, feelings, and actions we are trying to influence know better than we what will have such effects. We need to listen to them and enlist them into helping us.

This admonition is common in the education literature. But in practice it is rarely followed, despite the fact that it is one of the keys to truly effective communication.

All that I have discussed here is meant as a background to the speakers that follow, and each will, from his or her own perspective, examine various more specific aspects of communication as they relate to our fight against cancer. I would like to make an observation concerning processes of communication among us who are here today.

From a look at the list of professional and lay participants, there appear to be at least three distinct subgroups. One consists of those whose primary concern is with individual cancer victims and their families, that is, clinicians, nurses, volunteer workers, and so on. They probably view communication mostly in terms of an interpersonal process and of its direct effects on their clients. Then there are those among us whose primary concern is with achieving changes in the cancer-related behaviors of the public. Their interests are likely to be focused on the mass media and on their effectiveness in reaching and influencing large numbers of people. Finally, there are those whose primary concern is with communication itself and with the development of fruitful theories, and of effective methods and techniques of communication, whether or not these are used in relation to cancer, and other disease, or to health at all.

These three groups differ in the way they view communication processes, their purposes, their nature, their use, the criteria of their effectiveness, even the meaning ascribed to terms such as communication. For example, statistical data on the impact of the media on the public, demographic data on large media audiences, and theory and research dealing with communication are likely to be irrelevant to the first group, although they are vital tools for the other two, especially the third one. On the other hand, the highly personal problems of cancer patients and their families that are the daily experiences and concern of the first group are of little *professional* interest to the others, no matter how compassionate they may be.

All this gives rise to communication difficulties among the three groups whenever there is an interchange between them, and we must expect such difficulties at this conference as well. Yet, we are here for one shared purpose only: to evolve strategies, methods, and techniques to deal more effectively with one of the most devastating diseases. Each of the three groups deals with different dimensions of this problem, each approaches the fight from a different base, each brings a different understanding, and different skills and methods to it. None of them has all the answers. These differences are complementary, not conflicting. Ultimate success requires a cooperative, integrated multidisciplinary and multidimensional approach, a fusing of what each of the groups can bring to the problem.

To achieve this requires, in turn, that we listen to each other not only with an open mind but with an active, concerted effort to extract and incorporate whatever may be useful from the other's field into our own. Let the clinician learn and benefit from what the communication researcher and theorist have to offer, and let the sociologist and the media expert learn and benefit from understanding that the clinican, the volunteer worker, and the cancer victim himself can teach from their own perspectives.

If this volume achieves nothing else but the beginning of such meshing and of better communication and cooperation among us, it will have made a significant contribution.

Cancer: The Behavioral Dimensions, edited by J. W. Cullen, B. H. Fox, and R. N. Isom. Raven Press, New York © 1976.

The Impact of Mass Media on Cancer Control Programs

Irving I. Rimer

American Cancer Society, Inc., New York, New York 10019

Mass media must be viewed as narrow media. This nation of special publics has special media to reach them: magazines, radio, press, TV, blacks, Spanish speaking, academic, young. Although the networks do reach millions, most media, including the growing selection of bands on TV sets, can select and zero in on smaller segments. This is our advantage. Madison Avenue talks in terms of 60, 30, 10 special spots and ads. We talk about features, major articles, special films, programs, discussions in the media.

Veterans of the war against cancer are familiar with the significant gains made on the communications front. Until World War II the media sidestepped the area of cancer like a minefield. Editors and writers recoiled from the very use of the word that spelled death in boldface type. Consequently, the disease and any programs directed against it were kept under wraps by the press.

Of course, the media in any period reflect contemporary public tastes and attitudes. And because cancer was feared as a death sentence, the press responded by keeping a safe distance between itself and a distasteful subject.

The myths and taboos surrounding cancer run deep in our culture and society. Why else are patients still prey to gimmicks, gadgets, and glib prescriptions by quacks? Why else the concealment, the shame, and the guilt feelings which are more prevalent in this disease than in almost any other?

All of this is understandable when put into perspective. Since any real progress in the treatment of cancer began less than 50 years ago, it is not surprising that there should persist a deep-seated fear of a disease that until then was nearly always fatal. The recent successes have to compete in the public consciousness with centuries of fatalism toward a disease against which people had been almost totally defenseless. We have begun to correct this depressing view of cancer—this cultural lag—by moving public opinion toward a more realistic and simultaneously more hopeful outlook (1).

This more realistic, more hopeful outlook toward cancer is the guiding philosophy and strategy behind the American Cancer Society's (ACS) communication efforts. The ACS believes that effective use of media resources is as important to cancer control as the construction of medical centers for surgery, x-ray, and chemotherapy. We know cancer is preventable in some cases, and that it is most curable when found and treated by experts in the earliest stages. This is the platform for communications to the public.

Today the ACS packages its messages in specific action programs designed by the public education department; our public information department is devoted to promoting these programs. Each evolves from a careful assessment of medical and scientific evidence, and an intensive exchange of ideas and plans among physicians and educators translated into activities by people skilled in the art of mass communications. These people not only are the specialists on the ACS's staff but also writers, designers, film makers, and market research directors of advertising agencies—serving as volunteer creators of spots and ads.

Each of these programs demands a custom-tailored approach to specific audiences based on careful evaluation of their attitudes and behavior patterns, a determination of high-risk groups, a survey of community medical facilities, and a keen understanding of the attitudes and interests of the media managers. A campaign to persuade every woman to have a Pap test is quite different from a program to motivate women to practice breast self-examination at home month after month. A plan to encourage men and women to have a proctoscopic exam for cancer of the colon and rectum does not compare with an effort to influence the smoking behavior of teenagers or adults. And teaching people who live in certain geographic regions to protect themselves against the sun presents different problems than establishing the habit of regular checkups among the population.

But there are common elements to all—the value of early detection, early diagnosis, early treatment, and basic methods of prevention. Cancer is a personal responsibility. If people act in time, more lives will be saved. A hopeful, activist attitude is essential.

A potent way to emphasize this hope and action is by focusing on men and women cured of cancer. Stories of people take the newspaper or magazine reader or TV viewer behind the facts, behind the information. It puts them in contact with another person with whom they can immediately empathize and learn a vital lifesaving lesson in the bargain—cancer is curable.

The men and women who have had the courage and candor to share their stories with the public have made a vital contribution to cancer control. In turn, the discreet use of their experiences by writers, TV producers, and radio directors has developed inspiring, heartwarming lessons for millions of Americans. Yet, these good people sometimes confront the taboos still existing with respect to cancer. During "The Killers," a 90-minute TV special about cancer, a piano player related his experience with cancer of the colon and rectum. He explained in an informal way that his colostomy did not stop him from performing with a jazz combo. Shortly after, he reported that some musicians in his own group refused to take a glass of water from him. Old fables and myths of contagion die hard.

All media are vital to the society—the *New York Times* and *The National Enquirer, Harper's,* and *Playboy.* A sequence on the "Today" show is just as important as a plot on breast cancer incorporated into "All in the Family." We will work with Marcus Welby and Johnny Carson and always encourage Dear Abby or Ann Landers to bring a helpful message to their readers.

The ACS recognizes that the field of communications is composed of channels that reach specific groups of people and that each has its own points of view, biases, and approaches. In a diverse and pluralistic society every channel that reaches some group is worth the time, energy, and effort invested. The mass media is indeed the narrow media and should be thought of in those terms.

A strength in the ACS communications program is its commitment of local volunteers, many of whom are skilled in public information. These people have been advocates for positive cancer control programs, and it is their distribution of messages that has made the difference. How can we sum up the creative, imaginative programs on cancer which have been generated by these volunteers aided by a small corps of professional staff members? One word describes it—tremendous.

On the national level, the physicians and staff of the ACS have stimulated and provided in-depth news and information about cancer to the media. Because the ACS's credibility is established, it has been able to facilitate the acceptance of articles and features focusing on the hopeful aspects of cancer. The publishers and managers of networks are keenly aware that there has been a marked shift in the climate of public support and concern for greater action against cancer. Cancer is news, because of this perpetual, deep concern, and also because the conquest of cancer is now a national priority under the National Cancer Act. Things will never be the same again.

Every major consumer magazine has assigned writers to delve into the cancer story. Almost every network news director affords cancer a place on the programming schedules. But there are still some media directors who suffer from the social lag about cancer. It is up to us to convince them that their readers and viewers are willing to deal with the facts, if they are presented in a balanced way.

On a regular basis, news documentaries either include cancer in part or feature it entirely for their viewers in prime time. Giving cancer visibility in the context of the normal flow of news has had an important impact on the public's understanding and acceptance of cancer control measures. We recognize that television is a commercial medium that places a high value on the entertainment factor. Yet, by working with writers, producers, directors, a responsible message on cancer will result.

The capacity of the media to handle this complex and varied subject has benefited from the new generation of writers specialized in medical science writing. With their background in the biological and physical sciences they have raised the standards of reporting on health, and cancer specifically. This is a plus for the public because important scientific and medical advances are completely covered.

For close to 15 years the Society's Science Writers' Seminar has been a key source of news about cancer research. It has served two purposes. One, it has given the writers an opportunity to discuss advances and promises in research with leading scientists without the pressures of deadlines. Secondly, through these writers it has provided the public with a current analysis and sound perspective on a yearly basis of what is happening in the laboratories and medical centers. This has increased awareness of hopeful developments against the disease. This is important to the cancer control program.

Obviously, there is the danger of premature breakthroughs being reported and of promises that cannot be kept. But the advantages of this avenue of communications outweigh the risks. The scientist bears as much ethical responsibility as the writer. Sometimes in eagerness for a great award or a greater grant the scientist prematurely betrays an optimism for a project.

In its preparation of materials for the media as well as its extensive public education program, the ACS leans heavily on surveys and studies conducted on such diverse subjects as checkups, the Pap test, the procto, breast self-examination (BSE), smoking, and the warning signals. The key committees of the Board in this area have always sought the wise counsel of those engaged in market research as well as experts in behavioral research. The developers of spots, films, and special campaigns avidly seek and need this data.

These studies have involved pretesting of leaflets, evaluation of films before completion, follow-up to see how effective a TV special or series has been, or national random sampling studies of attitudes and behavior prior to the inception of new broad-scale programs. In each case, results have been incorporated into the public education and public information programs of the ACS.

Breast cancer points up the value of such studies and practices. This is a subject of deep emotional concern to women, their families, and the medical profession. Recently, a spate of magazine articles resulting from debates within the medical community focused on the subject of breast surgery. Interest has always been at a peak level in the media and the impact of these debates must not be minimized, particularly in view of the evolvement of patients' rights and women's equality. For example, Ann Landers, in one of her colums, recommended that her readers practice BSE. In fact, she pleaded with them to do so. She advised them to write the ACS for a folder on how to do breast self-examination. Some estimators of public response guessed that the column might draw 10,000 replies. One professional optimist claimed that a high of 40,000 might be reached. What happened? When the Post Office trucks finished unloading the mail, ACS's 300,000 requests for the folder had been received. What towering concern those letters represented! And what a demonstration of the impact of a writer whom readers trust and of the newspapers in which her column appeared.

The size and intensity of the reaction to the columns and to the magazine articles prompted our reexamination of women's attitudes and behavior toward breast cancer. We had an extensive program underway—a film on BSE, folders, posters, TV spots, special communications for minority and Spanish-speaking women, materials for leaders of discussion groups, and much more. But was this all working in behalf of the women of America?

A scientific survey of all aspects of breast cancer was carried out: knowledge of causes, knowledge and practice of BSE, attitudes toward surgery, and knowledge of rehabilitation programs such as "Reach to Recovery." The medical, public education, and public information departments participated in the formulation of the survey which was directed by the Gallup organization. Since a full summary of this survey is available to the professional community, let me share with you some highlights at this time (2).

We discovered that American women are more concerned about breast cancer than any other disease, and that this intense concern, coupled with some misconceptions about the incidence, cause, and treatment of the disease, prevent many from taking positive action which will enhance their chances of survival from this cancer. There are four reasons why women who are aware of breast cancer do not practice BSE regularly; in fact, only 18% do it regularly.

1. Only 12% realize that the monthly examination is essential.
2. Fear and anxiety: almost half the reasons for not doing self-exams were what are called "avoidance" responses—they did not have the time, or felt they did not need it. These same women also said that they would postpone seeing a doctor if they did find a breast lump.
3. Many women who know *about* BSE don't know how to do it.
4. Lack of confidence: Only 22% of all women who have ever practiced BSE feel confident that they could distinguish a lump from normal breast tissue.

In addition, the old wives' tales persist about bumps and injuries to the breast as well as some current fears about the birth control pill being a cause of this disease. To change these factors in a direction that will be most helpful to women, we obviously need a variety of approaches.

1. For the women ignorant of the value of regular self-examination, we must convince them how important it is.
2. We must reassure the "avoidance" people that finding a breast lump is no certainty of cancer but is the first step in a lifesaving procedure, and that to give themselves the best chance for survival they should tell their doctors about it immediately.
3. For those who lack information on the procedure, we can demonstrate how to do BSE.
4. For those who have no confidence in their self-detection of breast lumps, we need to persuade physicians to instruct them.

There is also the problem of treatment. Most women realize that mastectomy is the primary adequate treatment, but every woman is deeply worried about being less feminine after such surgery. This is a very serious deterrent in seeking help in examination and in treatment.

How did we handle these approaches? Two parallel tracks were undertaken. First, the public education department shifted its effort from emphasis on the importance of BSE to showing women how to do it and requesting a commitment to continue the practice. Over and above initiating major revisions in films and leaflets, the public education department has designed a program to achieve this objective by enlisting physicians and nurses in local communities to introduce and teach by using a realistic plastic model of the breast to give women a chance to feel the lumps.

Second, because knowledge of the BSE and how to do it were lacking, the ACS accelerated production of a film for television which would demonstrate with a live model all aspects of BSE. This was a breakthrough in television communications. To assure its acceptance, the ACS showed the Code Authority of the National Association of Broadcasters various photo approaches on the subject for approval. To their lasting credit, the Authority heartily endorsed the live model procedure for TV audiences. Their conclusion: Good medicine is never pornographic.

The film, which stars Jennifer O'Neill, is a thorough look at the problem of breast cancer. The viewers see how BSE is done, meet women who have had mastectomies, and learn how to cope with taboos and fears surrounding the disease. The use of this film by local stations has been phenomenal, a credit to their social responsibility.

A process was established to test the effectiveness of the film in 10 cities to determine whether women decided to practice BSE and felt more confident about doing it after viewing the film. The evidence is that many women moved from indifference to actual commitment after seeing this film on television.

The findings from the basic survey were placed in the hands of volunteer advertising agencies preparing ads and spots for the ACS. They felt free to explicitly demonstrate BSE in a TV spot and to use illustrations of the technique in ads designed to fill the gap in understanding and knowledge which the survey had disclosed.

Recently, women all over the world empathized with Mrs. Ford and Mrs. Rockefeller. The media coverage was overwhelming and prompted the presentation of BSE on television news and specials on the networks and local stations —all of which must have done much to lift the level of understanding. A few women wrote angry letters about this candid view of what they considered a private concern, but for most, it alleviated fear through frankness.

This is not to deny the problem of overcommunication in cancer. Shana Alexander, writing in *Newsweek,* took exception to the practice, headlining her article, "Breast Cancer and News Overkill" (3). But it was an incredible coincidence, with the President's wife and then the Vice President's wife requiring breast cancer surgery within 16 days of each other, which heightened the newsworthiness of these events.

I wish we had been able to take soundings of women's attitudes toward breast cancer during the height of this coverage. The phone calls and letters to our local offices, the long waiting lists established at breast cancer demonstration projects and clinics were all immediate responses. We have no way of knowing how deep-seated and long-lasting this interest and concern will be, but it certainly resulted from coverage by the mass media.

Another dramatic example of mass media impact is the antismoking campaign. From its beginnings in the 1950s until the early 1970s this was page-one news. The battle involving the voluntary health groups against a major industry—a David-and-Goliath situation—had something to do with this. But more important, this is a matter of life and death for more than 50 million smokers and their families.

The ACS and others made intensive use of studies on attitudes and behavior toward cigarette smoking. Conferences and symposia were held to determine the role of fear—whether it motivated or blocked action. Tests were run in specific cities to determine whether the authoritarian, fear, or make-up-your-own-mind approaches worked best for smokers and nonsmokers. Many of these assays were conducted by the ACS. Throughout, experts in communications, market research, behavioral science, and even psychoanalysis were involved in planning, consultation, and interviewing.

As we recall it now, a high point was the television campaign against smoking. Never before was so much time and visibility given to public service messages. A variety of approaches was used in the spots; some were straightforward warnings, some satirized cigarette commercials, many relied on humor. Some were expensive, some cost very little. For the 4 years when the spots were frequently used, broadcasters contributed an estimated $50 million of air time annually (4).

The results are as follows: Up to 1967, total cigarette consumption increased annually. Then there were major declines in 1968 and in 1969, the years when the spots had their greatest visibility. According to the National Clearinghouse on Smoking and Health, from 1966–1970, 10 million Americans quit smoking. While broadcasting does not claim all the credit, it deserves the lion's share. For the first time there was mass impact of public health messages. In all aspects of life people talked about them, and when people begin to talk about ideas, they begin to take action.

Today, there is a sharp drop in these spots and an upswing in per capita smoking, among both young people and adults. One can not prove cause and effect, but the relationship seems reasonable. Tom Whiteside said in his recent *New Yorker* article: "[The spots] made the greatest impression, it seems to me, when viewers were able to juxtapose them in their minds with the content of the cigarette commercials. Without the enemy there on the screen, too, the anti-smoking commercials tended to lose a bit of their anti-establishment quality—a quality that may have been cheering on a lot of long-suffering viewers" (5).

Certainly, this was a classic example of communication resulting in action, which has prompted other causes to look for the magic or secret ingredient. But fundamental to it was the vast involvement of governmental, voluntary interests, and a giant industry with millions of advertising dollars and a habit adopted by millions. How do you repeat that act?

From the breast cancer and antismoking campaigns, we have learned that when cancer is related to prominent personages or is a critical public issue the media will cover the story continuously and thoroughly. Our challenge is to use our creative capacities and skills to produce programs that warrant public attention and concern on a year-round basis.

Essentially, we are confronted with providing the public in a democratic society with information about a grave, but not inevitably lethal, disease, provided people can be motivated to take self-protective action. To our advantage, major advances are being made in the techniques of news dissemination. At the same time, we need assurance that our messages are truly making an impact, and that each one is stimulating people to take action. That is why we need the thoughts and active participation of this group. That is why this meeting is so important. I eagerly anticipate your recommendations for the associated enterprise of the ACS and the National Cancer Institute, so that together we can wipe out cancer in your lifetime.

REFERENCES

1. Wakefield, J. Learning to save lives. *World Health Magazine,* (February–March, 1970).
2. Women's attitudes regarding breast cancer. American Cancer Society, New York (1973).
3. Alexander, S. Breast cancer and news overkill. *Newsweek* (December 9, 1974).

4. Panel Discussion, The Role of the Mass Media, In *The Second World Conference on Smoking and Health*.
5. A reporter at large. *New Yorker Magazine* (November 18, 1974).

Discussion

Monaco: Earlier, Dr. Clark said, "We have to look at cancer with hope within a framework of reality." Unfortunately, I fear that too many of the communications about cancer are very simplistic and do not present the realities of the problems that we meet in cancer. For example, Mr. Rimer made the rather obvious slip, on more than one occasion, that cancer is curable. Many forms of cancer are curable through combinations of surgery, radiation, and chemotherapy. But more of the killers in cancer are the types of disease that can be controlled temporarily, but we have not reached a state where we can say that we can cure them. Slipping into that mistake is the same mistake that we see made by many of the reporters in the media who are looking at breakthroughs, as you mentioned, or are reporting cures. We all remember a couple of years ago when L-asparaginase came on the scene and the media wrote this up as the cure for leukemia. Then adriamycin comes along and that becomes the new potential cure for different forms of cancer.

When we talk about cures we may be turning off a large segment of the population who are interested in helping direct attention to proper funding for some of the studies that are needed to attack the cancers that are not currently curable. A number of the ACS volunteers I have talked to say that the word cure confronts them when they are going from door to door to solicit funds. I think that the media representatives relating to the ACS should look into this area.

A very important point that Dr. Hochbaum made is that you see an excellent list of warning signals covering the generalities with respect to cancer, but at the end it says "See your doctor." However, may people do not have a doctor and do not know where to go to get specialized cancer information. In the metropolitan Washington area, when I monitor the television commercials that deal with cancer problems, I see, "See your doctor," but I don't notice the focus on the black community that you mentioned was available, or the focus on the Spanish-speaking community that refers them to available clinical services. This lack is true for the local as well as the national stations. Could we not make sure that it says, "See your doctor, but if you don't have a doctor or if you want to know what specialized cancer centers and clinical facilities are available in your area, contact either the ACS regional office or contact the National Cancer Institute through a toll-free number." This additional information should be given so that we are not only warning people, but are giving them the tools, if they are motivated at that moment, to go to a phone and call the people that have the information. Of course, we have to make absolutely certain that the people we are referring them to will have truthful information to give them. If they call an ACS number in Washington, D.C., Lillian Horowitz is there and she has the right information. If people called her and said "Look, where should I call?" she would be able to give them several numbers to call or she would refer them to the Office of Cancer Communications at NCI.

Unfortunately, there are a lot of people and agencies who do not have the proper information. In fact, the *National Observer* recently did a study on this in Washington and called various voluntary agencies to ask where to go and what to do. The ignorance of at least 50% of the people called was appalling.

Another thing we should strive for is to include the elements of truth and reality in the information we are giving people. We do not want to scare them half to death, but we want to make sure that the information is realistic as well as accurate. The job that Georgia

Photopoulus is doing in that Cancer Call program is really fantastic. However, the literature relating to that program mentioned that chemotherapy was a simple practice and that the side effects of drugs were nausea and a few other things. It downplayed chemotherapy side effects. Anyone who has lived through chemotherapy with someone under treatment for cancer—leukemia, lymphomas, Hodgkin's disease, and the like—knows that many of the side effects are far more devastating than the disease itself at some points. Thus, when we give information to the public, we should be hopeful and give them all the tools they need to be hopeful with because things are constantly improving. However, we have to give that hope within a framework of reality, because it is the reality that holds the promise of people doing the things they need to change their behavior. It is reality that is going to establish the feeling of confidence and the feeling of trust in the communicator which may lead that person to continue doing the types of activities that could mean they will reach a good conclusion to their cancer problems. But if we are not realistic and if we are unsure of our data base, the moment that someone finds an error in our information, we lose our credibility. And the thing that we have to sell more than anything else to the general public is credibility in what we are telling them. I would like to know how you feel about the realities in the type of information that you are putting forth.

Photopoulus: Cancer and I discovered each other 6½ years ago when I was 34 years old. I would like to respond to Grace Monaco's comment about the chemotherapy guidelines. Credibility is probably the most important thing for me. I had to fight all the way to get even the chemotherapy guidelines in our CALL-PAC program—chemotherapy guidelines in a layman's language. They were prepared for us by the chief of medical oncology at Presbyterian-St. Luke's Hospital in Chicago, which is a major cancer center. And that was as far as we could go. The radiation guidelines were prepared by a very prominent radiation oncologist in Chicago. Our intent is not to frighten, not to alarm, but to let people know that it is not unusual to experience side effects or reactions. And it is further than we have ever been permitted to go before. I hope that I have the opportunity to speak later, because as a layman I believe I have some important contributions to make to this conference. I do not have medical credentials, but I feel that I, too, am a specialist in living and coping with cancer—surviving a catastrophic illness. I am not pronounced cured, I am not pronounced arrested, but I am free of symptoms today and am leading a full, productive, creative life.

L. Fink: Dr. Hochbaum mentioned in his presentation that we may be overdoing it. We may be turning off the smokers by overemphasizing the fear of cancer. I would like to ask why is it that we use the fear of cancer in our antismoking campaigns when we realize that the fear of cancer is a negative approach. It is something that everyone is afraid of and things that people are afraid of they turn away from. I offer this as a challenge to the behavioral scientists. Why not come up with some sort of positive approach that people will readily accept, such as, to name a few things, that there is an improvement in the senses of taste and smell after cessation of smoking? That would be a positive approach. We know that nothing smells worse than a dirty ashtray, especially when it is wet. There is nothing that smells worse to the mate of a smoker than his or her breath. The improvement of one's image is an improvement of life style and that would also be a positive approach which is more acceptable to the smoker than the fear of cancer.

Hochbaum: I think that there is enough evidence that the fear of cancer is quite an effective motivation for people to decide that they ought and want to quit. The problem arises not in getting people to realize they should quit, but in helping them to translate the decision into behavior. The kind of motive that leads to a decision to do something and what happens later are two different kinds of problems. At that point, probably, positive reinforcing kinds of appeals do occur. There is considerable evidence that the present impact of antismoking effects is less related to an increased fear of cancer than to the increase in social pressure that nonsmokers put on smokers in creating a different atmosphere, an antismoking culture, so to speak, which is a more positive kind of motive.

Rimer: The smoking problem is not just a matter of messages in cancer control. It is also a political problem. We are trying to get the Congress to take further action on the levels of tar and nicotine content of cigarettes. You are not going to get Congress excited about the smell and appearance of the smoker to achieve that objective. The only way you are going to move Congress to take action is to really convince the members of the House and the Senate that smoking actually does take the lives or threaten the lives of at least 300,000 Americans year after year.

Leventhal: I want to respond to Mr. Fink's comment on why we don't do something. As a matter of fact, we don't have a big data base but we have done some things. For example, the point that Dr. Hochbaum made about specific instructions on how to execute behaviors after a person is motivated has been made perhaps a half-dozen times, both in the psychological and public health literature. I feel somewhat responsible since I have made it in detail at meetings of the American Cancer Society, the American Heart Association, and other places. No one ever listens to what you say. You give example after example, and it just doesn't get through. Those of us who do research, which is my business, don't have the time to try to translate our findings or become full-time translators. But I would urge you to look at some of the limited data we have and see what we have found to stimulate your own thinking. You ask why we use fear appeals or why don't we invent something positive. Again, the literature shows that these things are not as negative as you think; in fact, they do have effects, but that does not mean that positive appeals would not have equally good effects. Richard Evans has done some exploring in this respect, but more needs to be done. If you would examine what little data there are, you would get ideas from it and you might stimulate us to raise new questions. In turn, we might be able to go ahead and do something. There needs to be a two-way street here.

Weisman: I think Mr. Rimer's concept of narrow media for limited audiences is brilliant. There is nothing more discouraging in any field than to try to be all things to all people at all times. Then we end up feeling guilty and accomplishing nothing. So, it is a good idea to combine research information plus public information, as exemplified yesterday by Dr. Antonovsky in his typology and certain other findings such as personality and otherwise about women who delay the longest in coming to the doctor for breast cancer. I wonder if he has done any work about targeting his narrow appeal to certain groups such as churches, funeral directors, athletic organizations, clubs that cater to certain kinds of interests. Because people differ so much, some women might be impressed by Betty Ford's experience, while others wouldn't be touched by it. Breast cancer has different significance to people. I would appreciate your comments on how you have tried to implement your concept of narrow media for limited audiences, tying it up with research information we have.

M. Brown: I am a lay person, and I have been feeling very frustrated by the constant remarks made about going to see your physician for a checkup. It seems to me that unless you have something clearly wrong with you, it takes a long time to make an appointment. When you go and all the results are negative, you are made to feel almost a hypochondriac by both the nurse and physician. Why are you coming here? What is wrong with you? I have what I consider a good physician, but every time I go I feel as if I am taking the time of someone who really should be there with a more serious illness. I feel very frustrated with the result, so, like most of my friends, keep on putting off annual checkups. Would it be better to establish clinics where we could go annually for just a Pap smear or a checkup, rather than a complete physical examination?

Hochbaum: My physician in Washington always started out by asking me, "What's the trouble?" An obvious way for him to greet every patient is not with "What's wrong, what's the trouble?" Rather, he should say, "I am glad you came in; I hope there is nothing wrong, that you just come for a good checkup." I think that ties in with what you are saying.

Evans: Mr. Fink more or less reflected, as a layman who is very interested in this topic, the kind of thing that I think we could see from another aspect. Let me relate to you experiences that I have had over a period of several years with the American Heart Association's Public Education Committee. I saw some of the problems of the so-called behavioral scientists (or whatever we are supposed to be called) trying to interact with a group of cardiologists and others who were also interested in some of these same issues, like smoking. One of the first things that I noticed is that people like Mr. Rimer and his counterpart working in agencies are caught up in a pretty tough situation. Even establishing what all these television spots and other types of mass communications are for is rather tricky. For example, rather honestly, one purpose is fund raising for the American Heart Association or for the American Cancer Society. In other words, you are trying to get the public concerned about cancer and heart disease, not so much to go out and try to prevent these diseases, but to get these messages on prime time television and succeed in a fund-raising effort. This is not bad but the messages are—they are not really that interested in trying to affect behavior. The behavior they are interested in is the kind that is involved in giving a certain amount of money to these fund-raising efforts, which is very good, but it might be specified a little better.

Another great confusion is the difference between an awareness campaign and one directed toward actually changing behavior. To illustrate, the government set up a task force on a new disease—at least most people never heard of periodontal disease—and they asked me to chair a subcommittee on mass communications. I brought together a group of people like Jules Bergman of ABC and *Time*, all the top media representatives, to try to take a new disease and get it across to the public. The discussions were fascinating because in every point there was confusion as to what should go into this campaign in terms of whether we were talking about awareness or trying to get them to change their behavior.

Among the problems with respect to the positive-vs.-fear appeal, there is no way that you can have any kind of message on cancer that already does not have a fear appeal. The word "cancer" triggers fear. The real question is what other appeals you can make. We have demonstrated through research that positive appeals are really rather effective—perhaps more effective than fear appeals—but, in themselves, they are not the whole answer. You are never talking about a nonfear message in cancer education. Automatically, you have a term that makes a lot of our academic research almost irrelevant because you are dealing with something that is already so emotionally charged. Another point is the plethora of agencies trying to reach the public. For example, take the antismoking spots—they were sponsored by the American Heart Association. Tuberculosis was doing some and Cancer was also using them. There was no coordination. People were confused—who was behind the spots? If they all directed people effectively toward antismoking—fine. The question one would have to ask is, "Would there not be some utility in coordinating these efforts?" Is there not a danger of overexposure, saturation, or confusing well-designed messages with poor messages? It looks like everybody is fighting for that broadcast time. The point that Irv Rimer made was that the networks welcome competition. But is this competition from the standpoint of planning serious efforts to acquaint the public with serious disease and how to deal with it? Can we afford the luxury of the network saying, "We like competition in the messages." Should there be some coordination? Has there at times been confusion in messages? Hasn't that very confusion affected the behaviors they might elicit? These are very complicated issues, and there is no way that they can be solved at this conference. But I would admonish whoever is interested in mass communication in these areas to look at the policy problems behind these efforts and perhaps try to recognize what could be done. Perhaps Mr. Rimer would like to comment as well.

Rimer: First of all, the American Cancer Society has always kept its antismoking campaign as far removed from the fund raising as it could. Since there are 12 months in a year, there is a limit as to how far you can remove it. Secondly, in the antismoking campaign, I really think we should stop talking about spots. We have got to start talking about programs; 30-minute programs, facts integrated into shows like "Good Times," "All in the Family," discussions on the "Today" program, the use of local personalities, and so on. We have to give it depth, weight, broad-scale understanding, and involvement in the local community. The days of the late 1960s and early 1970s when we received $50 million worth of free public service time from the networks and the stations are over. We have got to talk in terms of the National Cancer Institute and the American Cancer Society, which have programmed messages in depth to the American public on a vital, responsible subject.

Wendy Schain: As a clinical psychologist who has had two unilateral mastectomies, I feel very strongly that I want to respond to Mr. Rimer's desire to have specialized projects.

I am amazed at the absence of concern here for good empirical studies on aftercare for women who have had breast surgery. There is disproportionate emphasis now on detection and screening, but along with this increased awareness there are increases in cancer incidence and breast amputations. What happens to these women who have voiced to you, "We are concerned, we don't want to lose our breasts; we are afraid of a change in life style, a change in sexual gratification, a change in all kinds of relationships at home and with our loved ones." Few of these women have been reached postsurgery and actually asked what did happen. What was it like when they visualized their incision? With whom were they? Who helped give them information about appropriate and attractive kinds of prostheses? Whom did they go to for support? Reach to Recovery performs a very valuable service, but primarily it is a one- or two-time exposure to a woman who perhaps needs continuous exposure to somebody who has had the problem, and has effectively learned to cope with it. Betty Ford, Happy Rockefeller; we see a part of their exposure. We see them come out of the hospital and wave and say, "It didn't hurt a bit, girls." It does hurt. There are ways, though, to overcome it. There are ways to adapt to it. What we need to do is expose the realities, and to show women how to cope effectively with them. What are the processes of learning to defend against the fear of recurrence, the fear of death, the actual change in body image, and the possible consequences of mutilation?

There are needs for special projects, and I wonder if there couldn't be the possibility of including in a hospital, when a woman is faced with almost an assured likelihood of mastectomy, some kind of film or audiovisual about what she might be exposed to beginning with the time she wakes up in the recovery room with the drains and the bandages. Children who go in for heart surgery get a little doll and they know where tubes are going to be, they know the changes that are going to take place. I think the other thing that we really need to define clearly is what kinds of information we can communicate so that we arouse and not paralyze. I think our goal should be to reduce anxiety. We also need to explore carefully the timing, the amount of intervention, and the types of material most effective in helping women to deal with problems that they may live with for as long as 30 or 40 years. What about the possibility of periodic reinforcement clinics where women can go biannually or monthly, to share again at some emotional gut level what is going on, what the latest problems are, and some of the old angers that do recur, perhaps around anniversary times? There is no clinic I know of that is primarily devoted to coping with the symptoms of a mastectomy patient in addition to whatever other struggle she may be having. This is one of my ploys for specialized projects to a specialized population—those after the breast examination who have had amputation.

Hochbaum: In this discussion I hear at least three messages. One is that because I think our efforts in this area have a basic medical orientation, our efforts to change the thinking and the action of people usually focuses on a particular act that is desirable from the medical point of view. Get the person to quit smoking, get the person to come in for a checkup, get the person to undergo surgery, and so on. We forget that our goal in producing this kind of behavior may only be the beginning of the problems that the person faces. We have heard this story just now. The same holds true for the smoker and other people, but we feel that our job has been done when we have indoctrinated people with what we think they should know; when they have carried out the one act that we are concerned with, then we will forget about the patient or the person and go to another problem, to another person. I think it is very important to understand that the kind of actions required in the fight against cancer must bring about a rather fundamental change in the whole life style, in the feelings, in the personalities of the people concerned. It is something that we have not dealt with in our research and certainly not in practice.

That is one message that I got. The other is the importance of producing reliability in our messages. It is not necessary for everyone to know everything about the disease or the conditions involved. I don't think it is at all important. What is important is the person's point of view! What does he need and want to know in order to be encouraged and enabled to carry out certain actions that he sees are of benefit to him? That may or may not involve knowing exactly what kind of treatment is effective, under what conditions, with whom, or what kind of symptoms are associated with what kind of disease. Many of us are educated, intelligent, and aware of the health areas and the behavioral sciences. We are influenced by logic, reasoning, and facts. We like to think that we make our decisions based on this. But millions of people to whom we address ourselves in our communications are not like this or partially like this and many of these people do not need to know that much about the facts and reasons to make decisions and to act. I think that we have to be careful about this. The credibility to our audience is more important than what we tell them or how much detail we give. I want to respond to what Mr. Fink, Dr. Leventhal, and someone else mentioned. It is very strange and rather ironic that we are here to tell our colleagues in the health professions how to communicate effectively with and influence effectively the lay population. Yet we behavioral scientists constantly bemoan the fact that we are unable to influence the health professions, to communicate to them, and persuade them to change their behavior. Something about it is not quite right.

Cancer: The Behavioral Dimensions, edited by J. W. Cullen, B. H. Fox, and R. N. Isom. Raven Press, New York © 1976.

Introduction

Jack B. Haskins

University of Tennessee, Knoxville, Tennessee 37916

The mission of this section is twofold: to evaluate the impact of previous mass communications efforts to change health behavior, and to discuss how it might be used more effectively in future efforts.

To "evaluate the impact" of mass communications, or any other action, means to determine its effect. To determine the effect of any action, one must establish with a reasonable degree of certainty a cause-and-effect relationship between an independent variable (e.g., mass communications) and a dependent variable (e.g., health behavior). To establish such a cause-and-effect relationship, one must have a suitable research design (1). The research· design must be planned before the communication takes place; both the communication and the research should take place in a naturalistic real-life situation, preferably using unobtrusive measures of effect. There are other more detailed requirements of a suitable research design, but my point is that evaluating the impact of mass communications is not a haphazard subjective process.

To determine "how mass communications can be used more effectively in the future" implies that one has already evaluated the impact of previous mass communications efforts, that one has already determined the previous efforts are less than completely successful, that one has learned some general principles about what kinds of communication are successful and what kinds are unsuccessful, and that those principles will work in future communications campaigns.

Have previous cancer control communications campaigns been accompanied by the right kinds of research designs so that rigorous evidence about cause-and-effect is available? If so, how successful have those campaigns been? If some were successful, can we adequately pinpoint the communications techniques that worked as well as those that did not work?

If those questions cannot be answered satisfactorily, perhaps some answers are available from other sorts of health communications research, or from other sorts of public service communications research, or from advertising research. I do not believe that we can rely on evidence from previous cancer control communications campaigns. Having reviewed the state of the art regarding mass communications results on several other topics (e.g., fire prevention, drug abuse, drinking/driving, etc.), I assume that there is little if any acceptable evidence regarding cancer control communication per se.

I have prepared an "All-Purpose Review of What We Know about the Effect of Mass Communications on (INSERT ANY TOPIC)." I hope that the following chapters will make it necessary for me to scrap my all-purpose review in regard to cancer control communications.

AN ALL-PURPOSE REVIEW OF WHAT WE KNOW ABOUT THE EFFECTS OF MASS COMMUNICATIONS ON ANY SPECIFIC TOPIC

(Insert name of topic in blank spaces)

A review of the topical and research literature was undertaken to determine what is known about the effects of mass communications on _____. The findings are as follows:

(1)   A large number of education-information-communications campaigns aimed at changing _____ behavior have been conducted in the last few years.

(2)   On most of those _____ campaigns, no research at all was conducted to determine effectiveness.

(3)   Of those few campaigns where research was conducted, almost none used an adequate research design so that effects could be determined. Consequently, the principal conclusions from most was that "no conclusions can be drawn about communications effectiveness apart from other factors." Some of them drew unjustified conclusions based on wishful thinking, not evidence.

(4)   In three cases where adequate research was conducted, one showed positive effects of communication, one showed no effect, and one was counter-productive. However, it is impossible to determine just what aspects of the campaign produced success or failure.

(5)   Consequently, no clues are available to facilitate success of future communications campaigns to change _____ behavior.

I hope the state of the art in cancer control communications is better than the pessimistic picture just presented. But let us not be dismayed; looking over the whole scope of mass communications, not just cancer control or health behavior, a considerable body of evidence does exist.

A great deal of it, of course, comes from laboratory experiments on communications. And we can't always generalize from results obtained in the forced-exposure artificial environment of the laboratory to the real world of mass communications. However, in a monograph I prepared some years ago (2) concerning three dozen controlled field experiments on communications, a variety of topics were uncovered and there have been several others since then.

So, from the voluminous laboratory studies on communications, and more relevantly from the controlled field experiments, perhaps we now do have a basis of theory and fact on which cancer control communication efforts can proceed most efficiently and effectively. As Benjamin Franklin is reputed to have said, "The best physician is the one who knows the worthlessness of the most medicines."

Our speakers are here today as "communications physicians" to tell us about some things which have been found to be worthless and some which are worthwhile.

REFERENCES

1. Campbell, D. T., and Stanley, J. C. *Experimental and Quasi-Experimental Designs for Research*, Rand-McNally, Chicago, 1963.
2. Haskins, J. B. *How to Evaluate Mass Communications*, Advertising Research Foundation, New York, 1968.

Cancer: The Behavioral Dimensions, edited by J. W. Cullen,
B. H. Fox, and R. N. Isom. Raven Press, New York © 1976.

Mass Communications and Cancer Control

Harold Mendelsohn

University of Denver, Denver, Colorado 80210

To me, the current state of educational efforts in public health is frankly disappointing. I look at a recent finding from a national survey and learn with considerable shock that some three-quarters of the American public still do not know what the normal human body temperature is. I read reports from the National Safety Council that some $100 million in cash and donated space and time is spent annually in this country in mass communications efforts to control traffic accidents, and the very same reports indicate that the incidence of traffic fatalities in America persists at an alarming pace. I note that despite the concerted massive efforts of the responsible public health authorities throughout the land, the scientifically sound recommendation that communities fluoridate their drinking waters has met with stubborn and astonishingly effective public resistance.

Apparently my pessimism is shared by professionals in the area of cancer control as well. For example, the Report of the Conference Directors summing up the National Cancer Control Program Planning Conference notes that, "While public education has been one of the basic elements of cancer control for many years, it has not been markedly effective in the prevention of cancer. Moreover, the means of education concerning cancer have not been widely developed..." (p. 33).

There are many historical, sociological, and psychological reasons why current mass educational persuasion efforts in public health fall short of reflecting unmitigated successes. Time permits only a rough sketch of some of the more important ones.

Among the more obvious reasons for public education failures in cancer control are the emphases placed on "education" rather than on mass communications; the inability to articulate specific middle-range goals that are most amenable to mass communications processes; overemphasis on the presentation of anxiety-producing "facts" unaccompanied by reassurance and a sense of "hope"; rank amateurism at the hands of well-meaning though unsophisticated mass communications practitioners operating in the field; and an overall frightening lack of understanding of both the power and the shortcomings of mass communications in influencing human behavior.

If we are to become more effective in the future, we must introspect a bit and then apply ourselves to a more meaningful reorientation to the complex business of communicating health messages to the public in an effective manner. To do this, we must take note of four considerations I now offer for your attention.

1. *Social science has revolutionized our thinking about the power of mass communication's effectiveness.* The work of functionalists, such as Lazarsfeld, Merton, Riley and Riley, Klapper, Katz, and Mendelsohn, has seriously challenged the old behavioristic model of mass communication's effect as resulting from sheer exposure. No longer can effect be equated with simple exposure. Indeed, one can still produce this kind of phenomenon artificially in the laboratory by first exposing unsuspecting freshmen, for example, to speeches on buckwheat production in Bulgaria, and then measuring increments in so-called learning as a consequence. However, in real-life situations, this simply does not occur. As human beings, if we have no interest whatsoever in Bulgarian agriculture, we merely avoid being exposed to messages about it; or if we happen to come upon such messages by chance, we will ignore them or select only those things from them that may fit in with our prior prejudgments, interests, and likes; or we may simply forget everything about the subject to which we may have been forcibly exposed.

Additionally, the *new* social science approach to mass communications has demonstrated that factors of personality, social-economic position, prior interest and commitment, mass media habits, placement in informal networks of face-to-face communication, and individual motivation serve in varying complex ways to predispose people to mass media messages, and, at the same time, to intervene between what communicators intended to happen and what actually does happen in the communications situation.

In short, no longer can we cling to the old-fashioned notion that mass communication messages act directly and immediately upon individuals as if they had been injected with a powerful communications hypodermic needle. Rather than being a hypodermic needle, we now begin to look at mass communication as sort of an aerosol spray. As you spray it on the surface, some of it hits the target; most of it drifts away; and very little of it penetrates.

2. *The new orientation to mass communications sees the media as only one element in complex persuasive situations. This calls for the adoption of a new image of man that is suited to the new paradigm.* In our time, much of our mass communication efforts has been dominated by two basic images of man, neither of which serves as a viable model for effective mass communication in the cancer control area.

The predominant image of man sees him as a bundle of physiological needs and predispositions that are responsible for predetermined responses to external stimuli. Under this image of man, promulgated principally in the learning theories of behaviorist, stimulus-response psychologists, simple exposure to mass communications *is* equated with effect; that is, supposedly all one must do is expose people to messages under so-called rewarding circumstances and they will be influenced by these messages accordingly.

Given the fact that each of us encounters some 350 mass-communicated commercial messages daily plus countless public service and instrumental messages, we would become veritable perpetually bobbing yo-yos were we to be equally influenced by each and every one of these messages separately.

Obviously, we do not respond to every possible stimulus equally. All human beings are capable of selecting, discarding, modifying, distorting, ignoring, and avoiding the bombardment of messages to which we are all exposed every day of our lives.

Whether we react and how we react to messages are not only related to physiological "tissue" needs, but they are most importantly related to the widest array of social circumstances as well. Exposure may be a necessary variable in the mass communication process, but it is certainly not sufficient to guarantee called-for effect.

The second image of man is one we take great pride in—the image of *Homo sapiens*—man, the cognitive, thinking organism.

Within this rubric, man is seen primarily as a rational, discerning organism who acts in a "sensible" manner under most circumstances. In communicating with him, all we have to do is "educate" him to the "facts," and he will act prudently as a consequence. All we have to do, for example, is offer him data on the chemistry of fluorides, data on the incidence of dental caries infection in the population, and evidence of the effectiveness of fluorides in reducing dental caries among children, and *Homo sapiens,* being a "thinking" organism, will support fluoridation of public drinking waters as a consequence.

Yet, support for this apparent "rational" approach to a human disease has not been widespread, to say the least. Those "rational, *Homo sapiens* thinking" men who have been opposing community fluoridation have used irrational arguments such as: fluoridation causes kidney infections, mottled teeth, cancer of the mouth, and a variety of additional imagined ills; or that fluorides are poisons—poisons, by the way, that the Communists are using to take over America; or, from the opposite end of the political spectrum, the "rational" argument that fluoridation of community waters represents a serious threat to civil liberties by the unwarranted intrusion of government.

For me, the most telling illustration of the futility of relying solely on the cognitive image of man as a guideline for effective mass persuasion—and I am now speaking of *persuasion,* not education—is presented in the example of the man who, as he attentively peruses the Surgeon General's factual report of the correlation between cigarette smoking and lung cancer, becomes so tense that he lights a cigarette to ease his emerging anxiety.

If we are to be effective communicators, we must recognize that man is a complex organism who is partially rational and partially irrational; who sometimes responds to internal stimuli and at other times to external stimuli; and most of the time a combination of both. This complex man functions in complex social situations which he subjectively "defines" for himself in varied ways—no matter the amount of "facts" to which he may or may not have been exposed.

Because man is a complex actor-reactor in complex, ever-changing situations, we cannot pin him down and draw neat formulas about how we can affect him through the mass communication process. Alone, persuasive mass communications do not and cannot operate effectively without considerable institutional support.

Our image of man must be a dynamic one if we are to be effective communicators. Let us discard those handy but thoroughly misleading analogies between man, the complex human social organism, and simple-minded behavior-mod mechanistic models that compare him with laboratory rats or with thermostats, combustion engines, or with electronic systems.

3. *Too much of the mass communication efforts in public health are oriented to presenting factual information and to attempts at changing attitudes. Too little is devoted to the fundamental problems of altering socially derived perceptions and affording both insights into actual health threats and reassurance regarding their proper and effective control.* By now, it is almost a cliche that people's perceptions of what comprises a health threat are fundamentally a function of two interacting variables: *perceived* susceptibility plus *perceived* severity. Notice that we emphasize the *perceptions* of phenomena, rather than the objective existence of them. Health percepts, including those relating to cancer, are culturally rooted and defined. When an individual becomes aware of a health threat in terms of his own subjective estimates of susceptibility and severity, the specific actions he will take will be determined most often by his own private values, attitudes, and beliefs about amelioration rather than by the values that are promulgated by "outsider" health "authorities."

In my opinion, past public educational efforts in the cancer area have over-emphasized the matters of threat and severity and have produced what mass communications researchers call a dysfunctional boomerang effect—one that is antithetical to the objective intended. Rather than moving audiences to precautionary and ameliorative action, factual information overemphasizing the threats and severity of cancer have served to frighten them into immobility for the most part.

Because mass communications are capable of manipulating symbols, they have the potentiality of changing *perceptions* of the potentialities of cure and survival as well as information levels and attitudes. However, symbol manipulation requires a substantial amount of prior insight into their social determinants, their unique meanings for different persons, their functions in sustaining individuals and groups, and into their power either to implement or hinder change, before attempts at mass persuasion can become even moderately effective. In the area of cancer control, we must focus first on altering how various publics perceive the possibilities of cure and survival well before we attempt to change information levels and attitudes regarding the matter.

For many years, it was thought that we could change attitudes directly by communicating information directly to audiences. Even the pioneer work done by Hovland and his associates at Yale some 25 years ago demonstrated quite contrarily that changes in informational levels are not necessarily accompanied by changes in attitudes. This is particularly true where we attempt to alter those tenaciously held central core attitudes that we acquire, as one psychologist wag put it, "at our mother's knee and in various other joints."

Moreover, we no longer insist that attitudes are "predispositions to action." Instead, the modern approach to attitudes views them simply as psychological valuations that we place on persons, things, and ideas in hierarchical fashion. Some things we treat as more important than others; others we consider to be bad or not worthwhile. Our actions may or may not be governed by our attitudes. Consequently, changes in attitudes need not be accompanied always by changes in behavior.

Unfortunately, in the health area, we encounter vague unspecified kinds of attitudes and beliefs among various publics. Health is something that exists obscurely in the background, like motherhood and loyalty. It is something that people "ought" to be concerned with, but surprisingly few of us really seem to give a damn. There are far more important things from the psychological point of view as far as the public is concerned. The public is much more concerned with whether they are loved, whether they are powerful, whether they are socially accepted, whether they are attractive or beautiful, or whether they are successful. America's advertisements are the mirrors of America's major concerns—not our health education texts. These concerns are considerably more important to people than the hierarchy of self-attitudes relating to whether they are healthy or whether they are living in a clean, well-governed, wholesome community. Such matters require a lot of effort. To begin with, they are quite drab and unexciting. No glamour is attached to them, and in a cultural milieu that glorifies "fun," there really is very little fun that can be associated with such dull matters as cancer control. Not only is the matter of cancer dull, it is deadly frightening as well. Certainly, the endless statistics, graphs and charts, technical jargon, insipid slogans, and incessant admonitions that clutter up so much of our health communications do much to destroy even what little sense of excitement the public may generate on its own from time to time.

Why the lay public should be concerned about their health is a question we may all ask ourselves. Self-survival seems to be but one of the many reasons that makes common sense in this regard. Yet, as just one case in point, the facts on ever-mounting household, farm, industrial, and traffic accidents alone in this country do little to sustain the thesis that man is motivated primarily by self-survival.

Let us turn to another problem. Many people who use the mass media for education and persuasion have a quixotic notion that they can "modify" or change "bad" habits, alter "wrong" attitudes or correct "improper" behavior simply by promulgating a few "messages." In other words, there is a naive segment in the education-communication fraternity who continue to insist that conversion can be accomplished readily and painlessly through the mass communication process. A mountain of scientific evidence demonstrates that conversion rarely occurs and only under the most complex of psychological, sociological, and communications circumstances. Ask any missionary, politician, or psychotherapist.

Research evidence has shown that, rather than converting audiences, the mass media serve essentially to reinforce what they may already believe or do or what they would like to believe or do. Furthermore, the mass media reinforce, more often than not, what audiences already like or dislike, and they serve to underpin what audiences have already learned in the past.

To look at people merely from a rational point of view, to view them as being capable of altering their attitudes, habits, and action patterns drastically once they are merely communicated the "facts," will usually result in ineffective communication. It simply does not work. People are not interested in "the facts" by themselves, and frequently—most frequently—the public does not know what to do with the facts when they are given them, unless we as communicators tell them what to do, and then show them what to do and how to do it in an explicit, interesting, dramatic, and, most important, persuasive manner.

4. *We must end the confusion between mass education and mass persuasion in public health.* The health communicators not only have the obligation to give certain factual information to the public they seek to serve but, most importantly, they have the obligation to interpret and dramatize those facts so that they may be able to alter public perceptions of health threats realistically.

In mass communication, we often try to persuade people, rather than merely educate them, to get them to behave in a manner that will be not only ameliorative from the individual's point of view, but from the long-range social point of view as well. As persuasive communicators, we must drop the euphemistic "education" mantle. Let us leave education to the educators. Educators do not necessarily make persuasive, effective communicators. Nor do effective communicators necessarily make the best teachers. I think this is a most important distinction to keep in mind in laying down mass communication strategies for controlling cancer.

Education seeks simply to *expand* the intellectual horizons of the individual so that he ultimately can make *rational* choices from among alternatives—nothing more. It does not seek to change behavior per se, nor should it. Persuasion, on the other hand, tries to *limit* choices and control percepts to the degree that audiences begin to pursue only those goals that the communicator wants them to pursue, be it rationally or otherwise. In other words, where education enlightens, letting the chips fall where they may, persuasion, quite unabashedly, manipulates. If we are to be successful in our public health efforts, it is obvious that we must do both: enlighten and, like it or not, persuade.

Mass communications can be effective in the persuasive process as well as in the educational one. By themselves, however, mass communications cannot *create* a healthy population. Urging people to be healthy through the mass communications media is as inane and wasteful as prodding them to be "good," "unselfish," or to be "safe." Cajoling, moralizing, and nagging are not persuading. Much of what we see in so-called mass education in public health today is more often designed to please the whims of some well-meaning board members than it is to accomplish meaningful effects. Most of it comes from the fertile imaginations of sincere but totally unprofessional weekend sloganeers. The great majority of these efforts are generally relayed to the public without benefit of sound scientific rationales, careful pretesting, or objective systematic post hoc evaluation. All too often a bulging scrapbook is offered as evidence of effect rather than hard data on whether the communications had actually accomplished the changes and actions that were intended.

In their persuasive roles, the mass media can be of tremendous utility in producing insights into discrepancies that exist between the subjective estimates that various publics hold of certain health risks and the actual inherent risks. There is considerable evidence to indicate that such alignments of subjective and objective risk estimates can be accomplished more effectively through the devices of drama and storytelling than through sheer exposition of facts. The mass media are far more adept at using the former techniques for persuasion than they are at conveying bits of tasteless, dull, and unwanted information. Whether we like it or not, popular TV programs, such as "Medical Center" and "Marcus Welby, M.D.," are actually conveying insights into a wide range of health problems as they are entertaining their audiences.

It must be borne in mind that the media's principal powers, particularly that of television, lie in their ability to demonstrate, to interpret, and to dramatize, rather than to educate. Consider for a moment the positive impacts of actually seeing the smiling faces of Mrs. Ford and Mrs. Rockefeller emerging in high spirits from their respective mastectomies. Compare these images in terms of public impact with the countless pamphlets, brochures, posters, TV commercials, and the like offering factual information of the incidence, prevention, and treatment of breast cancer that have been aimed at the public over the past decades.

I must emphasize that I am not suggesting that "Marcus Welby, M.D.," or "Medical Center" are suitable vehicles for effective health communication in the area of cancer control. I am quite aware of their shortcomings as media for serious public health communication. What I mean to stress is that the mass media can be extremely powerful in involving audiences with the abstract matters of health in dramatic, personalized ways, and in so involving people they can become quite capable of affording insights that might ultimately produce ameliorative actions.

What we must do is make the most vigorous study of this power of mass communications so that it may be harnessed in the service of sustaining a sound public health situation. This is a particularly thorny task, because it means discarding a panoply of comfortable, hoary nostrums relating to so-called public service communication and mass health education. Instead of loping along with our trusty but usually ignored slogans, fact sheets, brochures, and annual reports, we must now turn to new vistas, to untried orientations, and to imaginative and novel communications techniques. This can be done only by bringing professional communicators together with communications scientists to work out these modes of mass persuasion empirically and in tandem—all oriented to the question, "What if information campaigns were designed to reflect empirically grounded mass communications theories and principles?"

What little empirical experience we have accumulated from the past suggests that public information campaigns have relatively high success potentials:

1. If they are planned around the assumption that most of the publics to which they will be addressed will be either only mildly interested or not at all interested in what is being communicated.
2. If explicitly stated, middle-range goals, which can be reasonably achieved as a consequence of exposure, are set up as specific objectives.
3. If, after middle-range objectives are set, careful consideration is given to

delineating specific targets in terms of their demographic and psychological attributes, their life styles, values and belief systems, and mass media habits. Here, it is important not only to determine the scope of prior indifference, but to uncover its roots as well.

4. If campaigns are grounded in sound scientific principles and are accompanied by systematic, formative, implemental, and evaluative effects research.

Our experience at the University of Denver in developing such highly successful Emmy-winning socially ameliorative public information efforts as the CBS *National Driver's Test* and *Cancion de la Raza* has convinced us that only from complex processes of research, creativity, and evaluation working together can innovative, meaningful, and effective mass communications guidelines for controlling health threats be developed. Hopefully, this kind of systematic approach can be applied successfully to the many complex problems to which this conference has addressed itself.

Cancer: The Behavioral Dimensions, edited by J. W. Cullen, B. H. Fox, and R. N. Isom. Raven Press, New York © 1976.

The Potential of Mass Communication and Interpersonal Communication for Cancer Control

Matilda Butler and William Paisley*

Applied Communication Research, Inc., Palo Alto, California 94300; and* Institute for Communication Research, Stanford University, Stanford, California 94305

Four major types of messages flow from mass communication media to the public. The types can be characterized either from the sender's perspective in terms of intent or from the receiver's perspective in terms of effect.

From the sender's perspective, the types are:

1. *Entertainment*—The sender asks for the receiver's attention on the premise, "This message will divert you, amuse you, make you sad, etc."
2. *Information*—The sender's premise is, "This message contains facts that will help you make decisions, look out for yourself, anticipate future developments, etc."
3. *News*—The sender's premise is, "This message concerns something 'news-worthy' that has happened. It is my responsibility to tell you about it, whether or not it entertains you or helps you personally in any way."
4. *Persuasion*—The sender's premise is, "This message concerns a change that you should make in your beliefs or behavior."

The effect of a message on the receiver may or may not be congruent with the sender's intent. A message intended to entertain may have the effect of informing. A message intended to persuade may have the effect of informing, entertaining, and so forth.

Indeed, in the flow of millions of messages through communications media, senders find it advantageous to combine message types in the same communication, so that information will appear to be entertainment, or persuasion will appear to be information, and so on. Receivers who cannot be reached under one premise are thus reached under another.

Many social institutions assume the role of sender in this process, each for its own reasons. Government agencies seek to explain and justify their activities. According to their mandates (e.g., to improve public health), they may also seek to change public beliefs and behavior. Political parties, lobbies, businesses, and labor unions join government agencies in informing and cajoling the public.

Communication media are themselves the chief producers of news and entertainment messages. They are less concerned than government, business, and so on, with "message as content" and more concerned with "message as commodity."

Messages disseminated by "public communication programs" generally combine informative and persuasive intents. Relative proportions of information and persuasion in such messages vary according to public knowledge and public beliefs/behaviors surrounding the topic of concern. Topics of major public communication programs of the present and recent past have included such causes as: smoking, cancer control, heart disease prevention, automobile safety, environmental protection, energy conservation, consumer economics, drug abuse, civil rights. In addition to these programs, which involve substantial information content, various agencies carry on programs that are essentially devoid of information content and extend over decades as slogan campaigns (an example is Smokey the Bear's campaign to prevent forest fires).

Early public communication programs were predicated on assumptions of direct mass communication effects on "target audiences." Particularly in the post-World War II period, communication researchers have recognized the minimal role that mass communication media can play by themselves, without reinforcement from interpersonal communication networks, in either informing or persuading the public. An understanding of the complementary roles of mass communication and interpersonal communication sets the stage for an era of "social communication engineering" that can be used to increase public knowledge and utilization of social benefits—health care, education, vocational opportunity, and so forth.

OBJECTIVES OF THE NATIONAL CANCER CONTROL PROGRAM

The overall goal of the National Cancer Institute's Cancer Control Program is "to reduce the incidence, disability, suffering, and mortality from cancer" (1). This goal is being addressed via five objectives (1):

PREVENTION, where knowledge of causative factors permits
SCREENING AND DETECTION, to avoid progression of the disease by finding it in the earliest possible stages
DIAGNOSIS AND TREATMENT, to accomplish the maximum in cure through the most modern techniques
REHABILITATION, for those in need of special restorative measures
CONTINUING CARE, for those who must live with cancer.

Each objective calls for action both from health professionals and from the public. The amount and type of action, the locus of initiative, and aspects of coordination and timing vary considerably, however, from one objective to another.

Some of the action steps that will be required to achieve these objectives were outlined by one of the Cancer Control Program's planning groups (2):

Prevention

1. Increase the understanding of the public and health professionals of measures that would reduce the risk of cancer
2. Motivate people to take steps to reduce the risk, morbidity, and mortality of cancer

Screening and Detection

3. Identify, field test, and evaluate screening tests that have the greatest potential for reducing morbidity and mortality
4. Demonstrate and promote the widespread application of practical and effective screening methods

Diagnosis and Pretreatment Evaluation

5. Aid professional groups in the assessment of current practices and in the development of principles for the optimal diagnosis and pretreatment evaluation of cancer
6. Field test, evaluate, demonstrate, and promote measures for the optimal diagnosis and pretreatment evaluation of persons with precancerous or cancerous lesions

Treatment

7. Promote optimal, comprehensive, and continuous treatment and follow-up care for each cancer patient

Rehabilitation

8. Identify, field test, evaluate, demonstrate, and promote widespread application of measures for the optimal rehabilitation of patients

Continuing Care

9. Identify, field test, evaluate, demonstrate, and promote widespread application of methods for the optimal continuing care of patients with recurrent or disseminated cancer.

Scattered throughout the nine action steps are initiatives that should be taken by cancer researchers, clinicians, educators, communicators, and the public. In all initiatives that involve the public, we find that conditions of knowledge, attitude, and behavior are implied. That is, the public should understand, accept, and adopt measures to reduce risk. The public should be aware of, accept, and seek out appropriate opportunities for screening. The public should understand, accept, and cooperate with the requirements of optimal diagnosis, pretreatment evaluation, treatment, rehabilitation, and continuing care. Particularly in rehabilitation and continuing care, the public should understand, accept, and carry out many self-care steps.

Thus, in addition to initiatives that researchers and clinicians should undertake, initiatives critical to the success of the Cancer Control Program lie with the public. Generally, the public neither understands, accepts, nor acts upon principles of risk reduction, early detection, prompt and full cooperation with treatment, and so on. The role of educators and communicators in the Cancer Control Program is chiefly to affect public knowledge, attitude, and behavior in such a way that cancer control opportunities created by researchers and clinicians are not impeded, but rather facilitated, by the public response to them.

THE ROLE OF COMMUNICATION IN IMPLEMENTING PUBLIC PROGRAMS

Communication is perhaps society's most fundamental process. Other essential processes, from political participation to the distribution of social benefits such as health care and education, depend on channels of communication that are open, free, and managed in the public interest.

Studies of mass and interpersonal communication, as well as the experience of professional communicators, attest to the subtle forces at work in effective communication. Despite any amount of money that may be spent on communication programs for the public benefit, the line between success and failure in such programs is a narrow one.

The outcomes of any public communication program are mixed. Subgroups of the public respond differently according to factors related to demography, knowledge and attitudes, prior experience, and so forth. An example of differential effect is provided in a letter to *Science* by Schneiderman and Peters of the National Cancer Institute (1972):

> Substantial progress has been made in preventing cancer. The antismoking campaigns have been much more effective than many people seem to be aware. So much so that if there is anything to the smoking-cancer link, we should soon see declines in lung cancer mortality in white males. From 1965 to 1970, 42 percent more men and 37 percent more women became 'former smokers.'

Counterbalancing these successes are the relative failures:

> However, the incidence of lung cancer in women and in blacks is increasing. Too many women smoke; too few are giving it up. At one time the ratio of male to female deaths from lung cancer was nearly 7:1. It is now 4:1, and not because male deaths have declined. The antismoking campaigns have not done as well as we would like among women, and among blacks.
> There is a need for a vigorous, well-directed, antismoking campaign that would appeal to blacks, to women, and to young people.

Why are some programs failures and some successes? Why have white males heeded the mass media antismoking programs while women, blacks, and young people have not heard or have not heeded the persuasive messages? Answers to these questions lie in the history of communication research.

Precursors of modern communication research were Lippmann, a journalist and "public philosopher," and Lasswell, a political scientist. Lippmann, in writing about "The World Outside and Pictures in Our Heads" (3), founded a tradition of research in which concepts of "stereotyping" and "imagery" have led to more rigorous theories of "subjective reality." Lasswell's "Propaganda Technique in the World War" (1927) was a cornerstone of pre-World War II communication theory, in which powerful and immediate effects of communication media on mass audiences were asserted. The "bullet theory" of communication effects introduced the concept of the "target audience;" these military metaphors are a not-accidental consequence of Lasswell's work.

Lazarsfeld, Merton, and their colleagues (4) at Columbia University must be credited with blunting the "bullet theory." In studies of communication behavior during the 1940 presidential election campaign, the Columbia researchers found little evidence of direct media effects on electoral attitude or behavior. Rather, it seemed that "opinion leaders" were attuned to the mass media and that they in turn influenced others in their social networks, but not necessarily in the directions that mass media were advocating.

The "two-step flow" theory that resulted from the Columbia research has survived in various permutations up to the present. Research that continued to find direct media effects, for example, Merton's study (5) of the outcomes of the Kate Smith war bond marathon has had to be interpreted in terms of unique aspects of communicator credibility, message appeal, audience readiness to respond, ease of response, and so forth.

Hyman and Sheatsley (6) published their now-famous article in 1947. The list of points they covered can still be found on the agenda of communication research:

Chronic "Know Nothings" in Relation to Information Campaigns
The Role of Interest in Increasing Exposure
Selective Exposure Produced by Prior Attitudes
Selective Interpretation Following Exposure
Differential Changes in Attitudes after Exposure.

Doubly upset by their egalitarian biases and by the limited success of communication programs that they have planned, communication researchers have been forced to agree with a conclusion drawn by Hyman and Sheatsley: "There is something about the uninformed that makes them harder to reach, no matter what the level or nature of the information."

In postwar communication research we see the "mass audience" concept of earlier research become more subtle and textured. Audience variables of prior knowledge and attitude as well as post-message interpretation become major predictors of attitude and behavior change.

A public education program was undertaken shortly after the Hyman and

Sheatsley article appeared. It is now well known as the Cincinnati Plan for the United Nations (Star and Hughes, 1948). The variable of interest proved crucial in determining why some people paid attention to the campaign while others did not. The authors write:

> A survey ... demonstrated that it is those already interested, even if poorly informed, who will welcome information, while the well informed, if not interested, pay little attention to it, and that the interested also tend to be favorably inclined toward the United Nations. Therefore, the recommendation was made that the campaign be planned so as to interest certain specified classes which were found to be the most in need of enlightenment. But a second survey made immediately after the campaign disclosed that the materials circulated by the plan, voluminous and ingenious though they were, reached few of these people. The principle derived from the experiment is that information, to be disseminated at all, must be functional, that is, interesting to the ordinary man because he has been made to see that it impinges upon his own affairs.

Three major studies published by the mid-1950s pointed to the next direction for communication research. Katz and Menzel, in a study of the diffusion of a new drug among physicians in four cities (8,9), expanded the "two-step flow" theory to any number of steps or nodes in the progress of a message through a social network. Rogers and Shoemaker state a current view of the "multistep flow" theory (10):

> It does not call for any particular number of steps nor does it specify that the message must emanate from a source by mass media channels. This model suggests that there are a variable number of relays in the communication flow from a source to a large audience. Some members will obtain the message directly through channels from the source, while others may be several times removed from the message origin. The exact number of steps in this process depends on the intent of the source, the availability of mass media and the extent of audience exposure, the nature of the message, and salience of the message to the receiving audience.

Zimmerman and Bauer (11) indicated that audiences remember message elements selectively, at least partly in accord with what they perceive to be interesting and acceptable information for audiences to whom they in turn will serve as communicators in the multistep flow.

The third work indicative of future directions was that of Cartwright (12). His research, now the basis of a major public communication program in three California communities (the SCOR heart disease prevention program coordinated by Stanford University), integrated concepts of media presentation and concepts of small-group dynamics.

Meanwhile, Hovland, after leaving the War Department's Information and Education Division, had established an attitude research laboratory at Yale. There he and his colleagues studied communicator, message, context, and audience variables under controlled conditions, achieving results so different from those of field studies that he found it necessary to address the difficult problem of "Reconciling Conflicting Results Derived from Experimental and Survey Studies of Attitude Change" (13), emphasizing personal and social factors that are dominant in field settings but largely suppressed in the laboratory.

Communication research in the 1960s was strongly influenced by two statements. Klapper's "The Effects of Mass Communication" (14) argued that the role of mass media was chiefly to reinforce attitudes and behavior patterns that the social network was initially responsible for creating. Klapper explored the limited circumstances in which mass media might change attitudes and behavior in themselves.

Bauer (15) summarized conclusions of persuasion research that were, in most cases, antitheses of the "bullet theory" of 30 years before. In a debunking vein, he reanalyzed data from the Kate Smith war bond marathon and wrote:

> I have made some computations on the famous Kate Smith war bond marathon, which elicited $39 million in pledges. Kate Smith moved apparently a maximum of 4 percent of her audience to pledge to buy bonds; the more realistic figure may be 2 percent.

Schramm (16) says about these early years of communication research that:

> ... the most dramatic change in general communication theory during the last 40 years has been the gradual abandonment of the idea of a passive audience, and its replacement by the concept of a highly active, highly selective audience, manipulated by a message—a full partner in the communication process.
>
> To appreciate the magnitude of this change, one must recall how frightening World War I propaganda, and later Communist and Nazi propaganda, were to many people. At that time, the audience was typically thought of as a sitting target; if a communicator could hit it, he would affect it. This became especially frightening because of the reach of the new mass media. The unsophisticated viewpoint was that if a person could be reached by the insidious forces of propaganda carried by the mighty power of the mass media, he could be changed and converted and controlled. So propaganda became a hate word, the media came to be regarded fearfully, and laws were passed and actions taken to protect "defenseless" people against "irresistible" communication.

The early 1970s bring signs of a balanced view that rejects both the "powerful media" and "obstinate audience" alternatives. Careful research reviews of the late 1960s, for example, Sears and Freedman on selective exposure to communication (17); Higbee on fear-arousal messages (18) showed configurations of interacting factors from which different effects on attitude and behavior might be predicted.

Symptomatic of the current view is Mendelsohn's (19) 26-year sequel to Hyman and Sheatsley. Mendelsohn criticized previous research that evaluated public communication programs in which no research-derived principles contributed to strategy or content. He argued that teams of researchers and communicators can plan and execute successful communication programs as long as:

1. They are planned around the assumption that most of the publics to which they will be addressed will be either only mildly interested or not at all interested in what is communicated
2. Middle-range goals which can be reasonably achieved as a consequence of exposure are set as specific objectives
3. Careful consideration is given to delineating specific targets in terms of their demographic and psychological attributes, their life styles, value and belief systems, and mass media habits.

Mendelsohn's success stories include the "CBS National Drivers' Test," a short film entitled "A Short History," and a 65-installment "Chicano information-giving soap opera series" designed for the Los Angeles area.

The 1970s are proving to be a decade in which earlier predictions of media effect are being borne out, in limited but useful ways, by communication programs that are designed "from the ground up" on the basis of research-derived principles. For example, in the SCOR heart disease prevention program coordinated by Stanford, the researchers have established three communication conditions in three California communities. One community receives specially designed mass media messages only. These messages emphasize smoking reduction, exercise, dietary changes, and so on. The second community receives the same mass media messages, but, in addition, small groups of high-risk males have been formed. They meet with speakers and consultants who help them understand the effects of diet, exercise, and smoking on their health. The third community, serving as the control, gets neither the specially designed media campaign nor the small groups. Results from the second year show a continuum of effects across the three communities with the control group showing some changes, primarily in the area of smoking reduction, the media-only community showing greater changes, and the media-small group communities registering quite significant changes. Changes in all three communities are measured physiologically, affectively, and cognitively. Some unobtrusive measures are used to check for food consumption pattern changes.

The past 40 years have taught us much about the use of mass media to inform and persuade. We have seen cases in which the media failed to help in the implementation of public programs and we have seen cases in which the media were quite effective. We now realize that more factors interact in determining the success of mass media programs than previous studies have encompassed.

THE HIERARCHY OF COMMUNICATION EFFECTS

Behavioral researchers distinguish among the effects of messages of knowledge, attitude, and behavior. It is clear from a half-century of communication research (beginning with Lippmann, 1922 and Lasswell, 1927) that these components of response, as they may be called, are differently affected by communication events that differ in source, channel (medium), message content, and so on. However, principles of differential effect and relationships among response components are far from clear.

Characteristics of communication events interact with characteristics of audiences to strengthen or diminish their effects on knowledge, attitude, and behavior. Channel differences (e.g., interpersonal channels, print media, electronic media) are related to exposure probabilities for different audiences. Sources regarded as credible for new knowledge may not be credible for new attitudes or behaviors. Sources credible to one audience may not be credible to another.

The sequence of response to communication (e.g., whether behavior change is preceded by attitude change and attitude change by knowledge change) is much debated by behavioral researchers. If a single sequence of responses, such as the common-sensical sequence of knowledge → attitude → behavior, always occurs, then a program can concentrate on addressing the first-occurring response component first, and so forth.

However, other plausible sequences of responses can be argued. From the perspective of dissonance theory (20), if behavior change can be induced for its own sake, then attitude and finally knowledge will change to become more consistent with the new behavior. An important variable in the dissonance-theory sequence of behavior → attitude → knowledge is each person's perceived latitude to comply or not to comply with the suggested behavior change. If the person perceives no alternative to compliance, then she or he will suffer no "cognitive dissonance" and require no compensating change in attitudes and knowledge. However, if the person perceives that compliance was freely chosen, then "cognitive dissonance" will trouble her or him to the extent that the new behavior is discrepant with behavior that would have been predicted from previously held attitudes and knowledge.

Conditions under which each of these effect sequences is likely to occur are explored in an important comparative analysis by Ray (21). He introduces, in fact, a third sequence, knowledge → behavior → attitude, as the probable outcome of Krugman's "learning without involvement" theory (22).

CONSTELLATORY NATURE OF COMMUNICATION EFFECTS

Mentalistic psychology, driven almost underground a half-century ago by behaviorism, shows new vigor in its applicability and adaptability to problems of psychosocial effect in complex, large-scale, field-based public communication programs. Nurtured by clinical psychologists, the mentalistic school offers relevant perspectives on motivation and effect. Nurtured by phenomenologists, the mentalistic school offers relevant perspectives on "pictures in the head" or "images" that, far more than demographic differences, divide the mass audience into individuals who receive different messages from the outside world according to their prior experiences and/or combine messages in new mental composites that are uniquely (i.e., phenomenologically) their own.

In the age of electronic media, "image" has come to mean a prepackaging or staging of impressions, a play upon audience pride or prejudice. In fact, however, the image has a more basic role in perception and cognition than advertising agencies and public relations firms conceive. Before there were media, there were images of people, places, times. Then, as now, a person's mental life consisted primarily of images.

In his landmark study (23), Boulding writes:

> As I sit at my desk, I know where I am. I see before me a window; beyond that some trees ... the roof tops which mark the town of Palo Alto ... the bare golden hills of the Hamilton Range. I know, however, more than I see. Behind me, although I am not looking in that direction, I know there is a window ... beyond that the Coast Range ... the Pacific Ocean. Looking ahead of me again, I know that beyond the mountains that close my present horizon there is a broad valley; beyond that a higher range of mountains....

After continuing to describe his sense of orientation in space, time, personal relations, and the world of nature, Boulding states:

> What I have been talking about is knowledge. Knowledge, perhaps, is not a good word for this. Perhaps one would rather say my "image" of the world. Knowledge has an implication of validity, of truth. What I am talking about is what I believe to be true; my subjective knowledge. It is this image that largely governs my behavior.

Boulding's "image" was the basis for a theoretical book by Miller, Galanter, and Pribram (24), that deals more with behavior sequences than with percepts or cognitions. The "plan" postulated by Miller and his colleagues has been formed from images, but it contains a dynamic or frankly purposive element that shapes a person's behavior ("purpose" was perhaps the mentalistic variable most often criticized by behaviorists). It is a small step from Miller's abstract "plan" to the "life management plan" that researchers now begin to recognize as an organizing principle behind the statements and behaviors of respondents in field studies.

Although it undoubtedly contains knowledge, attitude, and behavior elements, an individual's "life management plan" owes more to his or her images, or subjective reality, than to these perhaps artificially distinguished constructs. Basic psychosocial research is needed on the question of whether knowledge, attitude, and behavior have independent status as communication effects, or whether they represent inseparable aspects of a person's global image of himself or herself, other persons, space, time, nature, logic, and causality, and so on, that we are increasingly disposed to call the "life management plan."

If it is found that communication effects are more "constellatory" than separate, then the question of sequence becomes moot and empirical conditions under which one or another sequence seems to have occurred become conditions for eliciting one or another facet of an integral but partly hidden constellation.

FACTORING THE PREDICTORS OF EFFECT IN COMMUNICATION PROGRAMS

Figure 1 synthesizes some of the intrapersonal factors that communication research and basic psychological research reveal as important predictors of message effect. Because a person's early experience continuously interacts with later experience to form a subjective reality, "socialization influences" are shown on the periphery of the self. School, church, family, work, peers, and other socialization influences form the person's first and continuing "social construction of reality" [cf. Berger and Luckmann (25)]. Media are a lifelong socialization influence; with the rise of audiovisual media, audiences are shown explicitly how to react to an enormous variety of situations, including, for example, suspected illness and diagnosed illness.

Surrounding the person are factors from his or her past or present that filter incoming messages and shape the image that the person will retain from them. In this illustration, it is not important that these particular factors are the most significant set. Rather, all such factors are theoretical constructs; they belong to

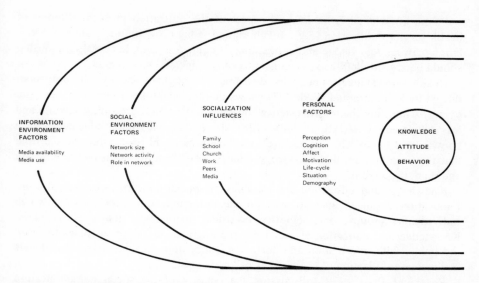

Fig. 1 Knowledge, attitude and behavior are created and reinforced through the interaction of personal factors (past and present), social environment factors, and information environment factors.

the mind of the researcher, not necessarily the mind of the person. They have only heuristic value; that is, by taking account of them, it may be possible to devise more effective public communication programs.

Additional factors reside in the social environment surrounding the person and in the information environment of sources, channels, and messages. Adopting the perspective of most public communication programs, that is, quite far away from individual members of the "target audience" both in psychological and physical terms, we can see why communication effects are elusive and unpredictable. From the time it is born as a concept within the communication program to the time it modifies a person's image in such a way as to produce desired outcomes, the message may have traveled over several networks and through many phases of transformation, some of them external to the person, the others internal.

COMMUNICATION RESEARCH AND SOCIAL COMMUNICATION ENGINEERING

Despite the obvious need for improvement in the availability and accessibility of cancer control services, it is true that public knowledge and utilization of such services lag considerably behind changes in their actual availability and accessibility. At a time when particularly rapid change is expected in the provision of services, important questions of public knowledge and utilization need to be addressed, both through research and through action programs.

Public knowledge is an integral aspect of the utilization problem. Studies of health services utilization [e.g., Eichhorn and Aday (26)] routinely show a correlation between knowledge and utilization. Of course, no simple causal relationship should be argued—utilization can lead to knowledge and vice versa.

Health knowledge is unequally distributed throughout society. A study conducted by Schramm and Wade (27) shows that the health knowledge "haves" are young, white, and better educated while the "have nots" are old, nonwhite and less educated. Utilization studies (28) show that the better-educated health knowledge "haves" in fact require little health care and readily receive the little that they require. Health knowledge "have nots" require extensive health care and do not receive it.

Knowledge and utilization are variables of special concern to the social communication engineer who focuses on the communication processes by which individuals, groups, and societies co-orient themselves and achieve goals. Knowledge and utilization also concern the engineer in her or his plans to reach the public with information and persuasion campaigns to raise knowledge levels and increase utilization of social services and benefits.

Rees and Paisley (29), discussing the concept of the social communication engineer in 1968, wrote:

> Our growing knowledge of the operation of communication systems, including information seeking and media use behavior, leads to communication strategies fitted to needs and dispositions of the target audience.
> This adaptive approach, based on message/channel/audience analysis, committed to objectives rather than institutions, might be called "social communication engineering." ... its success depends upon the best application of new knowledge in the development of innovative strategy.

The social communication engineer envisioned by Rees and Paisley is concerned with an interweaving cycle of research and action steps. Cyclically, the engineer needs answers to these six questions:

1. What is the current status of the problem (e.g., public delay in seeking cancer screening, diagnosis, or treatment)?
2. Drawing upon appropriate theories of communication behavior and health behavior, how can the problem be explicated into compensable and uncompensable aspects?
3. Given financial resources, medical backup, ethical and legal constraints, and so on, what is the range of alternative strategies that may deal effectively with the problem?
4. How can the most reasonable of these strategies be tested for effectiveness?
5. How can the strategy that "passes" be refined and extended to reach maximum effectiveness?
6. How can the short-term and long-term outcomes of the strategy be evaluated?

The social communication engineer answers the first question with system-status research. This phase provides data on problem-associated behaviors as well as on public knowledge, attitudes, contextual variables, and so forth.

The engineer answers the second question with problem-definition research. The second phase focuses precisely on interrelationships among problem associated behaviors and their probable antecedents. The engineer looks for enough evidence of a theoretically reasonable pattern to "get on with" an exploration of intervention points and related strategies.

The third question leads to strategy-formation research. This phase is marked by the systematic nomination and review of alternative strategies. The emphasis changes from "What is the problem?" (number 1), and "What causes the problem?" (number 2), to "What can be done about the problem?"

To answer the fourth question, the engineer designs an environment (laboratory or field setting) in which alternative strategies can be tested, with restrictions as necessary on the time period during which the alternatives are allowed to run and the size of population samples involved with each alternative. Carrying a single alternative into this phase—a common aspect of "nonengineered" programs—leaves only the binary possibilities of success or failure. Carrying multiple alternatives into this phase, even at the expense of the thoroughness with which each is tested, leaves the engineer with a range of choices for each criterion that the program is intended to meet. Multiple testing also allows for the serendipitous finding that two or more alternatives are equally successful but with different groups or in different contexts.

The fifth question leads to more precise study of the "winning strategy," so that it can be refined—"tuned" or "calibrated"—and extended in its application. Greater effect for lesser cost is the criterion of this phase.

The sixth question is by far the most difficult and controversial. An extensive research literature exists on "first-order effects," "second-order effects," "unanticipated effects," "spurious criteria of causality," and so on. It may take years of program operation before certain questions of effect can be answered reliably and validly.

In the meantime, evolution of the policymaker's and engineer's view of the original problem is likely to refocus attention on the first question and launch a new cycle of research and action.

Much of the sequence just described is hypothetical in the sense that social communication engineers scarcely exist and are generally not allowed to develop entire public communication programs from research-derived principles (at the expense of policymakers' hunches). However, no sequence of research and action steps less systematic than this can be justified on the basis of:

1. Our growing knowledge of effective communication strategies
2. Federal and other resources being committed to programs, such as cancer control, in which success ultimately depends on public knowledge and utilization
3. Present and future potential for major reduction in public suffering and loss.

APPENDIX 1. *Cancer public education programs of the past decade exhibit variety in cancer sites, target audiences, communication strategies, and program objectives[a]*

Program Name	Sponsor	Origin Site	Media Used[b]	
PREVENTION Project HEALTH	G. D. Searle	Skokie, IL	AV: PR: IP:	film monographs discussion groups
Smoke-Choke-Croak	American Cancer Society	Ft. Lauderdale, FL	AV:	film (videotape)
Youth Patient Panel Patient Panel	American Cancer Society	Los Angeles, CA	PR: IP:	posters, brochures, school newspaper articles panel
San Diego Smoking Research	National Clearing-house on Smoking and Health	San Diego, CA	AV: PR: IP:	films, slides, tapes (TEL-MED) via telephone pamphlets, work-books, catalog of resources peer counseling
Wisconsin Clini-cal Cancer Center	National Cancer Institute	Madison, WI	AV: PR: IP:	radio, TV psa spots brochures, news-paper articles telephone counseling
Philadelphia Em-ployee Education	American Cancer Society	Philadelphia, PA	AV: PR: IP:	ACS films ACS brochures discussion groups
Feeling Good	Children's Televi-sion Workshop	New York, NY	AV: PR:	television newspapers and magazines for publicity
Why You Smoke	American Cancer Society	New York, NY	AV: PR:	television newspapers for publicity
Sioux Indian Cancer Control	American Cancer Society	South Dakota	AV: PR: IP:	ACS films for Community Health Representatives (CHR) ACS brochures visits by CHR to homes
CAN-DIAL	Roswell Park Memori-al Institute and NCI	New York	AV: PR:	tapes via telephone brochures
Speakers Bureau	Roswell Park Memori-ial Institute	New York	IP:	speakers
Smoking Education	American Cancer Society	California	AV: PR: IP:	film (videotapes shown on UHF) booklets discussion groups

Leave It to Laurie	American Cancer Society	Washington	PR: IP:	play text drama presentation
Elementary School Curriculum Project	National Clearing-house on Smoking and Health	California	PR: IP:	classroom materials teacher training
The Big "C"	American Cancer Society	Philadelphia, PA	AV:	telethon using ACS films, guest stars
Poster Contest on Health Hazards of Smoking	American Cancer Society	Minnesota	AV: PR:	radio and TV used for publicity newspapers for publicity, posters
Sack Lunch Employee Education	American Cancer Society	Iowa	AV: PR: IP:	ACS films ACS brochures discussion groups
Breast Cancer: Where We Are	American Cancer Society	New York	AV: PR:	television newspapers, magazines for publicity
Medical Students Teach the Community "Lifeguard Program"	University of Southern California, School of Medicine	Los Angeles, CA	AV: PR: IP:	ACS films, slides ACS brochures medical students talk with lifeguards
Speakers Bureau	Mountain States Tumor Institute and NCI	Idaho	IP:	speakers
Cancer Prevention (Pap and BSE)	Public Health Service, Indian Health Service	Arizona and New Mexico	IP:	community health representatives receive training before visiting Indian homes
Study of Effectiveness of Alternative Mass Distribution Leaflets	American Cancer Society	CO, PA, MD, VA, OH, CA	PR: IP:	Leaflets in four versions Volunteer gives leaflets; phone follow-up of effectiveness
Study of the ACS Employee Education Program	American Cancer Society	Quaker Oats (IL) Central Wire & Steel (IL), Barnett Manufacturing Co. (FL)	AV: PR:	ACS films payroll stuffers, newspaper articles, pamphlets, posters
Study of a Six-Month ACS Employee Education Program	American Cancer Society	Container Corporation of America (IN)	AV: PR: IP:	ACS films literature distribution, payroll stuffers, newspaper articles, pamphlets, posters, exhibits medical speakers

SCREENING/DETECTION

Experimental Cytology	Public Health Service, Division of Community Health Services	Ohio	PR: IP:	statement read by worker community worker

Health Insurance Plan of Greater New York— Screening	Health Insurance Plan of Greater New York	Greater New York	PR: IP:	letter telephone
Operation Cancer Control	American Cancer Society	South Carolina	AV: PR: IP:	ACS films radio, TV for publicity newspapers, church bulletins, poster contest for public- ity and information/ education multiphasic screening
Cancer Control	Department of Health and Environmental Sciences—NCI	Montana	IP:	workshops, seminars
Pap Test Clinic and Education Demonstration	American Cancer Society	Spartanburg, SC	AV: PR: IP:	radio and TV for psa stories and interviews for publicity newspapers announce free clinic locations and times OEO representa- tives in Model Cities area
Motivation Tech- niques in Cancer Detection	Public Health Service, Division of Chronic Diseases	Pennsylvania	AV: PR: IP:	radio and TV for publicity postcards with information and appointment times newspapers and posters for publicity through agencies and health fair
CANSCREEN	Preventive Medicine Institute of NY and Fox Chase Center for Cancer and Medicine Science in Philadelphia	Philadelphia, PA	PR: IP:	letter of invita- tion, health history questionnaire counseling and screening
Cancer Education for Inner City Residents	American Cancer Society	Philadelphia, PA	AV: PR: IP:	ACS films for group leaders ACS brochures discussion groups
Have-a-check	American Cancer Society	Maryland	AV: PR: IP:	films and exhibits for publicity brochures and posters for publicity volunteer gives fascimile check

Community Cancer Demonstration Project	Public Health Service, Division of Chronic Diseases	Florida	PR: IP:	letters group meetings and opinion leaders
Multiphasic Health Screening Clinic	Department of Health & Environmental Sciences and NCI	Montana	IP:	group meetings
Workshops on Cancer Detection for Women	Department of Health & Environmental Sciences and NCI	Montana	IP:	group meetings
REHABILITATION Management of Intestinal Stomas	Regional Medical Program	Maryland	AV: PR:	films, slide-tapes manuals
Reach for Recovery	American Cancer Society	National	PR: IP:	brochures former mastectomy patients visit women just after operation
Ostomy Rehabilitation and Counseling	American Cancer Society	Georgia	IP:	former colostomy patients visit new patients

aSource: Ongoing project for the National Cancer Institute, *Review and Evaluation of Methods of Public Education in Cancer* (M. Butler-Paisley and W. Paisley-Butler, N01-CN-45041).
bKey: AV = audiovisual (film and electronic media); PR = print; IP = interpersonal.

SELECTED BIBLIOGRAPHY

Allen, T. H. Mass media use patterns in a Negro ghetto. *Journalism Q.* 45:525–527 (1968).

Allport, F. *Theories of Perception and the Concept of Structure,* Wiley, New York, 1955.

Alper, S. W., and Leidy, T. R. Impact of information transmission through television. *Public Opinion Q.* 33:556–562 (1969–1970).

Atkins, C. Instrumental Utilities and Information Seeking. In Clarke, P. (ed.): *New Models for Mass Communication Research,* Sage Publications, Beverly Hills.

Bagdikian, B. H. *The Information Machines: Their Impact on Men and the Media,* Harper & Row, New York, 1971.

Bauer, R. A. Communication as transaction. In Payne, D. E. (ed.): *The Obstinate Audience,* Foundation for Research on Human Behavior, Ann Arbor, pp. 3–12, 1965.

Beasley, J. D., et al. Attitudes and knowledge relevant to family planning among New Orleans Negro women. *Am. J. Public Health* 56:1847–1857 (1966).

Bellin, S. S., and Geiger, H. J. Actual public acceptance of neighborhood health centers by the urban poor. *JAMA* 214:2147–2153 (1970).

Bem, D. J. Beliefs, Attitudes, and Human Affairs, Brooks/Cole, Belmont, Calif., 1970.

Berelson, B., and Janowitz, M. *Reader In Public Opinion And Communication,* 2d ed., Free Press, New York, 1966.

Bergner, L., and Yerby, A. S. Low income and barriers to use of health services. *N. Engl. J. Med.* 278:541–546 (1968).

Birch, D., and Veroff, J. *Motivation: A Study of Action,* Brooks/Cole, Belmont, Calif., 1966.

Blake, R. R., et al. *Beliefs And Attitudes About Contraception Among The Poor,* Carolina Population Center, University of North Carolina, Chapel Hill, N.C., 1969.

Block, C. E. Communicating with the urban poor: An exploratory inquiry. *Journalism Q.* 47:3–11 (1970).

Bogue, D. J. (ed.): *Sociological Contributions to Family Planning Research,* University of Chicago, Community and Family Study Center, Chicago, 1967.

Boorstin, D. J. *The Image: A Guide To Pseudo-Events In America,* Atheneum, New York, 1973.

Booth, A., and Babchuk, N. Informal medical opinion leadership among the middle aged and elderly. *Public Opinion Q.* 36:87–94 (1972).

Bowen, R. O. Effect of informal dissemination of health information. *J. School Health* 42:342–344 (1972).

Brightman, I., et al. Knowledge and utilization of health resources by public assistance recipients. *Am. J. Public Health* 48:188–199 and 319–327 (1958).

Bruner, J. S., et al. *A Study Of Thinking,* Wiley, New York, 1956.

Burkett, D. W. *Writing Science News for the Mass Media,* Gulf Publishing Co., Houston, 1973.

Burns, E. L., et al. Detection of uterine cancer: Results of a community program of 17 years. *J. Cancer* 22: (1968).

Campbell, D. T. Methods for the experimenting society. A proposal to The Russell Sage Foundation, 1969.

Cauffman, J. G. Medical students teach the community. *J. Med. Educ.* 46:618–620 (1971).

Childers, T. *Knowledge/Information Needs of the Disadvantaged,* Drexel University, Graduate School of Library Science, Philadelphia, 1973.

Clarke, P. (ed.): *New Models For Mass Communication Research,* Sage Publications, Beverly Hills, Calif., 1973.

Davison, W. P., and Yu, F. T. C. (eds.): *Mass Communication Research: Major Issues And Future Directions,* Praeger, New York, 1974.

DeLarue, N. C. The anti-smoking clinic: Is it a potential community service? *Can. Med. Assoc. J.* 108 (1973).

Dervin, B. L., and Greenberg, B. S. *The Communication Environment of the Urban Poor,* Michigan State Univ., Department of Communication, East Lansing, Mich., 1972.

Dillehay, R. C. On the irrelevance of the classical negative evidence concerning the effect of attitudes on behavior. *Am. J. Psychol.* 28:887–891 (1973).

Donohew, L., and Palmgreen, P. A reappraisal of dissonance and the selective exposure hypothesis. *Journalism Q.* 48:412–420 (1971).

Donohew, L., and Tipton, L. A conceptual model of information processing, avoiding, and processing. In Clark, P. (ed.): *New Models for Mass Communication Research,* pp. 205–242, Sage Publications, Beverly Hills, Calif., 1974.

Downs, R. M. and Stea, D. (eds.): *Image And Environment: Cognitive Mapping and Spatial Behavior,* Aldine, Chicago, 1973.

Eichorn, R., and Aday, M. *The Utilization of Health Services: Indices and Correlates.* DHEW, Washington, D.C., National Center for Health Services Research and Development, 1972.

Edwards, W., and Tversky, A. (eds.): *Decision Making,* Penguin Books, Baltimore, Md., 1967.

Feather, N. T. Cigarette smoking and lung cancer: A study of cognitive dissonance. *Aust. J. Psychol.* 14:55–64 (1962).

Fejer, D., et al. Sources of information about drugs among high school students. *Public Opinion Q.* 35:235–241 (1971).

Feldman, J. *The Dissemination Of Health Information: A Case Study in Adult Learning,* Aldine, Chicago, 1966.

Fink, R., et al. The reluctant participant in a Breast Cancer Screening Program. *Public Health Rep.* 83 (1968).

Funkhauser, G. R., and Maccoby, N. *Communicating Science to Nonscientists,* Stanford University, Institute for Communication Research, Palo Alto, Calif., 1970–1971. Two volumes.

Funkhauser, G. R., and Maccobby, N. Communicating specialized science information to a lay audience. *J. Commun.* 21:57–71 (1971).

Gerbner, G. Communication and social environment. In *Communication: A Scientific American Book,* pp. 111–120, W. H. Freeman, San Francisco, 1972.

Gerbner, G., and Tannenbaum, P. Mass media censorship and the portrayal of mental illness. In *Studies of Innovation and of Communication to the Public,* Stanford University, Institute for Communication Research, Palo Alto, Calif., 1962.

Gillespie, D. K. Media source use for health information. *Res. Q. Am. Assoc. Health Phys. Educ.* 38:149–151 (1967).

Gombrich, E. H. The visual image. In *Communication: A Scientific American Book,* pp. 46–62, W. H. Freeman, San Francisco, 1972.

Gordon, J. Evaluation of communications media in two health projects in Baltimore. *Public Health Rep.* 82 (1967).

Green, L. W. Diffusion and Adoption of Innovations Related to Cardiovascular Risk Behavior in the Public. In *Proceedings of Conference on Applying Behavioral Science to Cardiovascular Risk,* American Heart Association, New York, 1974.

Green, L. W. Should health education abandon attitude change strategies? Perspectives from recent research. *Health Educ. Monogr.* 1:30 (1970).

Green, L. W., and Roberts, B. J. The research literature on why women delay in seeking medical care for breast symptoms. *Health Educ. Monogr.* 2:2 (1974).

Greenberg, B. S. On relating attitude change and information gain. *J. Commun.* 14:151–171 (1961).

Greenberg, B. S., and Dervin, B. L. Mass communication among the urban poor. *Public Opinion Q.* 34:224–235 (1970).

Greenberg, B. S., and Dervin, B. L. *Use of the Mass Media by the Urban Poor,* Praeger, New York, 1970.

Griffiths, W., and Knutson, A. L. The role of mass media in public health. *Am. J. Public Health* 50:515–523 (1960).

Haefner, D. P., et al. Motivational and behavioral effects of modifying health beliefs. *Public Health Rep.* 85:478–484 (1970).

Hammond, P. G., Turning off: the abuse of drug information. *Library J.* 98:1337–1341 (1973).

Hannerz, U. Gossip, networks and culture in a black American ghetto. *Ethnos* 32:35–60 (1967).

Hart, E. J. Effects of contrasting messages on cancer control: Behavior of females in lower socioeconomic conditions. *J. Sch. Health* 42:262–264 (1972).

Health and Welfare Council of Central Maryland. *Description and Operation of the Information and Referral Service, 1962–1971,* HWCCM, Baltimore, Md., 1971.

Heidt, S. Knowledge and its consequences: the impact of information on a family planning program. *Am. Behav. Sci.* 12:43–48 (1968).

Herman, M. W. The poor: Their medical needs and the health services available to them. In *Ann. Am. Acad. Polit. Soc. Sci.* 399:12–21 (1972).

Hillman, B., and Charney, E. A neighborhood health center: What the patients know and think of its operation. *Med. Care* 10:336–344 (1972).

Hoff, W. Why health programs are not reaching the unresponsive in our communities. *Public Health Rep.* 81:654–658 (1966).

Holder, L. Some theoretical and practical considerations in influencing health behavior. *Health Educ. Monogr.* 30:49–69 (1970).

Holleb, A. I. Status of knowledge about cancer relevant to public education. In *Proceedings of the Conference on Cancer Public Education, Health Educ. Monogr.* 1:3–10 (1973).

Horn, D. Man, cigarettes, and the abuse of gratification. *Int. J. Addict.* 4:471–479 (1969).

Horn, D. Public attitudes and beliefs relative to cancer prevention, cancer health care services and access thereto. In *Proceedings of the Conference on Cancer Public Education, Health Educ. Monogr.* 1:11–17 (1973).

Hovland, C. I. Reconciling conflicting results derived from experimental and survey studies of attitude change. *Am. Psychol.* 14:8–17 (1959).

Hovland, C. I., et al. *Experiments on Mass Communication,* Princeton University Press, Princeton, 1949.

Hovland, C. I., et al. *The Order of Presentation in Persuasion,* Yale University Press, New Haven, 1957.

Hulka, B. S. Detection of cervical cancer among the medically indigent. *Public Health* 81 (1966).

Hulka, B. S. Motivation techniques in a cancer detection program: Utilization of community resources. *Am. J. Public Health* 57:229–241 (1967).

Hunt, W. A., and Matarazzo, J. D. Recent developments in experimental modification of smoking behavior. *J. Abnorm. Psychol.* 81:107–114 (1973).

Ikard, F. F., and Tomkins, S. The experience of affect as a determinant of smoking behavior: A series of validity studies. *J. Abnorm. Psychol.* 81:172–181 (1973).

Is knowledge of most worth in drug abuse education? *J. Sch. Health* 40:453 (1970).

Isaacs, H. R. *Scratches on Our Minds: American Images of China and India,* John Day, New York, 1958.

Jackson, A. R. A model for determining information diffusion in a family planning program. *J. Marriage and Family* 34:503–513 (1972).

Janis, I. L., et al. *Personality and Persuasibility,* Yale University Press, New Haven, 1959.

Kariel, P. E. Social class, age, and educational group differences in childbirth information. *Marriage and Family Living* 25:335–353 (1963).

Katz, D. The functional approach to the study of attitudes. *Public Opinion Q.* 24:163–176 (1960).

Katz, E. Communication research and the image of society: Convergence of two research traditions. *Am. J. Sociol.* 65:435–440 (1960).

Katz, E., et al. Uses of mass communication by the individual. In Davison and Yu, T. T. C. (eds.): *Mass Communication Research: Major Issues and Future Directions,* pp. 11–35, Praeger, New York, 1974.

Kegeles, S. S. Attitudes and behavior of the public regarding cervical cytology: Current findings and new directions for research. *J. Chronic. Dis.* 20:911–922 (1967).

Kegeles, S. S. Behavioral science data and approaches relevant to the development of education programs in cancer. In *Proceedings of the Conference on Cancer Public Education, Health Educ. Monog.* 1:18–33 (1973).

Kegeles, S. S. Communications problems of experimental research in the ghetto. *Med. Care* 7:395–405 (1969).

Kegeles, S. S. A field experimental attempt to change beliefs and behavior of women in an urban ghetto. *J. Health Soc. Behav.* 10:115–124 (1969).

Kegeles, S. S., et al. Survey of beliefs about cancer detection and taking Papanicolaou tests. *Public Health Rep.* 80:815–823 (1965).

Kelly, G. A. *A Theory of Personality: The Psychology of Personal Constructs,* W. W. Norton, New York, 1963.

Kline, F. G. Media time budgeting as a function of demographics life style. *Journalism Q.* 48:211–221 (1971).

Kochen, M. Directory design for networks of information and referral centers. *Library Q.*

42:59–83 (1972).

Krugman, H. E. Mass media effectiveness: Some other points of view. In Payne, D. E. (ed.): *The Obstinate Audience*, pp. 13–24, Foundation for Research on Human Behavior, Ann Arbor, 1965.

Kuehl, P. G. *An Examination of the Influence of Family Life Cycle and Social Class on Information-Seeking in Self-Medication Behavior*, Unpublished Ph.D. dissertation. Ohio State University, Columbus, Ohio, 1970.

Lang, K., and Lang, G. The unique perspective of television. *Am. Sociol. Rev.* 18:3–12 (1953).

Lehmann, S. Personality and compliance: a study of anxiety and self-esteem in opinion and behavior change. *J. Pers. Soc. Psychol.* 15:76–86 (1970).

Lester, E., et al. Information and referral services for the chronically ill and aged. *Public Health Rep.* 83:295–302 (1968).

Leventhal, H. Fear appeals and persuasion: the differentiation of a motivational construct. *Am. J. Public Health* 61:1208–1224 (1961).

Logan, F. A. Self-Control as habit, drive, and incentive. *J. Abnorm. Psychol* 81:127–136 (1973).

Long, H. B. Information sources, dogmatism, and judgmental modifications. *Adult Educ.* 21:37–45 (1971).

Long, N., et al. Information and Referral Centers: A Functional Analysis, American Rehabilitation Foundation, Minneapolis, 1971.

Lynch, H. A New Approach to Cancer Screening and Detection. *Geriatrics* 28:152–157 (1973).

Maccoby, N. Arguments, counter-arguments and distractions. In Payne, D. E. (ed.), *The Obstinate Audience*, pp. 33–42, Foundation for Research on Human Behavior, Ann Arbor, 1965.

Maslow, A. H. The need to know and the fear of knowing. *J. Gen. Psychol.* 68:111–125 (1963).

Mausner, B. An ecological view of cigarette smoking. *J. Abnorm. Psychol.* 81:115–126 (1973).

Mendelsohn, H. What to say to whom in social amelioration programming. *Educ. Broadcasting Rev.* 3:19–26 (1969).

Mendelsohn, H. Which shall it be: Mass education or mass persuasion for health. *Am. J. Public Health* 58 (1968).

Mendelsohn, H., et al. *Operation Stop-Gap: A Study of the Application of Communications Techniques in Reaching the Unreachable Poor*, University of Denver, Denver, 1968. Two volumes.

Monk, M., et al. Evaluation of an antismoking program among high school students. *Am. J. Public Health* 55:904–1004 (1965).

Naguib, S. M., et al. Response to a program of screening for cervical cancer. *Public Health Rep.* 83:990–998 (1968).

New, P. K. An information service for the aging. *Geriatrics* 17:609–614 (1962).

Niemi, J. A., and Anderson, D. V. *Television: A Viable Channel for Educating Adults in Culturally Different Poverty Groups? A Literature Review*. ERIC Clearinghouse on Adult Education, Syracuse, N.Y., 1971.

Ogg, E. *Tell Me Where To Turn: The Growth of Information and Referral Services*, Public Affairs Committee, New York, 1969.

O'Keefe, M. T. The anti-smoking commercials: A study of television's impact on behavior. *Public Opinion Q.* 35:242–248 (1971).

Paisley, W. J., and Rees, M. B. *Social and Psychological Predictors of Information Seeking and Media Use: A Multivariate Re-analysis*. Stanford University, Institute for Communication Research, Palo Alto, Calif., 1967.

Palmore, J. The Chicago Snowball: a study of the flow and diffusion of family planning information. In Bogue, D. J. (ed.): *Sociological Contributions to Family Planning Research*, pp. 272–363, University of Chicago, Community and Family Study Center, Chicago (1967).

Parker, E. B. Implications of new information technology. In Davison, W. P., and Yu, F. T. C. (eds): *Mass Communications Research: Major Issues and Future Directions*, pp. 171–183, Praeger, New York, 1974.

Parker, E. B. Information utilities and mass communication. In Sackman, H., and Nie, N. (eds.): *The Information Utility and Social Choice*, pp. 51–70, American Federation of Information Processing, Montvale, N.J., 1970.

Parker, E. B., et al. *Patterns of Adult Information Seeking*, Stanford University, Institute for Communication Research, Palo Alto, Calif., 1966.

Payne, D. E. (ed.): *The Obstinate Audience*, Foundation for Research on Human Behavior, Ann Arbor, 1965.

Pomeroy, R., et al. *Studies in the Use of Health Services by Families on Welfare*, City University of New York, Baruch College, Center for the Study of Urban Problems, New York, 1969. Three volumes.

Proceedings of the Conference on Cancer Public Education. *Health Monogr.* 1:36 (1973).

Ray, M. L. Psychological theories and interpretations of learning. In Ward, S., and Robertson, T. S. (eds.): *Consumer Behavior*, pp. 45–117, Prentice-Hall, Englewood Cliffs, N.J., 1973.

Rieger, J. H., and Anderson, R. C. Information source and need hierarchies of adult population in five Michigan counties. *Adult Education* 18:155–175 (1968).

Roberto, E. Social marketing strategies for diffusing the adoption of family planning. *Soc. Sci. Q.* 53:33–51 (1972).

Roberts, D. F., and Maccoby, N. Information processing and persuasion: counterarguing behavior. In Clarke, P. (ed.): *New Models for Mass Communication Research*, pp. 269–307, Sage Publications, Beverly Hills, Calif., 1973.

Roemer, M. I., and Anzel, D. M. Health needs and services of the rural poor. *Med. Care Rev.* 25:371–390 and 461–491 (1968).

Rogers, V. *Guidelines for a Telephone Reassurance Service*, U.S. Govt. Print. Off., Washington, D.C., 1972.

Rokeach, M. *Beliefs, Attitudes, and Values*, Jossey-Bass, San Francisco, 1968.

Rokeach, M. Long-range experimental modification of values, attitudes, and behavior. *Am. Psychol.* 26:453–459 (1971).

Rokeach, M. *The Open and Closed Mind*, Basic Books, New York, 1960.

Rosenberg, M. J., et al. *Attitude Organization and Change*, Yale University Press, New Haven, 1960.

Rosenblatt, A., and Mayer, J. E. Help seeking for family problems: a survey of utilization and satisfaction. *Am. J. Psychiatry* 128:1136–1140 (1972).

Rosenstock, I. M. Why people use health services. *Millbank Mem. Fund Q.* 44:94–127 (1966).

Rosenstock, I. M., et al. Public knowledge, opinion, and action concerning three public health issues. *J. Health Soc. Behav.* 7 (1966).

Sackman, H., and Nie, N. (eds.): *The Information Utility and Social Choice*, American Federation of Information Processing Societies, Montvale, N.J., 1970.

Sadler, M. A pilot program in health education related to the hazards of cigarette smoking. *RI Med. J.* 52:36–38 (1969).

Samora, J., et al. Knowledge about specific diseases in four selected areas. *J. Health Soc. Behav.* 3:176–184 (1962).

Sarbin, T. R., and Nucci, L. P. Self-reconstitution processes: A proposal for reorganizing the conduct of confirmed smokers. *J. Abnorm. Psychol.* 81:182–195 (1973).

Sargent, L. W., and Stempel, G., III. Poverty, alienation, and mass media use. *Journalism Q.* 45:324–326 (1973).

Schatzman, L., and Strauss, A. Social class and modes of communication. *Am. J. Sociol.* 60:329–338 (1955).

Schulman, S., and Smith, A. M. The concept of 'health' among Spanish-speaking villagers of New Mexico and Colorado. *J. Health Soc. Behav.* 4:226–234 (1963).

Schwartz, J. L. A critical review and evaluation of smoking control methods. *Public Health Rep.* 84:483–506 (1969).

Seeman, M. Alienation and knowledge-seeking: a note on attitudes and action. *Social Problems* 20:3–17 (1972).

Sharp, L. J. *Health-Care Seeking Behavior of Project Head Start Families, Final Project Report,* University of Washington, Social Change Evaluation Project, Seattle, 1969. (NTIS PB 184 530)

Sherif, M., and Hovland, C. I. *Social Judgment,* Yale University Press, New Haven, 1961.

Simonds, S. K. Public opinion surveys about cancer: An overview. *Health Educ. Monogr.* 30:3–24 (1970).

Speidel, J. J. Knowledge of contraceptive techniques among a hospital population of low socio-economic status. *J. Sex Res.* 6:284–306 (1970).

Spitzer, S. P., and Denzin, N. K. Levels of knowledge in an emergent crisis. *Social Forces* 44:234–237 (1965).

Starch, K. Values and information source preferences. *J. Commun.* 23:74–85 (1973).

Stephens, L. F. Media exposure and modernization among the Appalachian poor. *Journalism Q.* 49:247–257 (1972).

Steinburg, S. S., and Richardson, C. E. *A Study of the Effectiveness of the Film "Time and Two Women" in Motivating Women to Secure the Pap Test for the Detection of Uterine Cancer,* presented at the 90th Annual Meeting of the American Public Health Association, October, 1962.

Stojanovic, E. J. The dissemination of information about Medicare to low-income rural residents. *Rural Sociol.* 37:253–260 (1972).

Stuteville, J. R. Psychic defenses against high fear appeals: A key marketing variable. *J. Marketing* 34:39–45 (1970).

Suchman, E. A. Social factors in medical deprivation. *Am. J. Public Health* 55:1725–1733 (1965).

Swinehart, J. W. Voluntary exposure to health communications. *Am. J. Public Health* 58:1265–1275 (1968).

Sykes, G. M. The differential distribution of community knowledge. *Social Forces* 29:376–382 (1951).

Tannenbaum, P. Communication of science information. *Science* 140:579–583 (1963).

Taylor, F. J. Adjusting the amount and level of information to one's audience. *Instructional Sci.* 1:211–245 (1972).

Taylor, W. Mental health content of the mass media. *Journalism Q.* 34:191–201 (1957).

Tesser, A., et al. On the reluctance to communicate undesirable messages (the MUM effect): A field study. *Psycholog. Rep.* 29:651–654 (1971).

Thistle, M. W. Popularizing Science. *Science* 127:951–955 (1958).

Tichenor, P. J., et al. Mass media flow and differential growth in knowledge. *Public Opinion Q.* 34:159–170 (1970).

Tolman, E. C. Cognitive maps in rats and men. *Psychol. Rev.* 55:189–208 (1948).

U.S. Department of Health, Education, and Welfare, Bureau of Health Services, Social Forces and the Nation's Health, U.S. Govt. Print. Off., Washington, D.C., 1968.

U.S. Department of Health, Education, and Welfare, Indian Health Service. A Prototype Indian Health Information System, U.S. Govt. Print. Off., Washington, D.C., 1969.

Vernon, D. T. Information seeking in a natural stress situation. *J. Appl. Psychol.* 55:359–363 (1971).

Wade, S., and Schramm, W. The mass media as sources of public health, science, and health information. *Public Opinion Q.* 33:197–209 (1969).

Wakefield, J. *Cancer and Public Education,* Pitman, London, 1962.

Wakefield, J. (ed.): *Seek Wisely to Prevent: Studies of Attitude and Action in a Cervical Cytology Programme,* Her Majesty's Stat. Off., London, 1972.

Weiss, W. Effects of the mass media of communication. In Lindzey, G., and Aronson, E. (eds.): *Handbook of Social Psychology,* Vol. 5, Addison-Wesley, Reading, Mass., 1969.

Westley, B. H. Communication and social change. *Am. Behav. Scien.* 14:719–744 (1971).

Westley, B. H., and Severin, W. J. A profile of the daily newspaper non-reader. *Journalism Q.* 41:45–50 (1964).

White, W. J. An index for determining the relative importance of information sources. *Public Opinion Q.* 33:607–610 (1969–1970).

Whitted, H. H. Early detection of cancer among low-income groups. *Arch. Environ. Health* 6:280–285 (1963).

Williams, F., and Lindsay, H. Ethnic and social class differences in communication habits and attitudes. *Journalism Q.* 48:672–678 (1971).

Wolpert, J. A regional simulation model of information diffusion. *Public Opinion Q.* 30:597–608 (1966).

Youmans, E. G. Health orientations of older rural and urban men. *Geriatrics* 22:139–147 (1967).

Young, M. A. C. Review of research and studies on the health education and related aspects of family planning (1967–1971): Communication, program planning and evaluation. *Health Educ. Monogr.* 1:35 (1973).

REFERENCES

1. Hammond, G. D., and Hilleboe, H. E. *National Cancer Control Program Planning Conference,* U.S. Department of Health, Education, and Welfare, National Cancer Institute, Washington, D.C., 1974.

2. Breslow, L. *Cancer Program Planning Conference: Summary Report of Working Group 8, Cancer Control.* U.S. Department of Health, Education, and Welfare, National Cancer Institute, Washington, D.C., 1974.

3. Lippmann, W. *Public Opinion,* Macmillan, New York, 1922.

4. Lazarsfeld, P. E., et al. *The People's Choice,* Columbia University Press, New York, 1948.

5. Merton, R. K. *Mass Persuasion,* Harper & Row, New York, 1946.

6. Hyman, H., and Sheatsley, P. B. Some reasons why information campaigns fail. *Public Opinion Q.* 11:412–423 (1947).

7. Star, S. A., and Hughes, H. M. Report on an educational campaign: The Cincinnati Plan for the United Nations. *Am. J. Sociol.* 55:335–361 (1950).

8. Katz, E., and Lazarsfeld, P. *Personal Influence,* Free Press, New York, 1955.

9. Menzel, H. Quasi-mass communication: A neglected area. *Public Opinion Q.* 35:406–409 (1971).

10. Rogers, E. M., and Shoemaker, F. F. *Communication of Innovations: A Cross-Cultural Approach,* Free Press, New York, 1971.

11. Zimmerman, C., and Bauer, R. A. The effect of an audience on what is remembered. *Public Opinion Q.* 20:238–248 (1956).

12. Cartwright, D. Achieving change in people: Some applications of group dynamics theory. *Hum. Relations* 4:381–392 (1951).

13. Hovland, C. I., et al. *Communication and Persuasion,* Yale University Press, New Haven, 1953.

14. Klapper, J. T. *The Effects of Mass Communication,* Free Press, New York, 1962.

15. Bauer, R. A. The obstinate audience: The influence process from the point of view of social communication. *Am. J. Psychol.* 19:319–328 (1964).

16. Schramm, W. The nature of communication between humans. In Schramm, W., and Roberts, D. F. (eds.): *The Process and Effects of Mass Communication,* rev. ed., pp. 3–53, University of Illinois Press, Urbana Ill., 1971.

17. Sears, D. O., and Freedman, J. L. Selective exposure to information: A critical review. *Public Opinion Q.* 31:194–213 (1967).

18. Higbee, K. L. Fifteen years of fear arousal: Research on threat appeals, 1953–1968. *Psychol. Bull.* 72:426–449 (1969).

19. Mendelsohn, H. Some reasons why information campaigns can succeed. *Public Opinion Q.* 37:50–61 (1973).

20. McGuire, W. J. The nature of attitudes and attitude change. In Lindzey, G., and Aronson, E. (eds.): *Handbook of Social Psychology,* vol. 3, pp. 136–314, Addison-Wesley, Reading, Mass., 1969.

21. Ray, M. L. Marketing communication and the hierarchy of effects. In Clarke, P. (ed.): *New Models for Mass Communication Research,* pp. 147–176, Sage Publications, Beverly Hills, Calif., 1973.

22. Krugman, H. E. The impact of television advertising: Learning without awareness. *Public Opinion Q.* 29:349–356 (1965).

23. Boulding, K. E. *The Image,* University of Michigan Press, Ann Arbor, 1956.

24. Miller, G. A., et al. *Plans and the Structure of Behavior,* Holt, Rinehart and Winston, New York, 1960.

25. Berger, P. L., and Luckmann, T. *The Social Construction of Reality,* Doubleday, Garden City, N.Y., 1966.

26. Eichorn, R., and Aday, M. *The Utilization of Health Services: Indices and Correlates.* DHEW, Washington, D.C., National Center for Health Services Research and Development, 1972.

27. Schramm, W., and Wade, S. *Knowledge and the Public Mind: A Preliminary Study of the Distribution and Sources of Science, Health and Public Affairs Knowledge in the American Public.* Stanford University, Institute for Communication Research, Palo Alto, Calif., 1967.

28. Anderson, O. W. *Health Service Use: National Trends and Variations, 1953*–1971. DHEW, National Center for Health Services Research and Development, Washington, D.C., 1972.

29. Rees, M. B., and Paisley, W. J. Social and psychological predictors of adult information seeking and media use. *Adult Education* 19:11–29 (1968).

Cancer: The Behavioral Dimensions, edited by J. W. Cullen, B. H. Fox, and R. N. Isom. Raven Press, New York © 1976.

Creative Use of Mass Media to Affect Health Behavior

James W. Swinehart

Children's Television Workshop, 1 Lincoln Plaza, New York, New York 10023

No one can guarantee creativity in the use of mass media, just as no one can guarantee creativity in science. However, we do know something about the conditions that favor innovative solutions to problems: Find people with imagination and a willingness to take risks, make sure they understand the needs to be met, then give them time and money and freedom to work. Presumably they will discover what has been tried before and develop a new approach that offers improved prospects for solving the problem. The odds are that they will have only partial success, but they will almost certainly learn something useful in the process.

This chapter looks at one major health education experiment in the context of health communications in general, describes its distinctive elements, and provides some examples of research findings from the effectiveness of health education in the mass media.

THE CONTEXT

Health education in the mass media is big business. More than $200 million a year is spent by government and voluntary agencies alone on health communications, and this is in addition to the much larger amounts spent for commercial advertising of tonics, headache remedies, toothpastes, and other products. Medical columns, news features, and straight news items on medical care, treatment, or diagnosis appear in hundreds of newspapers and magazines. Television has shown a number of information series such as "The Killers," "The Turned-On Crisis," "Inside Out," "Today's Health," "House Call," "The World of Medicine," "Medix"; several entertainment series such as "Emergency," "Medical Center," and "Marcus Welby, M.D."; occasional treatment of health topics on other entertainment series; many documentary specials such as "What Price Health," "Don't Get Sick in America," "How to Stay Alive," "An American Alcoholic," "The Right to Live," and "Heart Attack"; and public service announcements on a wide variety of topics—smoking, VD, vision, alcoholism, exercise, air pollution, seat belts, immunizations, breast cancer, and so on.

It is reasonable to expect that any new attempt to produce a health program for television would begin with a review of the evidence concerning the effects of previous efforts. In preparation for its "Feeling Good" series, planned as 26 1-hour programs, the Children's Television Workshop (CTW) made such an attempt but found little evidence to support the choice of one approach over another. Few studies of the impact of programs were found, and most of these dealt with a single program or mini-series and thus were of questionable relevance to a full series. Since 97% of the homes in this country now have TV sets, the review did serve as a reminder that most people have heard a great deal about health matters from television—and thus that any new series should seek to provide useful information in an attractive format if it is to have any hope of attracting viewers.

Many previous programs and films were designed only to explore an issue or to convey information; the CTW series was conceived as an attempt to do these things and also to influence behavior—and to do so in a highly competitive, prime-time broadcast period. Rather than being planned for an audience of people interested in health (as are most documentaries on health topics), it was initially designed for all adults, with special emphasis on young parents and on low-income families that often have difficulty obtaining good health care. This emphasis was chosen because of the need, and despite the fact that these segments of the population tend to be underrepresented in the public television audience.

Most studies of mass communications indicate that they are far more likely to reinforce than to change attitudes, beliefs, and behavior. The "Feeling Good" project was undertaken as an experiment to see whether this consistent finding could be modified, in part through the efforts described below.

In developing the CTW series, advice was sought from more than 300 health professionals and communications experts. Their frequent differences of opinion about themes and approaches were ultimately resolved by the production staff. Because the conclusions reached may prove useful to others responsible for designing health education programs, here are some elements of the series which are, to some extent, distinctive:

Use of stated objectives—A set of specific behavioral goals and information points to convey in support of these goals was developed for each topic to be treated in the series. After being checked by health professionals, this material was given to producers who then decided which formats to use in preparing the programs. Early specification of program content and objectives made it possible to design appropriate evaluation instruments for obtaining baseline data before the series began. Considerations in selecting the topics and objectives included the number of people affected by a given health problem, the seriousness of its consequences, the feasibility and efficacy of recommended actions, and the measurability of outcomes.

The recommended actions were later classified in terms of their purpose, frequency, and beneficiary; whether they involved seeking care or information (or neither) from providers; and appropriate target audiences. For each problem, we were concerned with audience perceptions of its prevalence, detectability, difficulty and cost of treatment, preventability, and seriousness of consequences.

Use of data on audiences—Data from surveys and other studies on what people know and do about their health have been used in selecting goals and appeals for several programs. The kinds of barriers noted below were identified from survey data and formed the basis for developing program content. This approach is commonly used in the advertising of commercial products, but has not been characteristic in many health campaigns.

Undermining barriers to action—Fear, apathy, and other barriers to action have been addressed specifically when it was felt appropriate to do so. A segment about breast cancer, for example, emphasized that most breast lumps are benign, that the cure rate after early detection is high, and that one can resume normal activities after a mastectomy. A segment on mental health attempted to counteract the beliefs that seeking psychiatric treatment is socially disapproved and that such treatment is costly and ineffective. In general, fear appeals have been avoided; the approach has been to stress the benefits of taking a recommended action rather than the consequences of failing to do so.

Use of motivational goals—The purpose of the programs has been to motivate rather than merely to inform. Some people need to be *informed*, but others need only to be *reminded*, and still others to be *persuaded* to take given actions. If a communication effort includes basic information for the first group, this may alienate the other groups who feel they already know what is being conveyed. Dramatic but real situations with which viewers can identify have been used in the hope of conveying information effectively to people in all three categories.

Multiple appeals—Whenever possible, a specific point is made in more than one way in a "cluster" of program segments to reinforce the message being given.

Use of entertainment—Through the use of guest stars, music, comedy, and drama we have tried to attract people who do not usually watch public television and people for whom health maintenance has a relatively low priority. In the latter group are those who would not choose to watch a documentary program on health, read medical columns in a newspaper, or request information from public or voluntary health agencies.

Recruiting influence agents—We have tried to use appeals to altruism as a means of getting people to reinforce the message through personal contact with a spouse, a child, or the person next door. This is an attempt to combine the *efficiency* of the TV series in reaching many people (currently about 1,500 adults each week) with the *effectiveness* of personal appeals for such actions as having a Pap test or a breast examination.

Concern about side effects—An ancient medical motto says "The first thing is to do no harm." This has not been a major concern of health education, but some recent studies of drug-abuse campaigns suggest that well-intentioned efforts to inform can have significant negative consequences. In selecting goals and content for programs, we have been aware of this danger—particularly when dealing with cancer, where increased perception of risk may be accompanied by denial and consequently by an avoidance of diagnosis.

Referral spots—Each program includes one or more "referral spots" which direct the viewer to a source of further information about a given health topic. The 250 stations of the Public Broadcasting Service are encouraged to identify local agencies which can respond to requests from viewers, and to broadcast phone numbers and addresses during each program. The hope is that the program will stimulate contact between the viewer and a local agency, which can supply detailed information and personal contact in response to interest generated by the broadcast.

Coordination—An effort has been made to schedule treatment of topics to coincide with campaigns being conducted by other organizations, for example, alcoholism during January (National Council on Alcoholism) and cancer during April (American Cancer Society). Such coordination makes it more difficult to assess the effects of the series, but increases the likelihood of raising public consciousness about particular health problems.

Community Education Services—This is a division of CTW that seeks to enlist the cooperation of local organizations and to promote viewing, particularly in low-income areas. Efforts to reach a variety of organizations and high-need populations are not normally associated with network television programs, but have produced important benefits in connection with all three series produced by CTW.

Testing of programs—Although production schedules have precluded testing of "Feeling Good" programs before they have been aired, each program is shown to test audiences as soon as it is completed so that later programs can be influenced by the results. Ideally, any material should be tested far enough in advance of use so that indicated changes can be made before it is shown to large numbers of people. Early testing, like early detection of health problems, often makes it possible to spot trouble while it can still be corrected. The four methods we use in testing material (questionnaires, observation of viewers, group interviews, and a program analyzer) usually produce results consistent with one another, and can be used with films as well as with television programs.

Evaluation of effects—A major investment is being made in evaluating the effects of the series. Four independent research organizations have contracted to conduct the research, which includes a field experiment with a low-income population in one city, repeated surveys with a selected population in four cities, four national sample surveys spaced throughout the series, and weekly viewership measures on another national sample. Most health education projects cannot undertake an evaluation on this scale, but the elements can and should be used elsewhere—assessments based on definite goals, using several complementary research methods and designs, conducted by outside contractors working in conjunction with the producing organization.

Process vs. product—As stated earlier, this project is an experiment. Some low-feasibility goals have been included in the series, in part because they deal with significant health problems and in part because we felt it important to try to stretch the boundaries of the possible despite the risks involved. The product of an experiment rarely fulfills all the expectations held for it, but the process itself has value in that it extends knowledge, and that is one of the two major purposes of the project.

It is impossible to summarize briefly the results from more than 20 studies conducted during the past year-and-a-half, but a sampling of conclusions may be helpful. Although the studies were done specifically for our series, some of the findings should be applicable to other programs and perhaps to other media. The usual cautions about generalizing should be kept in mind; care was taken to utilize samples of adequate size and diversity, but the findings should still be regarded as tentative.

1. Differential interest in topics overrides differences in themes or approaches to these topics; for example, programs about cancer elicit more interest than programs about other topics, regardless of whether the appeal is to altruism or self-interest and whether the theme is prevention or treatment.
2. Television segments using fear appeals are liked much less than those with attractive content such as a demonstration of correct behavior.
3. Segments with a strong emotional or fear appeal tend to be understood less well than those with a straight informational style, and the latter are more likely to be mentioned to others by viewers.
4. Appeal and comprehension are directly related; in general, the more a segment is liked, the greater are the chances that it will be remembered correctly. Both appeal and comprehension tend to be related to the perceived usefulness of the information conveyed.
5. Self-tests and other formats which involve the viewer directly rate high on both appeal and ability to convey information effectively.
6. The use of terms that denigrate persons with certain kinds of health problems (e.g., "fatso" or "drunk") are responded to negatively.
7. Viewers sometimes draw incorrect inferences from dramas or comedy sketches. Such segments frequently hold interest and score high on appeal, but some audiences have difficulty distinguishing factual material from statements made for comedic or dramatic purposes.
8. Believable dramatic situations can effectively convey information to diverse audiences, including those whose ethnic or other characteristics differ from those of the performers.
9. The use of a "laugh track" with televised comedy segments increases the number of people who find them appealing, but tends to decrease the number who understand the messages they contain.
10. In the context of a program with low information density, documentary segments and straightforward presentations of facts are usually far more effective than one might expect from their performance in isolation.
11. Songs are a high-risk format for conveying health information and inducing positive affect toward a recommended behavior. Some are regarded very favorably, while others are seen as inappropriate or foolish in the context of a health program.

12. Parody is a poor vehicle for conveying health messages, which are often misinterpreted—especially when viewers are unfamiliar with the basis for the parody.

These findings, together with those from surveys conducted as part of the evaluation of the series, have identified some of the problems in early programs and provided guidelines for subsequent selection and treatment of material. Modifications now being made in the series are based in part on research results obtained thus far, and testing will continue as new programs are produced. Many important questions remain unanswered, however, and most of these will have to be resolved by studies conducted elsewhere.

The basic need is for more detail and differentiation with regard to some things that are still conceptualized in a rather global way (e.g., fear and other barriers to action, target audiences, and motivational appeals of various kinds). For example, some people continue to ask whether fear appeals should be used, but it is more appropriate to ask *how much* fear or *what kind* should be used with *which audiences* under *what conditions*? Other relevant variables and questions:

Sequence of presentation—In a communication that uses both threat and reassurance, for example, should the threat come first (because it arouses concern and interest) or should the reassurance come first (because it may make the person more receptive to the message)?

Information persistence after learning—How long after a message is received should its effects be measured? As the interval increases, ability to recall learned information declines, but there is also greater opportunity for people to take a recommended action. We need to know more about the frequency and timing of reinforcing messages in order to produce both sustained knowledge gain and maximum adaptive actions.

Behavior thresholds—Identifying the thresholds at which information or motivational appeals produce actual behavior should be a relatively high-priority research task. Some people are prompted to act by low levels of information or motivation, while others resist even high levels. Greater knowledge of the nature and correlates of these individual differences should make it possible to design mass media programs that would be more effective as well as more efficient.

Density of information—The number of information points per unit of time or space can have important effects on attention, learning, recall, and action. A high density tends to decrease attention but produces greater learning in individuals who do attend. Experiments that manipulate information density as an independent variable, if they are to produce findings which can apply to the usual mass media situation, must provide an opportunity for subjects to avoid (i.e., not attend to) the material presented. Unfortunately, group experiments are seldom designed in this way.

Program design features—Which elements or formats produce the most learning and which produce the most behavior? The features that promote one sometimes undermine the other, and those that maximize both need to be identified.

Relative vs. absolute levels of perceived susceptibility to a disease and per-

ceived seriousness of its consequences—Is there some level for these variables (e.g., 90% certainty of experiencing "extremely serious" effects) which almost invariably produces behavior change, or does this threshold vary with circumstances? What are the effects of various combinations and levels of the four elements in the health beliefs mode—perceptions of susceptibility, severity, benefits of action, and barriers to action?

Variable interactions and distributions—In what ways do psychological variables (such as risk-taking propensity and tolerance of ambiguity) interact with experiential variables such as media usage and health behaviors? How much influence do they have on such decisions as postponing the diagnosis of a symptom? How are the relevant psychological variables distributed in high-need target populations and across standard demographic categories?

Message/recipient interactions—More studies are needed that use as independent variables the state produced in a person by a message, rather than the characteristics of the message itself or those of the recipient. Particularly in experiments on very serious disease topics, the appropriate analytic variable is not the amount of threat applied but the amount of fear produced.

Risk and uncertainty as positive values—For many people, a warning of risk (such as the hazards of smoking) has reward properties; the excitement of danger is a source of gratification. In this circumstance, efforts to maintain uncertainty (e.g., by delaying a checkup) may be increased rather than decreased by a message about health risks, thus producing an effect opposite to the one intended.

Familial determinants of health decisions—We still know too little about the circumstances that enable one family member (spouse or child) to influence the health behavior of another. The same is true of "third parties" such as neighbors, friends, or employers.

Use of indirect appeals—"Indirect" here refers to nonhealth-related values (such as saving money, gaining social approval, or fulfilling parental role expectations) which can be invoked as inducements to take preventive health actions. Most people want to avoid being seen as hypochondriacal or too self-protective, and providing alternative reasons for following medical recommendations might be more effective with them than the commonly used health appeals.

Conflict resolution—The decision about whether or not to have a possible cancer symptom diagnosed typically involves an approach-avoidance conflict, because the diagnosis may resolve the ambiguity either favorably or unfavorably. It would be helpful to know how communications about cancer could be designed to reduce this conflict and thus increase subsequent willingness to seek diagnostic tests. Providing reassurance (such as by emphasizing the efficacy of treatment) is the most commonly used approach, but its effectiveness may be limited by the presence of other factors not yet identified.

Seriousness and utility—To what extent is receptivity to information about a health problem influenced by the perceived seriousness of the disease and the perceived usefulness of the information provided? Some research indicates that there are striking individual differences in the relationship between these factors, and that for some people the availability of useful information on ways to handle a threat may actually increase rather than decrease the impact of that threat.

Comparison of appeals—What is the relative effectiveness of various appeals in altering the anxiety value of disease topics? In the case of cancer, for example, is it easier to reduce anxiety by emphasizing the value of early detection, the efficacy of treatment, or other appeals?

Consequences of "informedness"—Is there something intrinsic to the possession of health knowledge which predisposes people to seek more knowledge? If so, is the converse true of a lack of knowledge? If felt ignorance maintains itself by prompting avoidance of information, this is an additional barrier to raising the currently low level of knowledge among some population groups. On the other hand, an awareness of ignorance about health matters (relative to what others are believed to know, or to what one should know) probably motivates some people to seek information. The question for public health practice is: As a means of inducing people to seek health information, is it more effective to make them feel relatively ignorant or relatively informed?

The answers to questions like these will provide no assurance that health communications will become either more creative or more effective. They should provide the opportunity for both, however, and perhaps that is all we should expect.

REFERENCES

Becker, M. H., Drachman, R. H., and Kirscht, J. P. Motivations as predictors of health behavior. *Health Serv. Rep.* 852–862 (1972).

Booth, A., and Babchuk, N. Informal medical opinion leadership among the middle aged and elderly. *Public Opinion Q.* 87–94 (1972).

Cox, D. F. Clues for advertising strategists. In Dexter, L. A., and White, D. M. (eds.): *People, Society, and Mass Communications,* pp. 359–393, Free Press, New York, 1964.

Evans, R. I., et al. Fear arousal, persuasion, and actual versus implied behavioral change: new perspective utilizing a real-life dental hygiene program. *J. Pers. Soc. Psychol.* 16:220–227, 1970.

Higbee, K. L. Fifteen years of fear arousal: research on threat appeals, 1953–1968. *Psychol. Bull.* 72:426–444 (1969).

Kalmer, H. (ed.): Reviews of research and studies related to delay in seeking diagnosis of cancer. *Health Education Monogr.* 2: No. 2 (Summer 1974).

Leventhal, H. Findings and theory in the study of fear communications. *Advances in Experimental Social Psychology,* vol. 5, pp. 119–186, Academic Press, New York (1970).

Mendelsohn, H. Some reasons why information campaigns can succeed. *Public Opinion Q.*:50–61 (1973).

O'Keefe, M. T. The anti-smoking commercials: a study of television's impact on behavior. *Public Opinion Q.* 35:242–248 (1971).

Reder, G. G., and Schwartz, D. Developing patients' knowledge of health. *Hospitals* 47:111–114 (1973).

Simonds, S. K. (ed.): Strategies for Planning and Evaluating Cancer Education. *Health Education Monogr.* No. 30 (1970).

Smith, F. A., et al. Health information during a week of television. *N. Engl. J. Med.* 9:516–520 (1972).

Steuart, G. W. Planning and evaluation in health education. *Int. J. Health Education* 65–76 (1969).

Swinehart, J. W. Voluntary exposure to health communications. *Am. J. Public Health* 1265–1275 (1968).

Tennant, F. S., Weaver, S. C., and Lewis, C. E. Outcomes of drug education: four case studies. *Pediatrics* 215–246 (1973).

Young, M. A. C. Review of research and studies related to health education practice: what people know, believe and do about health. *Health Education Monogr.* No. 23 (1967).

Cancer: The Behavioral Dimensions, edited by J. W. Cullen, B. H. Fox, and R. N. Isom. Raven Press, New York © 1976.

Respondent

Walter G. James

American Cancer Society New York, New York 10019

Before responding to the foregoing chapters in this section, I would like to draw your attention again to several very important statements Dr. Bernard Fox made concerning cancer control. He said we had achieved some successes in our cancer control programs, mentioning cigarette smoking and the Pap test as examples. He is correct. Cigarette smoking is a minority habit among adults in America today. Of our adult population, 37% now smoke cigarettes, a big decrease from late 1958 and 1959 when approximately 60% of adults smoked cigarettes. The major reason this decrease is not larger lies in the fact that more women in America are smoking now than ever before, and are starting to smoke younger.

In the Pap test area, a recent special study done for us by the Gallup organization indicated that 78% of the women over 20 in America say they have had a Pap test. I almost had a stroke when someone criticized the validity of studies based on the reported action of individuals. I was returned to a state of reasonably good health by someone in the audience who took up the banner for evaluation based on the individual's reported action. Of course, we have not completed the job regarding uterine cancer by any means, but our health education programs have made the women of America aware of the Pap test, what it can do in cancer control, and most women have started the habit of getting one. But a major percentage of adult women do not get the annual Pap test as the American Cancer Society recommends and we have specific high-risk groups of women that have yet to have their first Pap test.

Two other cancer sites should be mentioned—cancer of the breast and colon/rectum. There have been successes here, too. All is not as dismal as some of your previous speakers would imply. There are many lives to be saved through earlier diagnosis in breast cancer. With the advent of mammography, which physicians warn us needs to be accompanied by a clinical breast examination and followed with monthly breast self-examination, we have the opportunity to bring women to treatment at the time when a high percentage of the cancers are curable.

The Gallup study indicated that only 23% of women examine their breasts with the regularity ACS recommends (up from 14% in 1970). Of this number, only 22% feel confident that they could identify a lump from normal breast tissue.

We are far from our Pap test success with the public in the breast program, and our medical leadership reminds us that BSE is still the most effective early detection technique in breast cancer accessible to a large percentage of the public.

In control of cancer of the colon/rectum, we are still seeking a more proficient and economic screening test for the public. It has not been easy to "sell" adults on the proctoscopic examination using the proctosigmoidoscope. While each study we conducted indicates an increasing number of both men and women are aware of the procto examination, only 24% have ever had one such exam.

We are presently conducting demonstration projects regarding screening for occult blood in the stool, which many believe is a much more realistic approach to screening for this site of cancer. We are conducting studies to ascertain the most effective health education techniques to employ in persuading people to adhere to the diet regimen that is necessary for effective guaiac testing, and also how to persuade them to take the samples necessary and mail them in to a central facility for analysis. This program offers so many opportunities in the area of cancer control it is hard to resist taking more time to describe what we are now doing in this public education area.

I have mentioned these four sites of cancer because I was distressed by the general tenor of the previous discussions. I thought I heard some who were emphasizing the negative, who were dealers of doom. This is not an honest evaluation of the present situation regarding cancer control. While no knowledgeable person will say that all cancers are curable, or even all cancers of the four specific sites I have referred to are curable, a very high percentage of the cancers in these four sites are curable. There are thousands of lives that could be saved through early diagnosis and prompt treatment now.

Put yourself in the position of a program planner such as I. It will be obvious that you would continue to conduct programs which offer an opportunity to save lives. We would do this while waiting for further medical research to provide an opportunity to save an increasing number of lives. Now, lest I be accused of taking on a religious fervor about public education and cancer control, I will respond to the chapters on communications and cancer control.

I decided it might be best for me to share with you what I thought our panelists would say, then discuss any significant differences in their points of view and mine.

I thought their chapters would say: Good communications planners will use both mass communications and personal communications methods, capitalizing on the assets of each. A cancer education planner is what Bill Paisley refers to as a "communications engineer." Mass media represents a one-way communications process. Large audiences are reached faster through their use than with personal communications. Mass media can get public attention more effectively than personal communication and are important in setting the pace for a campaign type of educational program. Mass media provides the program, and the organization conducting the program provides the credibility so many have discussed during our sessions.

I thought our panel would also report that personal communications, face-to-face encounters, group discussions (two-way communications), are more effective than mass media in persuading people to act and to change established health habits. Personal communications capitalize on the warmth of the individual communicator. Opportunities vary from programs involving physicians talking with people to lay volunteers speaking with their friends and neighbors. Personal communications provide opportunities for questions and answers, for the expression of fears, and for discussions regarding accessibility of facilities. Personal communications are also much more effective than mass media with those segments of the population with an average or less-than-average education. The mass media are attitude builders, conditions of the public for more effective face-to-face or group approach.

I wish there were time for us to discuss how to develop projects using the personal approach. They are not as easily delivered as mass media, but are worth the time and effort that it takes to develop them.

Now, how does this compare with some of the previous chapters? I was impressed with Dr. Hochbaum's chapter and his comments regarding the teachable moment. We have referred to the teachable moment in school education for some time. He thought that we had that teachable moment in taking full advantage of the timing of the illness of our President's and Vice President's wives. I must admit, however, that I cannot agree with him in his estimate that any great number of people have been going to their doctors because of this publicity. Perhaps he knows something I don't know, but it is not sufficient to me to say that the present facilities are jammed because of this publicity. Facilities are limited at the present time. I would submit that the present publicity will be transitory and we must continue to rely on more effective health education techniques.

Dr. Mendelsohn disturbed me a bit in his appraisal of what health education is and what he thinks are the differences between education, information, and persuasion. I agree with his statement that health education is not only spreading information but is a program requiring strong support for more personal communications. Perhaps I heard him wrong, but I disagree quite emphatically with his implication that we may be able to persuade people to do things without knowing what they were doing, if what we were persuading them to do was good for them. This smacks of the hidden persuader concept and I don't think it has any place in the health field. We are interested in the development of lifesaving health habits, not one-time actions. We are concerned with people not starting to smoke; stopping smoking and staying off; examining their breasts, not once, but every month for a lifetime; having a Pap test every year. I can't believe we can do these things by drum beating and handing them a carrot. Perhaps I misjudged what was said but I believe those were the implications.

I agree with Dr. Mendelsohn's thought that educational programs should not only inform people about what they ought to do, but should also show them how to do it. Recently we brought together 15 top psychologists, educators, health educators, and others, and asked that they look at our program and make recommendations for the future. We were informed that our program was still information oriented, and the group recommended that we do more to help the public start the lifesaving health habit by doing it a first time—help them get the first Pap test, show them how to examine their breasts, help them give up cigarette smoking via group discussion. The Paisleys presented a historical review of communications research which is exactly what I thought they would do, and what they said is similar to my earlier remarks.

There was considerable talk about the effectiveness of school health education programs. I thought earlier comments concerning school health education were a bad rap and not warranted. School health education has never been given the financial support it needs to provide well-trained school health educators. There is a real need for long-term evaluation of school health education. Research is needed in the area of cancer fear and the relative effect of fear-arousing cancer education programs. We also need more research in the area of cancer education in general.

Sketchy studies among college students, and the like, are not very useful. We need much more profound studies among the general public and with special population groups. The role of the family in cancer education also needs much research. Very little has been done in this area.

Cancer: The Behavioral Dimensions, edited by J. W. Cullen,
B. H. Fox, and R. N. Isom. Raven Press, New York © 1976.

Adoption of Innovations Related to Cancer Control Techniques

Gerald E. Klonglan and Joe M. Bohlen

Iowa State University, Ames, Iowa 50010

Interest in social change during the past few decades has increased. The processes by which new technical and social ideas and products diffuse from one individual, group, or society to another are of special concern to social scientists. Also of interest are the decision-making processes through which individuals, organizations, and communities adopt or reject the new ideas.

The innovations we are concerned with are myriad. On the technological side they include: transportation systems—railways, automobiles, highways, and airplanes; communication technology—printing processes, telephones, radio, and television; agricultural production systems—improved strains of plants and animals, fertilizers, chemical pest control agents; and health and medical innovations—miracle drugs, contraceptives, and nutritional practices. The diffusion of social innovations, for example, the spread of specific ideas in education such as kindergarten, modern math and, in business, new management strategies, is also of interest.

Research scientists would like to understand and explain how and why such change occurs and also the factors that speed up or hinder the utilization of innovations. To date, more than 1,500 empirical studies of adoption and diffusion processes have been completed in the fields of anthropology, sociology, medical sociology, education, communication, and marketing (1). Nearly half the work concerned the diffusion of agricultural innovations. Six universities—Iowa State, Wisconsin, Michigan State, Missouri, Kentucky, and North Carolina State—served as centers for much of this activity. During the past decade there has been a rapid growth in the cross-cultural testing of adoption-diffusion concepts.

This chapter discusses the utility of some of the concepts and models generated in past adoption-diffusion research that may help increase the adoption of cancer control techniques by the general public, by health providers, by organizations, and by local communities.

This chapter focuses on the adoption of innovations, with almost no attention given to the diffusion of innovations. This distinction between the adoption versus the diffusion of innovations is very important.

Adoption generally refers to the behavior of an individual or group as it decides to accept a new innovation (idea, practice, or product). For example, we would study how one woman decides to adopt a breast self-examination (BSE) practice. Diffusion generally refers to the process in which the adoption of an innovation spreads through a group or client (system) for whom the innovation is intended. For example, we would study the process of women adopting BSE among the patients of one doctor or health clinic, or among all the people in one city, county, state, or nation.

Six major concepts are useful in understanding adoption behavior.

1. Change agency or change agent refers to any group or individual that attempts to influence the decision of others regarding new ideas, practices, and products in a direction believed to be desirable by the change agent.

Examples of cancer control change agencies and change agents are government agencies such as the National Cancer Institute's Cancer Control Program, and state and local departments of health; voluntary agencies such as the American Cancer Society; and private individuals and organizations such as local doctors and medical centers.

A change agent confronting an adoption situation may ask a series of questions about that situation. An initial question would be: "What is it that I am promoting?" Related to this question is the concept of innovation.

2. Innovation refers to an idea, practice, or product that is perceived as new by the individual or group for whom it is intended. Examples of innovations in our society are: oral contraceptives, computers, plaque control techniques, and community dental health clinics. Specific cancer control innovations include prevention ideas such as not smoking and avoiding the sun, and diagnostic ideas such as BSE, the Pap test, and proctoscopic examinations.

A change agent, having delineated his innovation, may next ask: "Who is it I want to have make a decision regarding this innovation?" Related to this question is the concept of adoption unit.

3. Adoption unit refers to the individual or group that makes the decision to adopt or accept an innovation. There may be several different levels of adoption units for a given innovation; for example, one level of adoption unit for a cancer control innovation may be an individual, another level adoption unit may be a group such as a clinic that allows new cancer control practices to be used, a third level may be a community that adopts a comprehensive cancer control program. Adoption units may vary from one innovation to another.

The change agent that identifies his innovation, and the appropriate adoption unit(s) may next ask: "What do I want these adoption units to do in regard to this innovation?" Related to this question is the concept of adoption behavior.

4. Adoption behavior refers to the actions that the adoption unit takes with regard to the innovation. The adoption of some innovations may involve the purchase of a new product. The adoption of other innovations will not involve a new product, but perhaps will involve a new way of doing some task, such as brushing one's teeth.

After the change agent has identified his innovation, adoption unit(s), and desired adoption behavior, he may then ask: "What decision-making will the adoption units go through with regard to the adoption of the innovation?" Related to this question is the concept of adoption process.

5. Adoption process refers to the process through which an adoption unit passes from the first hearing about an innovation to accepting (or rejecting) the innovation. This process is composed of a series of decisions rather than a single decision.

6. Sources of information refer to the various communication media that adoption units utilize in the adoption process. The majority of individuals use different sources of information at different stages in the adoption process. Various types of mass media and interpersonal communications are important.

These major concepts are discussed in more detail in the following sections. As each concept area is discussed, research findings based on cancer control innovations are presented. We will begin our elaboration by focusing on the adoption process. The other concepts: innovation, adoption behavior, adoption unit, and sources of information will then be discussed as key variables that can affect the rate at which individuals go through the adoption process, that is, can speed up or slow down the acceptance of new cancer control techniques.

ADOPTION PROCESS

Although the adoption process is concerned with the behavior of one adoption unit, this behavior occurs in a community context and is subject to various influences and restraints from elements in the community. Six stages in the adoption process may be delineated. At the unaware stage the adoption unit: (1) knows about the innovation but (2) lacks details about the innovation. At the information stage the adoption unit: (1) develops interest in the innovation, (2) gets facts about it, and (3) sees possibilities of its use. At the evaluation stage the adoption unit: (1) mentally tries the innovation, (2) weighs alternatives, (3) asks, "Can I (we) do it?", that is, "Do I (we) know how to use this innovation?", and (4) decides to try the innovation. At the trial state the adoption unit: (1) uses the innovation on a small scale and (2) deals with the problem of how to use the innovation. At the adoption stage the adoption unit (1) decides to use the innovation continuously and on a large scale and (2) finds satisfaction in using the innovation.

Research indicates that for innovations of major consequence, people usually go through a decision-making process in this general order. In some cases there is vacillation between the stages—especially between information gathering and evaluation. One of the outcomes of evaluation may be, "I need more information." If the innovation is cheap and is not of major consequence, for example, a new brand of toothpaste, they may proceed directly from awareness to trial. The trial serves as the major information base and provides serious evaluation for continued usage following the trial. We realize that this conference is concerned with things of greater consequence than the decision between two brands of toothpaste.

The stages in the adoption process are used to present the current state of adoption of selected cancer control techniques. Data are from 1970 and 1974 studies conducted for the American Cancer Society by the Gallup organization (2). These studies provide the percentage of adults in the awareness and trial stages, but do not provide complete data for the percent in information, evaluation, and adoption stages. (The Gallup questions were not designed to "test" the adoption process.)

The inclusion of 1970 and 1974 percentages makes it possible to see the degree to which the population of the United States has moved (or not moved) from one stage to another during the past 4 years.

TABLE 1. *Adoption Process and Selected Cancer Control Techniques*

Cancer control techniques (innovations)	Una-ware (%)	Stages in the adoption process				
		Aware (%)	Infor-mation	Evalu-ation	Trial (%)	Adop-tion
Pap test						
1970 Women	10	90			53	
1974 Women	12	88			78	
Breast self-examination						
1970 Women	30	70			49	
1974 Women	17	83			66	
Proctoscopy						
1970 Women	34	66			18	
1974 Women	38	62			22	
1970 Men	44	56			17	
1974 Men	44	56			24	

Several points can be made from an analysis of the data in Table 1.

1. In 1970, while 90% of adult women in the Unites States were aware of the Pap test, only 53% had ever had one. And since only 71% had had a test in 1968, it appears that very few women had adopted the idea of having a Pap test every year. One conclusion from these percentages is that in 1970 cancer change agents needed to move some 40% of U.S. women from awareness to trial (and hopefully then to adoption) and to convince another 40% who had tried a Pap test to adopt its use on a continuing yearly basis. Cancer change agents do not need to devote many resources to make women *aware* of the Pap test, but rather to invest their resources in getting action, that is, trial and adoption. Education strategies should be evaluated to determine the function (awareness, information, evaluation, trial, or adoption) they are trying to accomplish.

2. A comparison of 1970 and 1974 percentages indicates approximately one-fourth more women had had the Pap test by 1974 (78% vs 53%). The awareness figure did not change. (Given the percentage of women who become 21 years old each year, change agents need to make millions of women aware of the Pap test each year just to "stay even"; similarly with trial.)

3. When one compares 1970 and 1974 percentages for BSE, one sees an increase in awareness (83% vs. 70%) and in trial (66% vs. 49%).

4. One can also compare the adoption status of different innovations in Table 1. In 1974, more women were aware of the Pap test (88%) than BSE (83%) or proctoscopic (66%). The trial percentages for women across innovations are even more varied (78% Pap vs. 66% BSE vs. 22% procto). Cancer control change agents obviously need different educational programs for different cancer control innovations.

The stages of adoption framework have also been used to analyze the discontinuance of smoking cigarettes (3,4).

The time it takes people to go through the adoption process varies: some may go from awareness to adoption in 1 to 2 years, others may take 5 to 7 years. A major objective of the cancer change agent is to shorten the time between awareness and adoption of cancer innovations.

ADOPTION BEHAVIOR

Change agents need to be aware of the different kinds of adoption behavior they expect of adoption units. Some educational programs fail because change agents do not clearly specify what they want the adoption unit to do. Three possible types of adoption can be illustrated.

Direct action occurs when the adoption unit has adopted both the idea and object level of the innovation. The innovation sounds good, and the adoption unit wants to use it—a woman wants to do BSE, a man wants to stop smoking, a woman wants a Pap test.

Anticipatory adoption behavior occurs when an adoption unit adopts the idea level of an innovation and also decides to use or practice the innovation whenever the need should arise, that is, it anticipates using the innovation when it is needed. For example, a high-school girl may learn that she should start a Pap test yearly when she reaches 20 years of age.

Symbolic adoption occurs when an individual or group adopts the idea level of an innovation that may have no immediate or clear-cut object reference. Many preventive health-measure innovations are symbolic in nature. For example, the change agent may want people to guard themselves from the sun or not start smoking cigarettes.

ADOPTION UNIT

As stated earlier, an adoption unit may be an individual or a group such as a family, formal organization, or community. If the focus is on an individual as an adoption unit, various characteristics of the individual become important. These characteristics have often been analyzed by adoption researchers and have implications for the perception of the innovation held by the adoption unit and the adoption unit's behavior in the adoption process. Personal characteristics, including age, education, income, marital status, and so on, affect adoption behavior. The amount of knowledge, general and specific, held by the adoption unit is important. The *attitudes,* including those about the change agency or change agent, about the innovation, and about the adoption situation, will also affect the degree of adoption.

The 1974 Gallup study shows that individual characteristics are related to differential awareness and trial of cancer control innovations. Table 2 presents a summary of differential awareness and trial of the Pap test by age cohort, education level, region of the United States, occupation, size of community, and family income.

TABLE 2.   *Adoption Unit Characteristics Related to the Awareness and Trial of the Pap Test (1974)*

Age (yr)		20–34	35–49	50 & over	
Aware (%)		94	92	79	
Trial (%)		89	85	66	
Education		College	High school	Grade school	
Aware(%)		94	92	64	
Trial (%)		83	81	55	
U.S. region		East	Midwest	South	West
Aware (%)		83	92	83	93
Trial (%)		71	79	74	86
Occupation	Prof. & Bus.	Cler. & Sales	Manual	Farmer	Non-labor
Aware (%)	94	95	90	68	75
Trial (%)	85	83	83	62	58
Size of Community	1 million & over	250,000– 1 million	50,000– 250,000	2,500– 50,000	Under 2,500
Aware (%)	82	92	93	87	82
Trial (%)	71	79	85	73	75
Family Income		$15,000 & over	$10,000– 14,999	$5,000– 9,999	Under $5,000
Aware (%)		95	92	87	75
Trial (%)		84	85	80	60

There are significant differences in awareness and trial across different levels of each of these variables. For example, women over 50 are less aware of the Pap test and have had it less frequently than younger women. Those with grade-school education are less aware and have not had the Pap test to the extent high-school and college graduates have. Women in the West and Midwest are slightly more aware and have more likely had the Pap test than women in the East and South. Women in professional business, clerical-sales, and manual occupations are more aware of and have more likely had a Pap test than farm women and women not in the labor force. Women in large cities (over 1 million) and in small towns (under 2,500) are less aware and have had the Pap test less than women in middle-sized cities. And women with lower incomes are less aware of and have not had the Pap test as often as women in higher-income families.

Social class was found by Hill (5) to be a factor in the use of the Pap smear test. Over 54% of the wives of professionals, executives, and self-employed businessmen had had the tests, whereas only 41% of the wives of white-collar and skilled workers and about 34% of the wives of semiskilled and unskilled workers had had them. Nearly 46% of the women living in high-status residential areas had had the tests, whereas only 28% of those living in low-status areas had done so. Two factors tend to explain these data: (1) There is a high correlation between social class position and place of residence; (2) as explained by Wakefield (6), more of those doctors who defined their clientele as high class had tried persuasion and taken smears. About 57% of those doctors defining clientele as middle class had followed this procedure, but only 30% of the doctors who defined clientele as lower class had done so.

Cancer change agents have many individual adoption units. The general public may be the first adoption unit to come to mind. However, there are many other important individuals who must adopt cancer control innovations if there is to be a successful cancer control program. These include doctors, nurses, teachers, school administrators, volunteers, legislators, community leaders, and many more key decision-makers.

Groups or firms as adoption units also have characteristics that affect the acceptance or rejection of innovations. Some of these characteristics are the goals of the organization, the roles in the organization, and the relative authority or power that people have in these roles. For example: How do cancer control representatives approach an industry to encourage it to adopt a cancer control program? To whom do they go—management, labor, the workers? Who has the authority? Who sets the goals? A recent book by Zaltman et al. (7) applies many of the adoption-diffusion concepts to organizations as adoption units.

Cancer change agents have specified many groups (social systems) as adoption units. These include businesses and industries, medical schools, public schools, hospitals, civic clubs, health planning councils at state and local levels, insurance companies, and so on. It is important that the change agent clearly identify the adoption unit (individual, group, or community) before he designs specific educational and action programs.

Sometimes the community is the adoption unit of an innovation. Federal and state law often require a vote of the people before a new school, library, or hospital facility (innovation) can be adopted. Some of the relevant concepts here include the community power structure, the system linkages, both vertical (extra community) and horizontal (within the community), between organizations in the community, and the importance of various subsystems in effecting innovation decisions. An example of research focusing on the community as the adoption unit is Aiken and Alford's (8) study of 582 American cities regarding their adopting urban renewal programs.

INNOVATION

The change agent asks: "What are the characteristics of my innovation?" As in a communication setting, the sender (change agent) and the receiver (adoption unit) of a message will each have perceptions of that message. The change agent's perception of the innovation and the adoption unit's perception of the innovation must both be understood. Often, however, these two perceptions are different. Thus, the change agent must ask: "What are the characteristics of the innovation as perceived by the change agent?" and "What are the characteristics of the innovation as perceived by the adoption unit?"

Two general characteristics of an innovation are the idea level and the object level. An innovation always involves a new idea, that is, it has an idea level. Some innovations also involve a new object such as practice or product. The innovation can be dealt with at the "idea" or abstract level and also at the practice level, which involves what a person does to his teeth each day.

There are more specific characteristics of an innovation to be considered by the change agent as he tries to get adoption units to accept his innovations.

Complexity refers to the degree to which an innovation is relatively difficult to understand and to use. The less complex the innovation, the greater the possibility of its being adopted by the adoption unit.

Divisibility refers to the degree to which an innovation may be tried on a limited basis. Smokers who try to reduce smoking may stop completely or reduce their smoking from three packs to two packs a day. The greater the divisibility, the greater chance for adoption.

Visibility refers to the degree to which the results of an innovation can be observed. The results of some innovations, such as weed spray, can be readily seen (the plants die), but the results of other innovations, preventive vaccinations, are not as visible, that is, the person is no more healthy after the "shot" than he was before. The greater the visibility of the innovation, the greater the adoption potential.

Compatibility refers to the degree to which an innovation is consistent with existing values and past experiences of the adoption units. For example, a woman who has had a physical each year will be more likely to request a Pap test than a woman who has not had regular physical exams. The greater the compatibility, the greater the chance for adoption.

In a research study, Sansom et al. (9) found that more women who had a regular physical examination were having Pap smear tests. They found that 9% of the women who had had the test (based on their medical records) did not even know they had had it. Although it is more important for women over 40 years of age to have regular tests, Hill (5) found that 50% of the women under 40 years of age had had smear tests, whereas only 30 % of those over 40 years of age had done so. One factor in this higher percentage among the more nubile women was the fact that the smear was included as a routine in postnatal physical examination—the compatibility factor.

Relative advantage refers to the degree to which an innovation is superior to ideas that preceded it. Three subconcepts of relative advantage are: economic costs, the direct purchase value; usefulness, the degree to which it meets a real need of the adoption unit; payoff time, the length of time it takes to see results from trying the innovation. The greater the relative advantage of an innovation, the more likely it will be adopted.

Accessibility-availability refers to the degree to which an adoption unit has opportunity to use the innovation. Some innovations such as fluoridation of water may be desired by some people, but if their community decides not to adopt fluoridation, the innovation is not as available or accessible as it would be to adoption units that experience fluoride in the water.

Almost no research has been done on analyzing the effect of innovation characteristics on the adoption of cancer control innovations. There appears to be a need to make a comprehensive list of all cancer control innovations and to clearly identify the characteristics of each innovation. It may be desirable to categorize the innovations in different functional categories, that is, prevention innovations (not smoke, avoid sun, etc.), diagnosis innovations (Pap test, BSE, procto, etc.), treatment innovations, and rehabilitation innovations.

SOURCES OF INFORMATION

Many researchers have studied the sources of information that people use at each stage of the adoption process. Most studies find that most people use more than one source of information at each stage in the adoption process. Another finding is that mass media sources (TV, radio, newspapers, magazines, etc.) are more important at the awareness and information stages, whereas interpersonal communication with neighbors, friends, and commercial (business) or professional people (doctors) tend to be more important sources of information at the evaluation, trial, and adoption stages.

There is a paucity of data regarding the relative importance of various sources of information at the different stages of adoption for cancer control innovations. The studies that have obtained source-of-information data have usually focused on the awareness stage, that is, "Where did you first hear about the Pap test?"

Wakefield (6) found that 10% of the women in his study had first heard about the Pap smear test (he calls it the "cervical cytology test") from a poster in their doctor's office. Sansom et al. (9) found that 39% of the patients obtained their first information regarding the Pap smear test from mass media; 37% from doctors; 11% from neighbors, friends, and relatives; and 5% from clinics.

The quality of the information varied greatly by information source (9). Approximately 25% of the respondents (all had had Pap tests) were unaware of or uncertain of the need to have regular tests. Where they had first heard of the tests seemed to be related to their awareness of the necessity of having repeated tests. Nearly 91% of those who had first heard about tests from a clinic or mass media knew of the necessity to repeat the test. Nearly 89% of those who heard from neighbors, friends, or relatives knew the test should be repeated, but only 54% of those who first heard from a doctor knew of this necessity.

Communication regarding the outcomes of the test was varied. About 50% of the women were notified of the results by the doctor, either on a face-to-face basis or via telephone or letter; about 25% were told that if they did not hear, they could assume the test indicated no abnormalities; about 17% had to take the initiative and contact the doctor; and about 5% never learned the results. One might conclude that in about half of the cases the doctors were missing an opportunity to educate and provide peace of mind to their patients.

Lieberman (10), studying the impact of distributed leaflets in the "Crusade for Cancer," found that 50% of the people who had been given leaflets had read them. Among those who had read the leaflets, there was a significantly greater awareness of the seven danger signals than among a control group. The intriguing and unexplained aspect of these data is the differential awareness of the individual signals. Among those who had received and read the leaflets, 60% recognized a lump or thickening in the breast as a danger signal (50% in the control group), but only 19% recognized a persistent hoarseness (8% of control) as a danger signal.

Because these leaflets were distributed door-to-door, there were two communication sets involved: the leaflet itself, and the interaction between the person who answered the door and the person dispensing the leaflet.

Lieberman found that if the volunteer who distributed the leaflet had encouraged the household to read it, 72% had read some; only 40% had read the leaflet when not encouraged by the dispenser to do so.

This finding is closely related to another. If the people receiving the leaflet felt that the dispenser was dedicated and involved in doing his job, 65% had read the leaflet, whereas only 47% who read it thought that the dispenser was doing a job for which he was paid and did not necessarily believe in what he was doing.

Dispensing leaflets by ringing doorbells has some definite limitations. Over 86% of those contacted in this manner were women. In addition to men being underrepresented, so were those under 30 years of age and the lower classes.

The 1974 Gallup study asked each woman who had had a Pap smear to state the reasons why she had her first Pap test (trial stage). The responses are summarized in Table 3.

Bond (11) compared two interpersonal sources of information settings, group discussion versus traditional lectures, to encourage breast examinations. She conducted 42 discussion groups and 33 lectures with 933 women. She found that women in the group discussion meetings had a higher rate of physician visits for breast examination than the women in the traditional lecture sessions. She also found that a larger portion of the women in the group discussion developed the habit of BSE and a greater percentage reported to a physician to demonstrate their BSE technique.

The answers do not clearly reflect the relative importance of various sources of information. However, over one-fifth said a doctor had suggested the test.

There appears to be social class differences in the use of sources of information. In a five-class categorization (6), more than 56% of the women in Class I and Class II had first heard about the Pap smear test via mass media, whereas only about one-third of those in the lower classes had first heard through this means.

TABLE 3. *Reasons Why Women First Have a Pap Test (Trial Stage)*

Women who have had a Pap test	
Reason	%
Part of routine physical	29
Suggested by doctor	23
Personal safety	12
Was having physical problems	11
Any contraceptive mentioned	5
Routine for pregnant women	4
Advertising influenced me	3
Routine after childbirth	2
Employment requirement	2
Miscellaneous	2
Undesignated	11

Another way of interpreting the Wakefield data, which define the task of the change agent more clearly, is the evidence that, in a census distribution of the area studied, only 2.6% of the women were in Social Class I, but they comprised 7.7% of all the women who had had a smear test. Nearly 34% of the women were in Social Classes IV and V, but they comprised only 15% of the women who had had the tests.

The few cancer-related source-of-information studies seem consistent with other research, that is, there is an important role for both mass media and interpersonal communication to play in affecting people's adoption process.

SUMMARY

This chapter reported some of the conceptual frameworks developed over the past 25 years by researchers studying the adoption of innovations. Cancer-related research studies were discussed to illustrate the potential use of the adoption framework in helping cancer control change plan and implement priority education and action programs. The five-step adoption process and some key factors affecting the rate of adoption were briefly discussed.

REFERENCES

1. Rogers, E. M., and Shoemaker, F. F. *Communication of Innovations: A Cross Cultural Approach,* Free Press, New York, 1971.
2. Gallup Organization, Inc. *The Public's Awareness and Use of Cancer Detection Tests,* The Gallup Organization, Inc. Princeton, 1970.
3. Warren, R., Klonglan, G. E., and Winkelpleck, J. M. Application of an adoption model to smoking and health. Paper presented at the Third World Congress for Rural Sociology, Baton Rouge, 1972.
4. Green, L. W. Diffusion and adoption of innovations related to cardiovascular risk behavior in the public. Paper presented at the American Heart Association Conference on Applying Behavioral Science to Cardiovascular Risk, Seattle, 1974.
5. Hill, J. *Attitudes and Behavior Related to the Cervical Cytology Test,* Neoplasm UICC Report Series, Vol. 9 (1972).

6. Wakefield, J. The family doctor: Key figure in screening by cervical cytology. *Health Trends* 3:25 (1971).
7. Zaltman, G., Duncan, R. and Holbek, J. *Innovations and Organizations,* John Wiley, New York, 1973.
8. Aiken, M., and Alford, R. R. Community structure and innovation: The case of urban renewal. *Am. Sociol. Rev.* 35:650–665 (1970).
9. Sansom, C. D., Wakefield, J., and Pinnock, K. M. Chance or chance? How women come to have a cytotest done by their family doctor. *Int. J. Health Education* 14:127 (1971).
10. Lieberman, S. Annual Crusade for Cancer: Opportunity for mass education. Paper presented at *New Jersey Division, American Cancer Society,* December 4, 1971.
11. Bond, B. *Group Discussion–Decision: An Appraisal of its Use in Health Education,* Minnesota Department of Health, 1956.

Cancer: The Behavioral Dimensions, edited by J. W. Cullen, B. H. Fox, and R. N. Isom. Raven Press, New York © 1976.

Cancer Call-PAC—People Against Cancer

Georgia Photopoulos

I am a cancer patient involved in person-to-person, patient-to-patient communication in the vast area of human need. In a sense, I feel I represent the countless thousands of cancer patients; the unheard voices pleading for an empathetic ear, a measure of understanding, and a sense of direction.

We have discussed mass media communications, but so far this volume has not touched on the urgent need for patient-to-patient and doctor-to-patient communication for the cancer patient.

I was 34 years old when I discovered I had cancer. By the grace of God and with the help of medical science, I am still alive, but I am also fighting to stay alive. I have had to draw on every ounce of energy at my command to wage this 6-year battle. During this time I have undergone bilateral mastectomies, with metastasis to the lymph nodes, a recurrence of the original malignancy, 120 treatments of cobalt and deep X-ray therapy, many localized excisions in the throat, right axilla, ribs, an oophorectomy, and a medical hysterectomy following additional complications. In addition to losing both breasts, most of my hair, and most of the sensation in my right hand and arm, I suffer from a variety of serious complications; a degenerative joint disease, continual bladder aggravation, and lymphedema.

In destroying the disease that invaded my body and threatens me daily, medical science has also destroyed other vital systems within my body. Healthy tissue was cut away with the diseased—muscles were severed—nerves were injured. The damage to my body will be with me forever.

The pain has been great. But it has not been mine alone. My husband, who has never wavered from my side, and two small adopted children also have suffered, and are suffering pain, mental anguish, and fear; all of this while tottering on the brink of financial disaster as more and more of our income is expended on medical and medically related expenses.

These past 6 years have been years of pain, doubt, fear, and anguish, but years of hope, too. I've learned there are only two ways of coping with cancer—either you fight it and give yourself a chance to live or you surrender to it. I decided to fight it. In so doing, I discovered that fear is the biggest enemy. Fearing cancer is harder than having it. Fear is what makes you delay in seeking treatment, fear is what cripples your ability to deal with it, and fear ultimately can be fatal.

Because I knew from my own experiences and those of many others that cancer brings not only physical but emotional suffering, I began to develop in my mind a program through which cancer patients themselves could help one another through their times of crisis and fear.

When I first was asked to lecture and share my battle with cancer, my private thoughts, family reactions, curiosity and denial encountered from friends, supportive measures that could assist other cancer victims, and the urgent need for communication between patients and caregivers, I decided to speak candidly.

The reaction that followed overwhelmed me. Demands for speeches, lectures, newspaper articles, radio and television appearances, interviews, and consultations with various hospital personnel poured in. But even more significant was the response from the general public, cancer patients and their families—people from all walks of life. I found people willing to listen because of my own experiences with cancer.

When called upon to give speeches, I used every opportunity to urge the American Cancer Society to begin a 24-hour-a-day telephone service—a hotline—for cancer patients. In my speeches, in newspaper interviews, on television, I kept repeating the need for such a program, not only for the patient, but for the family as well, to have a friendly, sympathetic, well-informed person who had been through it to talk with, whatever the hour, whenever there was a need.

The Chicago Unit of the Illinois Division of the American Cancer Society asked me to develop such a program as a pilot project to meet the nonphysical needs of cancer patients. It has been operating in the Chicago area and is known as CANCER CALL-PAC—People Against Cancer.

It has been incorporated as an ongoing service provided by the Chicago unit. This unique pilot program originated in the Chicago area over 19 months ago and is designed to help cancer patients and their families, via telephone, on a 24-hour basis, recognizing the fact that fear cannot be confined to a Monday through Friday, 9-to-5 basis. Offering emotional support, understanding and a sharing of supportive measures can often be the turning point in one's decision not to give up but to keep on fighting with all the resources he or she can muster.

PAC is not designed to interfere with the medical team or to intrude on the doctor-patient relationship. The service is designed to help patients and to help their families cope with many emotional burdens brought on by cancer.

I am delighted that PAC has been awarded a merit citation by a National Honors Committee of the American Cancer Society...because of the uniqueness of service offered to cancer patients and its high degree of volunteer involvement.

Many people have called for this service and they often mask their true reason for seeking someone to speak with. Some patients call in a state of anxiety the day they receive that much dreaded diagnosis. Calls have come from young children who want to know how to help a mother or father who is a cancer victim. Calls come from friends of patients asking: How do you talk to a cancer patient? How do you listen to a cancer patient? Help me convey that I understand. In what way can I offer assistance?

Calls such as "I can cope with my cancer diagnosis but since I've lost my hair, when I look into a mirror I literally scream. I need a wig. For me it's a necessity. Tell me where to go."

One caller, a young mother of four, was able to accept her diagnosis of terminal cancer of the pancreas. Her urgent need, as she expressed it, was to have the privilege of selecting a homemaker to come into her home to raise her children after her death. Her weakened condition would not permit her the luxury of interviewing 20 or 30 people. Her question—would we please, under her stipulations, narrow the list to three—and make it possible for her to put her house in order before she died.

Sometimes callers have needed assurance that it is not unusual to experience weakness and nausea following radiation. The knowledge that this is a possible side effect has a tremendous calming influence upon the caller who might feel that it was the cancer that was spreading and causing the distress.

Often, patients have been the victims of unkind remarks about the dreaded type of illness that has afflicted them. Some say they have been shunned, ostracized, insulted, and verbally attacked by unknowledgeable and superstitious people. Knowing that many of us have also been victims of the same attacks has given them a sense of relief. Others want a sympathetic ear because they are reluctant to discuss what is troubling them with the people closest to them because they are afraid their own friends or relatives might humiliate them or fail to understand.

One mastectomy patient called and said her intentions were to offer me some emotional support. I thanked her very much for thinking of me and after several minutes of conversation I tried to terminate the call. At that point her tone and mood changed. She poured out a tale of fear, anxiety, and a sense of guilt. She then admitted that she really had called for help for herself. She had lost two sisters and her mother to cancer. She lived in constant fear of dying. Her husband had refused intimacy with her. When she lost her second sister and couldn't bring herself to attend the funeral, she suffered a profound sense of guilt. The conversation continued for a very long time, and, step by step, we listed all of her immediate problems. The woman was very receptive to many suggestions, including a referral to a pastoral counselor to help her deal with her sense of guilt.

Apparently, with two phone calls, we were able to offer this troubled woman a sense of direction because she later took the time to write the Cancer Society to thank them for providing a service such as PAC. This feedback was valuable to us.

A young woman with advanced metastatic disease confined to bed in a hospital because of numerous fractures called for help. She said her need was very personal. As luck would have it, she was a patient in the same hospital I go to for physical therapy, so I suggested a visit with her in person.

The chemotherapy treatment she was receiving caused her blood count to become so low that the doctors had placed her in isolation. Her problems were many: Her mother had died of cancer in a hospital; her father had died of cancer at home; no family left; never married; no insurance.

Her time was limited. But, now, at age 36, she finally had acquired her first boyfriend. This overwhelmed her because he was sincere and attentive and loved her enough to visit her daily and go through all of the precautionary requirements needed to visit a patient in isolation. No one ever had lavished attention on her before. Those were the massive problems that confronted this frail young woman.

But her urgent need, which she felt was too humiliating for a dying woman to share with doctors, nurses, or with the hospital chaplains who visited her daily, was to be released from the hospital to live with this very special person she had just found. If she had 4 weeks to live if hospitalized, or just 1 or 2 weeks if released to go home, she preferred to bargain for less time with the man she loved than for more time spent in isolation. This very poignant need was what she wished me to convey to the hospital staff. A very big order, but she felt that "as another cancer patient" I would not ridicule the desire she couldn't share with nonpatients. Her wishes were granted and her friend was at home beside her when death came.

I think that doctors and nurses could do a lot to help cancer patients accept and deal with their diagnosis by explaining things a little better. They should explain what procedures will be followed, that pain is normal following surgery, that it takes a long time for the body to adjust to major surgery, and in some cases that certain chemical as well as physical changes will take place. I think that sometimes doctors withhold information from patients on the assumption that they might not be able to take it, or they assume that someone else will explain the hard facts of the case to the patient. Following my first mastectomy, whenever I had questions concerning the surgery, my gynecologist referred me to the surgeon, who in turn referred me back to the gynecologist, and then on to the radiologist. It was only by accident that I stumbled onto the information that there had been metastasis in the underarm lymph nodes, although I had assumed as much. It actually was a relief just to know for sure. At least the guessing game was over.

It is the patient's right to know where the trouble is, what it is, and what has to be done to provide a cure. The doctor should be able to tell the patient in clear terms why surgery is necessary. The term inoperable should be more clearly defined so that when there is a diagnosis of cancer, the patient will know that, although surgery cannot be performed in his particular situation, there are other avenues of treatment such as radiation, therapy, or chemotherapy. When not defined, a patient can hear the word inoperable and in his own mind believe that this means no surgery, no hope, fini!

It is difficult for people to continuously ask for help. It takes a good listener to hear what a cancer patient or his family is saying because frequently they mask the truth. In fact, patients may not understand their own problem well enough to know what help they might need. Frequently they need a sense of direction. Compassion alone is not enough. In my case, the family was a tremendous instrument that assisted me in coping with my stress and my problems. But after several thousand days of battling cancer, the stress and the burden of living with this disease has taken its toll on all of us. The enormity of this struggle and the problems it has wrought upon my family, the physical, psychological, emotional, and financial burdens it has imposed upon me and my loved ones, have caused me to suffer a profound sense of guilt. To compensate for this intrusion in our lives I have tried to be all things to all people.

I have learned that when you come face-to-face with an enemy such as cancer, when you are overwhelmed with physical pain and limitations, emotional, psychological problems, what you don't need is to be totally wiped out financially.

I have spoken with cancer patients from all walks of life, and what they want most is hope, understanding, and a sense of direction and dignity in the face of personal catastrophe. I have learned that they are willing to fight to stay alive, pay any price, go anywhere to seek a cure.

While doctors are expert at treating disease and experts in the behavioral sciences—others are expert at research, and still others are expert at fund raising—I feel that I am an expert in coping with and living with a catastrophic illness while being a full-time wife and mother living a full, productive, and creative life.

Cancer: The Behavioral Dimensions, edited by J. W. Cullen,
B. H. Fox, and R. N. Isom. Raven Press, New York © 1976.

Discussion

Hochbaum: As I was listening, it occurred to me that Mrs. Photopoulos has really said almost everything or has touched on almost everything we have discussed. Somehow I think · she has communicated these issues much more effectively than any statistics or research finding that I could cite. It may be that the one thing I learned is that we should not talk so much about how can we communicate what to whom, but how can we be more sensitive to the people to whom we want to communicate and discover what they want and need. Maybe we should turn the next session around and look at the whole problem from the other side. This is my own reaction.

Goldstein: I believe like you, Dr. Hochbaum, that that was a succinct summary of what we are doing here. My interest again is in behavior change. I am concerned that there is almost an "amen" that comes with the chapters and comments here, and since these proceedings do have serious implications for policy, I want to make the following response. At the end of Mr. James' comments and others there seems to be an almost flippant response that you don't change behavior with carrots. I suggest that we need to be concerned with behavior change and not theory. But the need for hard empirical ways of looking at behavior change on the part of business has been found in the mass media; they are experts at sickness. For example, Doctor Stein and I were looking at the Sunday *Times* and were thrilled to see the following advertisement—that if you behave in the following new way you will get a 50-cent check signed by Benny Goodman, or if you behave in this way, you will get a mirror poster from 1912, or if you behave in this way, you will get a Benny Goodman (which I gather is a very exciting and reinforcing item these days) solid sterling silver, music silver ingot. I am not sure of the value of these reinforcers to the population, but I do know that in the board rooms of Madison Avenue people are cooking up for the Sunday *Times* ways to pay off behaviors new and old. That's the behavior that Dr. Stein and I saw. We were shocked at the very effective use of behavior control by the mass media while we sit here and talk about not affecting change with carrots. They do it extremely well.

Evans: Dr. Goldstein seems to be making responses based on his feeling that behavioral modification is being attacked. He may know about the book I did with Fred Skinner, and I have this strange feeling that if Fred were sitting here, he would not have gotten up with Dr. Goldstein because he would be figuring out some way of attempting to handle this group rather than having aversive control. I don't think anybody I have heard here would suggest that we do away with behavior modification. The whole issue here is which of several types of strategy will work. I do not feel that there is any unjustified criticism of behavioral modification in the sense that he is suggesting. I really believe it has a definite place in the behavioral field and I think some of us who do research recognize that it does. By the same token, I hope he is open-minded enough to recognize that diffusion of innovation may be a factor and it is also very possible that some of the communication models that the Paisleys talked about may be factors, or the elegant analysis of communication that Mendelsohn talked about may also be a factor. I hope he recognized that, because I think it would be an incorrect impression to say that there is a concerted attack on behavior modification.

Mendelsohn: Apparently Mr. James thinks I am a believer in hidden persuasion. I can assure him I don't even know what hidden persuasion is. What I was trying to say is that

261

we should be overt persuaders, and most communications research people believe that the most powerful overt propaganda we can use is the truth.

Cancer: The Behavioral Dimensions, edited by J. W. Cullen, B. H. Fox, and R. N. Isom. Raven Press, New York © 1976.

Coping with Cancer: A Challenge to the Behavioral Sciences

Jimmie C. B. Holland

Albert Einstein College of Medicine, Bronx, New York 10461; and Montefiore Hospital and Medical Center, Bronx, New York 10467

Many challenging psychological issues are raised by a study of how the patient, his family, and the physician and medical staff cope with cancer. The stresses imposed by the disease upon all concerned and ways of coping with these stresses form the core of these psychological and psychosocial issues (1). Each patient's social, psychological, and medical situation is unique, yet a frame of reference is needed to compare one patient's reaction with those of others. Three clearly defined challenges exist for behavioral scientists:(a) to determine the spectrum of normal, adaptive responses to cancer and its treatment in patient, family, and physician; (b) to determine the origin and range of maladaptive responses; and (c) to search for early, effective, and economically feasible psychosocial interventions for the maladaptive responses (2).

The response to cancer is a continually changing adaptation based on stresses imposed by the disease itself. There are some critical points during the diagnosis and treatment of cancer, and psychological management at these junctures may either enhance or hinder a healthy adaptation. The three chapters on coping with cancer deal with three critical transitional periods: the time of diagnosis, the progression of the disease, and the terminal stage.

DIAGNOSIS OF CANCER

When the primary physician receives the pathological reports indicating cancer, he must begin to plan treatment and to deal with the matter of informing the patient. His own feelings about cancer and about the particular patient involved may lead him to shield the patient excessively or to blurt out the truth without correctly assessing the patient's capacity for accepting the information. These two extremes are characterized by: "There's nothing seriously wrong with you; you'll be well in no time," on the one hand, and: "You have cancer; there's nothing more I can do for you," on the other. The first response is improper because lies have no place in medical management; the other extreme reaction causes the patient to feel abandoned. Both extremes represent problems in the doctor's attitude that will result in the patient's distrust of him. Between these two extremes is the physician's constructive response in which he evaluates each patient's ability to deal with the information and therefore selects the most appropriate and empathic way to impart it (2). Dr. Krant elaborates on some of the doctor's problems that lead to his maladaptive responses and result in added distress for the patient.

Although it is diminishing, ingrained attitudes do not change easily, and for most people the word "cancer" alone produces fear. The fears are several: (a) threat of death; (b) uncertainty concerning the future; (c) fear of pain; (d) fear of losing a body part or function; (e) fear of losing family and work; (f) fear of dependency and costly medical care: and (g) fear of alienation from others (3).

All of these fears are exacerbated by knowing that one has cancer, no matter how sensitively the doctor has presented the diagnosis. An acute grief reaction may ensue as a normal reaction to the shocking news. This is similar to that noted in individuals informed of a disaster or of great personal loss (4).

An initial period of disbelief is followed by one of anger and depression but usually with gradual acceptance of the reality. The presence of anxiety, insomnia, anorexia, inability to concentrate, and irritability is normal at this time. Resolution of the acute reaction occurs when a feeling of alliance with the doctor develops, and a treatment plan is initiated (5). This normal reaction may be replaced by a spectrum of maladaptive responses. One response is total denial of the information, evidenced by the patient's refusal of further medical care. A search for other and less threatening medical opinions or even quack cures may ensue. Another extreme response is a fatalistic refusal to accept treatment because the patient feels that he will die anyway. These responses are detrimental to good care and must be tagged early by the doctor in order to provide optimal medical treatment and psychological support. JoAnn Vettese discusses the patient's problems in more depth.

The family's response at this point is crucial in enhancing the patient's opportunity for optimal care and in promoting the psychological support he can gain through close cooperation of family with physician. Since the doctor may choose to give the diagnosis to a spouse or other family member first, the patient may be isolated by a family response such as: "You mustn't tell him. He couldn't bear to know." More often than not, this response actually means that the family cannot bear to know. The complexities of "conspiracies of silence" (2) can reach extraordinary proportions in which the patient continues the pretense of not knowing and bears the lonely burden to protect his family. Early identification of a family member who shows a maladaptive response is essential.

TREATMENT OF CANCER

The treatments for cancer are sometimes as formidable as the disease itself. Surgical procedures are particularly frightening, and preparation for the loss of a body part or function should be an essential part of presurgical workup. Volunteers who have survived similar losses successfully constitute a great, untapped, psychosocial resource for patients undergoing cancer surgery. The medical profession's suspicion of nonprofessional volunteers has delayed optimal use of these individuals. They are particularly effective in the colostomy, laryngectomy, and mastectomy groups. By their visible survival and return to full function, they give hope to those confronting the same type of surgical procedures.

Before undergoing radiotherapy, patients need psychological preparation in order to correct misconceptions concerning radiation and its side effects. We are currently involved in a study of patient adjustment to treatment after he receives defined pretreatment orientation given by the radiotherapist. The patient meets the radiotherapy technician, sees the treatment room and machine that will treat him, and asks any questions that disturb him before coming for the first treatment. Levels of adjustment to the stress are compared with those patients receiving standard management, with little if any preparation.

Chemotherapy poses many psychological stresses. It is usually associated in a patient's mind with the phrase: "there isn't much left to be done for me." The threat of death is compounded by the unpleasant side effects of certain drugs. These effects include alopecia, life-threatening infections, and the mood changes associated with steroids. Some drugs have profound neurological effects. We have recently studied L-asparaginase, which causes profound loss of cognitive function. The deficit is corrected by infusion of asparagine, the essential amino acid which it blocks (6). Studying effects of the several classes of chemotherapeutic drugs, particularly antimetabolites, may lead to considerable information concerning normal brain function.

The great stress of loneliness is induced by the inability to touch family or others during the long period of enforced, total, physical isolation in germfree environments (7). Importance of physical contact in comforting the ill patient has been shown in a study of these patients, who actually tolerated their isolation quite well. This may be attributable to the highly specialized nursing care they received.

The stressful treatments outlined here must of necessity be given by skilled specialists, each of whom administers one treatment as consultant, usually assuming only temporary responsibility for the patient. The fragmentation of care in cancer may result in sequential management of the cancer patient by surgeon, radiotherapist, and oncologist, each responsible for a brief period. Better psychological support of the patient is obtained when there is one physician or medical person on whom the patient can rely and who explains the various treatments given by multiple specialists. The internist oncologist may by personality and training emerge as the best physician for the patient, although he deals infrequently with cancer and often finds it difficult to do so. Both surgeon and radiotherapist, accustomed to more clearly time-limited patient responsibility, are usually not interested in assuming continuing care of the patient. Use of a team approach, which shares responsibility but does not allow fragmentation of care and which provides for more participation of nurse and social worker, is preferable.

CLINICAL COURSES OF CANCER

Psychological studies of patients with cancer have focused largely on the mental adjustment to progressive incurable cancer and to death. As people live longer and more are actually cured of cancer, or as they live for longer periods with arrested disease, the focus must broaden to include reactions of groups suffering from quite different psychological stresses. These reactions can be outlined better by defining stress in relation to the course of the disease (5).

The clinical course leading to probable cure is described as one characterized by an early diagnosis and treatment aimed at curing by a surgical procedure, radiotherapy, or chemotherapy. The stress of almost any treatment or the loss of a body part can be tolerated if the patient believes a cure can be effected. When a positive response is sustained with time, a probable cure may be assumed. This time period varies but is usually thought to be 5 years. Most patients return to normal coping patterns, although the fear of recurrence is always present. Maladaptive responses can result, however, in the patient whose cancer is cured but who remains a psychological cripple or in one in whom fear of exacerbation precludes normal functioning.

The second clinical course shares the early pattern of the previous one in which treatment either results in a positive response that may be sustained for years or in which there are disabling or slowly progressing symptoms of chronic disease with the specter of exacerbation always present. Psychological problems for this group are those associated with chronic disease. Adaptive responses adjust to the symptoms and promote rehabilitative efforts to reach maximal functional capacity. Maladaptive responses to chronic disease, with excessive dependency, anger, and an uncooperative attitude toward rehabilitation, have all been studied. These responses are not different in any way from those of cancer patients whose illness also represents chronic, arrested disease.

The acute grief reaction seen at the time of diagnosis is exaggerated when recurrent metastasis occurs, and there are many more severe depressive symptoms as life is increasingly threatened. Optimal psychological management and emotional support by the physician are critical for the patient at this point. An altered treatment plan in the face of new evidence of disease must also emphasize the physician's commitment to continuing care of his patient, who may fear abandonment. The stresses of progressive and terminal disease are great for all concerned. They vary according to whether or not the patient's illness becomes uncontrolled in the second course, after long remission; or in the next course, the third one, in which no response is effected by treatment; or in the last and fourth course in which no treatment can even be attempted after the diagnosis is made. These clinical courses raise great ethical issues and strain. Strain upon all involved is examined in the second section. Ethical and psychological issues in terminal stage care are explored in the last section.

Depression in patients with cancer is a challenge confronting those in the behavioral sciences. It is difficult to determine the limits of a ''normal'' anticipatory grieving, particularly in progressive, uncontrolled disease, and once a depression demanding treatment has developed.

It is of great importance to identify those patients whose depressive symptoms are severe enough to require intervention. Several studies estimate depression (better defined as depressive symptoms) in from 20 to 58% of patients with cancer. Using a self-report, Craig recently found that half of 30 patients were moderately to markedly depressed (8). Of cancer patients referred for psychiatric consultation, 49% had diagnoses of depression (1). Of 100 cancer patients attending an outpatient clinic in Helsinki, 58% were depressed (9). In a study of 80 advanced cancer patients compared with 80 patients who were physically healthy but who had attempted suicide, we found 22.5% at depressed levels by Beck inventory self-report and 32% by the interviewer-rated data. In the patient with cachexia or advanced cancer, the symptoms of anorexia, insomnia, fatigue, weight loss, and apathy are expected, but they also represent the vegetative symptoms of depression. Regarding these vegetative symptoms, the cancer patients in our study were indistinguishable from patients who had attempted suicide. When we looked at psychological symptoms of depression, however, there was a marked difference—patients with cancer scored much lower on the presence of diminished self-esteem and on feelings of worthlessness and self-blame. We may have to rely more on these parameters in patients with cancer than on the less useful vegetative signs. When and how to intervene because of depressive symptoms are practical problems that often confront the oncologist and his psychiatric consultant. Psychotherapy, antidepressant drugs, and, in some instances, somatic treatment must all be considered part of the armamentarium for depressions exceeding the reactive form and requiring vigorous treatments.

Depression in patients with cancer is clearly a challenge to the behavioral scientists. When is a grief reaction no longer within normal limits? What characterizes severe depression and concomitant suicidal risk from reactive depression? When does it originate in character rather than in disease? When are the symptoms of advanced cancer confused with those of depression, or when is depression missed by assuming that the symptoms are those of advanced cancer? Does a patient's poor outlook on the future and his severely depressed feelings have any effect upon the course of his illness?

Questions far exceed answers at present. These sections concerned with the problems of patient, family, and medical staff in coping with cancer help to clarify the questions that should be asked by future psychological studies and to define the challenges from which answers may yet be found.

REFERENCES

1. Hinton, J. Bearing cancer. *Br. J. Med. Psychol.* 46:105 (1973).
2. Weisman, A., and Hackett, T. Predilection to death. *Psychosom Med.* 23:232 (1961).
3. Spikes, J., and Holland, J. C. The care of the patient with potentially fatal disease. In Strain, J., and Grossman, S. (eds.): *Principles of Liaison Psychiatry,* Appleton-Century-Crofts, New York, 1975 *(in press).*
4. Lindermann, E. Symptomatology and management of acute grief. *Am. J. Psychiatry* 101:141 (1944).

5. Holland, J. C. Psychological aspects of cancer. In Holland, J. F., and Frei, E., III (eds.): *Cancer Medicine,* Lea & Febiger, Philadelphia, 1973.
6. Holland, J. C., Fasanello, A., and Ohnuma, T. Psychiatric symptoms associated with L-asparaginase administration. *J. Psychiatr. Res.* 10:105 (1974)
7. Holland, J. C. Acute leukemia: Psychological aspects of treatment. In Elkerbout, F., Thomas, P., and Zwaveling, A. (eds.): *Cancer Chemotherapy,* Leyden University Press, Leyden, 1971.
8. Craig, T., and Abeloff, M. Psychiatric symptomatology among hospitalized cancer patients. *Am. J. Psychiatry* 131:1323 (1974).
9. Achté and Vauhkonen. M. Cancer and the psyche. *Monographs from the Psychiatric Clinic of the Helsinki University Central Hospital,* 1, 1970.

Cancer: The Behavioral Dimensions, edited by J. W. Cullen, B. H. Fox, and R. N. Isom. Raven Press, New York © 1976.

Problems of the Physician in Presenting the Patient with the Diagnosis

Melvin J. Krant

Lemuel Shattuck Hospital, Jamaica Plain, Massachusetts 02130

The physician involved in the care of the patient with cancer is one human being linked to another through fate. The relationship is not formed through normal agencies of social contact but is brought about through the professionalization of one life and the intrusion of a disease process in the other. The setting is that of the doctor-patient relationship, although it is never only that because both the physician and patient as people are subject to certain moral and ethical imperatives and constraints derived from the society or the culture that has nurtured them, and they respond to psychological "sets" inherent in the process involved. The role of physician imposes certain requisites and obligations for action. The more these obligations are contained within measurable and rigid compartments, the easier it is to standardize and to then judge the nature of the physician's work. Physicians are more comfortable when they have precise strategies for making an appropriate diagnosis and initiating appropriate treatment than they are when they are wallowing in what they define as poorly delineated cultural, ethical, or psychological areas. Yet these are the areas that constitute, at least in part, human interrelations. Virtually any well-trained physician can find a commonality of judgment concerning whether he or another physician acted appropriately in the technical management of a cancer problem. It is in the vague areas called "medical arts" that accountable behavior is difficult to measure, but it is in these same areas that the major problems besetting the physician exist.

We can examine these problems in two respects: (a) What are the problems that doctors have as human beings in dealing with cancer? (b) What problems do they have in dealing with patient responses to cancer? In this chapter, we do not deal with technical-decisional problems, as important as they are to the medical care of cancer patients.

There is a general feeling that the physician has a number of special problems when facing the patient with cancer, and we know from limited documentation but from vast anecdotal material coming from patient and family sources, medical staff sources, and other sources that there is often less than a satisfactory human interaction between physicians and their patients.

In our Tufts Psychosocial Cancer Unit's present investigation into the psycho-social dimensions of terminal cancer, we have asked several hundred patients and family members in three Boston hospitals to give us their reactions concerning the caliber of medical care that they are receiving. Virtually 98% of patients and their families believe that the individual patient, even though failing and close to death, has received and is receiving excellent technical medical care. However, well over 60% of these individuals state that the patients' needs are not being met by their physicians, and that when the going gets rough, they cannot lean on their physicians (nor upon their ministers, if that is any consolation to the physicians).

I will try to elaborate on where and why these problems exist, drawing from my own experience and from some of our research data gathered from medical staffs, from multiple conversations with oncologists of various ages and dispositions, and from the writings of a number of people. I will separate the problems into three areas: (a) attitudinal (what the physicians' biases and assumptions are); (b) cognitive (what he does and does not know regarding cancer management); and (c) psychological (what may motivate his behavior without his recognizing it).

We begin this discussion with the following indisputable fact: of all the biological conditions the Western world is heir to, the most terrifying is cancer. In a recent interview with a newly retired executive, in which the advantages and the disadvantages of growing older were explored, the *New York Times* quoted the gentleman as saying that an older person should come into his retirement with sufficient money, sufficient status, reasonably good health, and with fingers crossed to avoid the big "C." There was no mention of stroke, heart disease, lung disease, or an infinite variety of biological difficulties. Cancer is equated with more than death; it is equated with a manner of living and dying in chronic and endless debility accompanied by loss of muscular power and control. It is equated with a withering away of life's essential elements, and is associated with foul smells, feelings of dirtiness, hopeless irrevocability, severe and relentless pain, and eventual death after weeks and months of this suffering. It is associated with fears of being a burden and fears of being abandoned. Many discussions have analyzed the question of why cancer strikes such terror, but this is not the purpose of our present study. The feelings about cancer are there for all human beings, including physicians. Although the American Cancer Society and other organizations attempt to create a dispassionate image of a disease that requires simply attention rather than an emotional response, and although such agencies have attempted to desensitize people to the horror associated with the illness, cancer still strikes that horror.

One of the overriding problems, therefore, for the physician addressing the cancer patient is that he is cast in the role of condemner of the flesh and spirit, and ultimately executioner, when he gives the diagnosis of the disease to the patient. The role of the bearer of bad news has never been a comfortable one. In ancient times, the messenger returning from the battlefront with news of defeat was frequently made responsible for the defeat itself and executed on the spot. Such an attitude still exists; the physician in announcing to the patient that he has cancer is held responsible for the disease. He looks upon himself, and may be looked upon, as being the creator of the event rather than merely its reporter. If, in addition, the physician's attitude toward that cancer (not necessarily toward all cancer, but toward a particular cancer problem in a particular patient) is one of fatalism and futility, then this guilt in being the condemner may easily interfere with his ability to order a logical course of treatment and management. A sense of hopelessness prevails, fostering a feeling of defeat and inevitability in both the patient and the physician. The problem then becomes one of whether to tell the patient the truth or not, of whether the physician should "condemn" a human being. A physician unfettered by guilt, or one who sees his role as one of caring rather than curing, is in a better position to support a patient through a logical system of planned actions.

Dr. Charles Wahl, among others, has emphasized in his writings that, although young people go into medicine for a number of reasons, the fear of death seems to be greater among medical students than among other students. He tells us that such a fear causes a person to identify with aggressive or curative forces and arouses the feeling that one must fight to eradicate death, and avoid evidence of failure. Robert Senescu takes a tactic emphasizing the quality of omnipotence that can emerge in a physician in his relationships with sick people. Serious illness may create a regressive need in the patient for an omnipotent, protecting, parental physician, and this can produce an inappropriate sensation of power not only in physicians but also in other health-care personnel. Certain patients may want their physicians to be bigger than life, and some physicians like to believe that they are indeed the moral and intellectual giants their patients imagine them to be. Such physicians have difficulties when the omnipotent position is threatened by a failing patient, and they may either blame the patient for not responding to treatment or simply avoid seeing him again. In either case, the doctor proves to be a rotten "parent."

The interlocking of these phenomena, namely, an attitude of pessimism or fatalism in the management of cancer cases, especially those not amenable to primary curative therapy, and the threat to omnipotence, can easily provoke great anxiety in certain physicians, forcing them to effectively abandon their patients through avoidance tactics, such as referral to another physician. In essence, the physician simply is not there to deal with the needs of patients and their families because these needs arouse in him too much anxiety and a sense of helplessness. Helplessness implies not knowing what to do next. In attempting to compensate for such feelings of helplessness, the physician may rush into too many experimental tasks and tests and this in turn may lead to three-way problems with patients, families, and medical staff.

In a recent editorial in the *Annals of Internal Medicine*, Dr. Olsen pointed out that there are many cancer centers in the United States, but that for the most part these have developed independently of general hospitals and medical schools and have therefore maintained only a sketchy relationship with the educational design of the medical school. In the past, medical students have had little exposure to the multifaceted care of the cancer patient. Until recently, therefore, most internists, pediatricians, and general practitioners have regarded cancer as a surgical or radiotherapeutic problem, rather than one of general medicine. This has produced not only a lack of understanding of medical modalities of treatment but also a lack of training in caring for the cancer patient over and above the rendering of certain surgical procedures. Much of what constitutes good medical care lies in following an intense cognitive system of rules and regulations in patient management. Since the rules of managing psychological, social, economic, familial, and other consequences of cancer have neither been laid out in the medical-school educational system nor revealed to the student systematically through patient contact, it is not surprising when the physician feels awkward in addressing himself to the multifaceted dimensions of cancer care. Add to this the modern medical burden of technical expertise and the great medical advances in cure, and one can understand why the concept of "caring for the patient" has disappeared as a major educative goal. The physician is frequently placed in a rather helpless position when beset with difficult psychological, socioeconomic, familial, and other consequences of cancer. His response has frequently been to ignore them. Furthermore, the medical student is not trained to cooperate with other health-care people in the management of cancer problems. His education is primarily technical and biological. He has rather primitive psychological mechanisms operating within him concerning his choice of career. The education system of which he is a part may accentuate his feeling of uniqueness and isolation and foster a sense of omnipotence and fatalism. It is no wonder then that he often finds it difficult to acknowledge his ineptness in a certain field such as patient care.

This lack of knowledge is further accentuated when patients "react" to their disease or their treatment, to hospital conditions, to families, or to any of a number of conditions and people. By reacting, I am referring to anger, withdrawal, refusal to come for treatment, breaking of appointments, incessant phone calls, and other manifestations of depression. There is little trouble when a patient acts as he should, when he is "good" and complies with the doctor's wishes. When a patient acts differently, however, trouble arises. Physicians, in general, feel threatened by such behavior, but a large part of the threat seems to lie in their now knowing "how" to respond, and therefore feeling attacked. Most physicians receive little training in coping mechanisms, and therefore tend to react merely to the situation itself, showing little understanding of its underlying causes. Needless to say, the more these reactions embarrass or threaten, the more intense is the physician's response, usually serving to worsen the situation, and to promote maladaptive behavior, such as resentment. Resentment is a common reaction of other staff personnel when their feelings are hurt. How many times have we heard accusations that a certain physician is arrogant, insensitive, cruel, or worse? These responses are related, at least in part, to a lack of understanding of how to appropriately assess and respond to another's behavior.

Most medical education to date has taken the position that there is no need for the physician to know himself. Little attention indeed is paid to working through prejudices, poor attitudes, and negative feelings regarding other human beings. The failure to explore, even at a superficial level, some of the deep-seated feelings that physicians bring to medicine may well solidify certain attitudes behind great defensive walls. Such defended biases and perspectives, although not seen as problems by the physician, certainly produce an endless series of problems for the patient and his family. Ironically, of course, it is the doctor who is at the center of patient care and therefore at the center of the problem. If one adds to this the fact that his education is institutionalized and hospital-centered, it is not surprising that the physician has little awareness of how to deal with the world of men and women existing beyond the gray walls of institutional order.

Individual physicians who offer surgical or radiotherapeutic strategies, or both, for the cancer problem often find themselves with a set of problems similar to those already discussed. The surgeon or radiotherapist is often not the condemner—he is the rescuer. The more evil the condition, the more powerful the rescuer feels. If one identifies with the role of a dragon slayer, then rescuing somebody from so great an evil as cancer should entitle one to all kinds of awards, including the hand of the symbolic princess. Since the dragon is of such ferocity, then clearly radical therapies are permitted. It is no wonder that a surgeon can justify radical surgery in the name of rescue, and feel totally justified in demanding the patient's gratitude rather than see himself as the initiator of a new set of psychological problems.

Clearly, there are many such individuals in surgery, and even in radiotherapy, who proclaim their omnipotence through their rescue efforts and who do not deign to recognize the new set of problems that emerges as a result of their work. Moreover, why should such powerful individuals pay attention to the quibblings of other human beings, such as nurses, social workers, and especially psychiatrists and psychologists, who from sheer malevolence wish to indict the heroes? Here again, however, standard medical education fosters this alienation by presenting cancer as a surgical disorder rather than as a multifaceted problem. It discourages the young surgeon from a creative approach to the understanding of his own needs as well as those produced by cancer and cancer therapy. The heroic position does not take challenge well. Recently, the *Journal of the American Medical Association* printed a debate between a surgeon attempting to stratify data outcomes of radical mastectomy against the results of another surgeon who had been emphasizing simple or modified operations. The physician practicing his radical arts approached the topic in a gentlemanly and scholarly fashion but shortly thereafter initiated an attack upon the honesty and integrity of the other surgeon.

The problems of the physician in caring for the postoperative patient must be placed in a cognitive-educative context. A volunteer worker in the "Reach to Recovery" program recently described the efforts of the program in "opening the eyes" of surgeons who did not realize the enormous extent of the psychological and physical disablement accompanying mastectomy. The worker claimed that by demonstrating the benefits of the program to the doctor, especially by having several patients telephone their doctors, such physicians quickly became aware of "Reach for Recovery" work. Some physicians seem to have a simple lack of information that could help their patients. Once these doctors understand what can be done and the potential rewards for their patients, they are apt to use such programs. When made aware of the talents and functions of others in the health-care system, and when this awareness is brought about in an unthreatening and supportive fashion, doctors are more likely to use these talents. Such an education helps a physician to understand the aims in total management of the patient and to sympathize with them. Too many physicians, however, still feel that their patients are doing fine, that new programs are unnecessary, and that they themselves can (and do) do everything that is required. Such physicians obviously cannot "see," and their defensive attitude precludes a healthy change in their approach to patients.

I think it will be difficult for physicians who have been practicing for a number of years to tolerate a learning experience aimed at changing their attitudes toward the care of the cancer patient and his family. I do think, however, that an effort can bring about great changes in medical education not only for the student but also for the house-officer regarding an honest examination of biases, prejudices, and attitudes in dealing with the psychosocial problems of the cancer patient. We must emphasize the interpersonal dimensions in cancer care and develop a deeper appreciation for that which constitutes the motivated self and the afflicted other. We must address ourselves to the differences between "caring" and "curing," and to restate the goals of medicine so as to comprehend both "care" and "cure" within one system. We are certainly talking about a "humane" physician, but one who must be grounded in certain cultural, or if he wishes, "value-laden" objectives with understanding of how to practice his art in a systematic fashion.

Cancer: The Behavioral Dimensions, edited by J. W. Cullen,
B. H. Fox, and R. N. Isom. Raven Press, New York © 1976.

Problems of the Patient Confronting the Diagnosis of Cancer

JoAnn M. Vettese

Michigan Cancer Foundation, Detroit, Michigan 48200

The topic of this chapter is far more encompassing than it might at first appear. The patient faced with a diagnosis of cancer is confronted with problems that not only infringe on his own life but also on the lives of his family members and his close associates. Cancer will not only affect him physically but it will also affect his psychosocial equilibrium and certainly, as with any catastrophic disease, have tremendous financial impact. It is important, therefore, to use a multifaceted approach in trying to understand the consequences of a diagnosis of cancer for the patient and for his family. To study the impact of diagnosis as an isolated incident would be too limiting. It would be like considering the tail without the dog, for just as the tail is often an indicator of what the dog might do in a given situation, so too is the diagnosis (type of cancer, extent, prescribed treatment) a possible indicator of patient response. It is important to understand that diagnosis is an ongoing process, unique to each cancer patient.

According to American Cancer Society statistics, in 1975, 665,000 men, women, and children would be confronted with a diagnosis of cancer (1). For more than one-third of these Americans, their disease will be curable. For the other two-thirds, the diagnosis will mean eventual death caused by factors directly related to the disease. Cancer does not discriminate in its effects on age, race, and socioeconomic groups.

Whatever the course of the disease, be it treatment and cure or progression and death, the patient, his family, and the medical-care personnel charged with the responsibility for ongoing medical services are aware that even if the cancer appears to be in remission, there is always a possibility of a recurrence or another primary. In most cases, the patient is no longer operating under the delusion that "it will never happen to me." The possibility of recurrence and all its ramifications looms ever present.

For many patients, the confirmation of metastatic disease is much easier to handle than the constant anxiety caused by the existential question of if and when their disease will recur. The cancer patient is faced not only with diagnosis, treatment, and possible recovery but also with a chronic disease process demanding constant medical surveillance in order that any recurrence or progression can be identified in time to implement treatment.

In order for treatment and maximum rehabilitation to be effective, trust must be established between the patient and his physician. This relationship should be one ''in which both the doctor and the patient feel comfortable and confident in terms of the practical demands put on them'' (2). Successful communication is the most essential ingredient in this relationship.

For many patients facing the diagnosis of cancer, the treatment processes and the struggle for rehabilitation, the ultimate goal is to reach a true reconciliation with their fate.

> The way in which a man accepts his fate and all the suffering it entails...gives him ample opportunity—even under the most difficult circumstances—to add deeper meaning to his life [3].

Confirmation of the initial diagnosis causes the immediate profound trauma to the patient's psyche. Many patients react with shock and disbelief, others with anger or denial, and some with intellectualization. To what is the patient reacting when told that he has a malignant disease? For some, it is the immediate thought of death; for others, it may be hope of a cure; but for all, it is the deep mystery surrounding the new event in their lives.

The reaction of each patient will, to a great degree, be determined by (a) his own ego strengths and weaknesses prior to diagnosis:

> The patient whose will to live is very weak in a catastrophic situation...is almost invariably an individual whose will to live was weak before he became ill [4];

and (b) the innate meaning the diagnosis has for the patient, his family, and others close to him:

> initial responses are more intense when the illness is more than a physical threat and amounts to a social catastrophe [5].

Even if the patient suspects a serious problem because of some symptomatic evidence, e.g., pain, bleeding, hoarseness, a lump, and so forth, he will still experience the same fear, anxiety, and loss of control upon confirmation of the diagnosis. Given emotional support and proper information concerning his disease, the patient can better adjust to the new circumstances of his life and still find quality and meaning within them. Most patients who develop adequate coping mechanisms are able to adjust to truth and to fact more readily than to uncertainty and question.

The way in which the diagnosis is presented to the patient will determine in large measure the quality of his response:

> Truth telling can be barbaric, painful and nonsupportive and can destroy an individual quite easily....Those responsible for giving information to a patient must also bear the responsibility of an ongoing affective relationship with that patient [6].

The patient must understand that he is neither alone nor without hope:

> If a doctor can speak freely with his patient about the diagnosis of malignancy without equating it necessarily with impending death, he will do the patient a great service. He should at the same time

leave the door open for hope, namely new drugs, treatments, chances of new techniques and new research. The main thing is that he communicate to the patient that all is not lost; that he is not giving him up because of a certain diagnosis; that it is a battle they are going to fight together—patient, family and doctor—no matter what the results. Such a patient will not fear isolation, deceit, rejection, but will continue to have confidence [7].

There may be greater need for counseling and psychological support if the diagnosis is made in the absence of apparent symptoms or if it threatens an immediate, meaningful goal in an individual's life. In such cases, the denial phase is apt to be extended.

Whatever the circumstances surrounding the diagnosis, the need for psychosocial support for the cancer patient is, as Beatrix Cobb so aptly states, "implicit on two counts:"

First, if the patient survives the onslaught of the cancerous growth, he requires assistance toward an emotional acceptance of the disease and the threat it involves to his life and happiness, and consequent adjustments to disabilities or limitations. Second, if the patient succumbs early or late the ironic goal reversal arising so often in cancer is indicated wherein the counsellor's purpose becomes one of assisting the patient toward an acceptance of the sure approach of death and the separations and adjustments this event portends [8].

The family, like the patient, is often traumatized by the diagnosis of cancer.

They play a significant role during the time of illness and their reactions will contribute a lot to the patient's response to his illness [9].

Families of cancer patients sometimes subject the patient to criticism and impose a sense of guilt because of their own feelings of frustration and helplessness. It is as though

the responsibility for one's personal health resides in the activities and behavior of the individual himself, so that if he does get ill, especially with a fatal illness, in some way he bears responsibility for such illness, as if it were not in nature's domain for natural illness to occur at all [10].

The potential and actual abilities of a family to cope with the pressure, fear, confusion, disorganization, and disruption that accompany cancer will depend to a great extent on how the family members functioned and related to one another in the past. Only preexisting and continuing unity, love, and strength enable families to cope with the stresses created by a catastrophic disease, such as cancer. The patient's greatest need from his family is that of open and honest communication.

Communication with members of the family can have real benefit if they are willing to enter into conversation, expose their feelings and work through the problems *with* the patient. It is often a reassurance to the patient to know that there are some questions that do not have quick and easy answers and that we all stand before death (and life) aware of our inadequacy (11).

The fear, anxiety, and loss of self-determination created by the diagnosis of cancer are often increased by treatment procedures and their effects on the body, personality, and social image. Hope is more readily engendered by those treatments used to cure rather than those used merely to mitigate the effects of the disease or to prevent functional complications. The greatest anxiety for patients comes during the experimental course of their treatment when diagnostic and other procedures are used to determine the extent of the disease or its response to a specific treatment protocol.

At this time there are three standard procedures used for both curative and palliative measures in the treatment of cancer patients: surgery, radiation therapy, and chemotherapy.

The basic concerns for patients who undergo surgery are: fear of the loss of normal body function, as with a colostomy or laryngectomy; fear of mutilation or amputation, as with breast cancer or sarcoma; and fear of the extent to which the disease has invaded the body, as is determined by exploratory laparotomy in lymphoma patients.

In addition to fear and anxiety, there will be intense anticipatory grief associated with loss of a body part or function and the need for profound psychological readjustment if a productive, complete life is to be maintained.

> Grief is the emotion that is involved in the work of mourning, whereby a person seeks to disengage himself from the demanding relationship that has existed and to reinvest his emotional capital in new and productive directions for the health and welfare of his future life (12).

Grief is more overt in cases of cancer surgery, such as mastectomies, head and neck operations, and amputations; however, it is often just as intense with gynecological and genitourinary surgery where there is a fear of loss of fertility or of impotency. All cancer surgery tends to produce negative self-imagery and loss of self-esteem.

Radiotherapy and chemotherapy are often used in conjunction with surgery in attempting to arrest the cancer. Radiotherapy machinery and chemotherapy equipment and protocols are often frightening because of their complexity. The fear and apprehension a patient experiences when subjected to them can be greatly alleviated by a simple explanation from the physician. The treatment modalities of both chemo- and radiotherapy should be explained thoroughly so that the patient understands the procedures and is prepared for any of the possible side effects, such as radiation burn, nausea, vomiting, loss of hair, and peripheral neuropathy. For some patients, particularly those with lymphomas and leukemias, the treatment sometimes causes far more physical discomfort than the disease itself.

In the text *Cancer Medicine,* Dr. Jimmie Holland notes the necessity of a caring, communicative disposition on the part of the radiotherapist. These same qualities in the chemotherapist are vital:

> ...Reassurance can be very helpful, but does not substitute for the humanism of the radiotherapist in his fearsome surroundings of powerful machines. He must sensitively discuss the objectives of the treatment, whether for cure of the disease, local eradication, or pain control....The patient must not feel abandoned...careful explanation is necessary about the side effects of treatment and their regression after completion of treatment. A therapy clinic profits from a social worker who is familiar enough with therapy to be able to extend the doctor's explanation and listen intelligently [13].

Physicians can sometimes be overheard when they remark that a particular patient "failed" on MOPP or "regressed" after receiving 12,000 rads of radiation. These kinds of statements and the attitudes they reflect only serve to promote feelings of guilt in patients who already feel responsible for the fact that they have cancer. When evaluating all forms of treatment modalities, consideration should be given to the fact that it is not the patient's failure if the surgery, radiotherapy, or chemotherapy does not arrest the cancer.

Because of the focus on prevention and cure in the treatment of cancer in recent years, an area that has been greatly neglected is that of rehabilitation:

> Why is a previously dynamic corporation president confined to a wheelchair, with nurse in attendance—ten years after successful cancer surgery?...Why is a fifty year old woman "a prisoner in my bathroom," compulsively (and unnecessarily) irrigating a colostomy for twelve hours every other day, six years after successful cancer surgery? [14].

When reactions such as these are the outcome of successful cancer surgery, it is necessary to look at the wider implications that the diagnosis holds for the patient if success is to be achieved in rehabilitation. These examples quoted from the book *Where Medicine Fails* may appear to be isolated ones but in reality they represent reactions common to cancer patients everywhere.

It is vital that we, the professionals charged with the responsibility of assisting cancer patients who now, because of new and competent therapeutic techniques, live longer and potentially more productive lives than ever before, be aware that such patients struggle with serious physical, psychosocial, spiritual, and financial problems that they cannot handle alone.

To attempt to intervene therapeutically in one of these areas without consideration of all the other areas is to forget that the patient is a whole, integrated person and must be assisted as such.

> One major development in rehabilitation...has been the utilization of the team approach in which the various disciplines—medicine, psychology, sociology and economics—are brought together through the medium of a group of professionally trained persons who focus their skills and abilities on the individual as a whole in terms of his total environment and his total problems [15].

A program designed for total patient rehabilitation should begin with the diagnosis. If each team member works with the patient and his family toward this common goal, and plans for physical, psychosocial, and financial needs, then the impact of the catastrophic disease process should be minimized and the outcome of the diagnosis itself confronted in a more positive manner.

> Patients who are able to cope successfully with the emotional stress involved in the diagnosis and treatment are more likely to live longer and more productive lives following the diagnosis of cancer.

Existence without purpose or meaning is mere survival; it is certainly not full life. Our concern must not be limited to prolonging survival but must include enhancement of the quality of life for cancer patients.

The quality of a patient's life will be a determining factor in the choices he makes regarding his present circumstances and the future possibilities for himself and for those he loves. It is of ultimate importance that the patient receive assistance in becoming self-determining in the face of these life decisions.

During the 1960s and early 1970s, behaviorists have been preoccupied with the process of death and dying. The knowledge that has been attained is invaluable; however, this specialized area of inquiry has often neglected the fact that for the cancer patient the most important reality is the process of *living* with a dread and devastating disease.

The time of diagnosis is one of reassessment for the patient. He will now have to adjust to a changing body image, to anxiety and even fear regarding the outcome of treatment, to his changing role and self-esteem in relation to his family and friends, and to his own sense of personal productivity.

No matter what action the patient elects to take regarding his medical, psycho-social, or financial future, he will often feel like the patient Lawrence LeShan quoted as saying: "If the rock drops on the egg—poor egg! If the egg drops on the rock—poor egg!" (17).

Life decisions are based not only on the patient's self-image but also on his perception of how others see him. The decisions are not made independently, but with consideration of what their effects will be on the patient's family, friends, employer, and even the objective medical-care system that will, to a greater or lesser degree, determine the routine of the patient's life for several months or years.

In his book *Dying and Denying,* Avery Weisman delineates three distinct psychosocial phases that a patient with a fatal disease confronts:

> Stage I, Primary Recognition, covers the period from a patient's first awareness that something is amiss to the time of definite diagnosis. Stage II, Established Disease, is an intermediate phase which embraces events between a patient's initial response to the diagnosis and his reactions prior to the onset of the terminal period. Stage II also pertains to the periodicity of illness, its relapses, remissions, progress and periods of arrest. Stage III, Final Decline, begins when a patient undergoes unmistakable decline towards death (18).

The cancer patient will ponder possible life decisions in Stage I, but the most definitive action will be taken in Stage II. It is very important that the patient receive honest and supportive communication during this latter period, so that the same degree of self-determination and ability to make realistic and meaningful life decisions continues throughout Stage III.

Some patients are locked into the illusion that death will never occur. "There will always be treatment or a new medical technique" (19). For these patients, death often comes before realistic alternatives to present life circumstances are chosen.

The patient's family plays a crucial role in facilitating the patient's ability to make rewarding alternate life decisions without feeling a tremendous burden of guilt. However, many families attempting to be supportive and feeling that the diagnosis of cancer means a swift and certain death begin to expend all available energies to make those last days just what the patient wants and to neglect their own needs. Family members who respond in this manner need assistance, so that they "handle their energies economically and not exert themselves to a point that they collapse when they are most needed" (20).

The environment in which the patient and his family find themselves and the one that places the greatest restrictions on the capacity to make self-determining life decisions is that of the hospital. Hospital rules, regulations, and routines are organized for the convenience of the staff, and the system tends to keep the patient in a state of childlike dependency and to isolate the family in the care process:

> Hospitalization engenders feelings of helplessness. Subjected to awesome and impersonal hospital routines, cut off from the usual sources of emotional gratifications and placed in a dependent, powerless situation, the patient finds anticipation solidifying (21).

It is also in this same environment that patients spend the closing moments of their lives, not free to express their anger or to work through their grief. How unfortunate that we should forget that the only thing most patients want is to take part in the decision-making process that determines how they live and certainly how they die.

During his fight with cancer 4 years ago, the late Sam Manser developed guidelines for patient rights based on his own experience. He summarizes the feelings and needs of the cancer patient with keenness and sensitivity, and his effort provides us with extraordinary insight into the problems of the patient facing the diagnosis of cancer:

> The patient must understand his condition, its consequences, what can be done to help him and how, and how much it costs in time, energy, pain and money. And when the patient understands the doctor's recommendations and the reasons for them, then he can cooperate with them.
>
> Unless there is this flow of information, the patient is confused and frightened, unaware of any alternatives, thus trapped which leads to panic, a paralyzing fear.
>
> Should the patient embark on a serious medical enterprise in this condition, he will most likely fare worse than no action at all even though no action may mean quick death.
>
> Without being respected—as an individual person—the patient will heal very slowly and laboriously, and sometimes not at all.
>
> The patient will be subdued to a statistical event, a number, a single punchcard, a nobody lost-in-the-crowd. He will resent the treatment he's getting from the system and he will eventually rebel.
>
> He will die internally for having compromised with a tyrant, for having submitted to expediency at the cost of self-respect.
>
> The more courtesy, respect, even real affection the patient receives: (1) the faster the patient will heal; (2) the more quickly and attentively the patient will comply with the wishes of the medical system; (3) the less emotional friction there will be; and (4) the more humor will reign and the easier the overload of work will be to bear.
>
> But this will not work unless the system initiates and perpetuates it as a policy. It's the patient who needs the help and the system which is supposed to be capable of providing it.
>
> The staff is supposed to help the patient by first treating for shock, especially psychological shock. Every trip to the hospital is a shock. The staff must be competent in handling unreasonable patients reasonably.
>
> Most patients want a little attention and don't need much—just enough to assure them they are not abandoned like a helpless infant. Some need to know what's going to happen next. This assures them they have not completely lost control of their life, body and person.
>
> Others need to be left quietly alone by all except those who are the patient's professional staff so they can be assured of more personal service.
>
> This system should not be just an idealist's dream, but a reality...Love heals. I don't "believe" this, I know it [22].

REFERENCES

1. American Cancer Society, '75 Cancer Facts and Figures, p. 1, American Cancer Society, New York, 1974.
2. Somers, R. *Health Care in Transition: Directions for the Future,* p. 91, Hospital Research and Educational Trust, Chicago, 1971.
3. Frankl, V. E. *Man's Search for Meaning,* p. 107, Beacon Press, Boston, 1963.
4. LeShan, L. Psychotherapy and the dying patient. In Pearson, L. (ed.): *Death and Dying,* p. 31, Western Reserve University Press, Cleveland, 1969.
5. Weisman, A. D. *On Dying and Denying,* p. 110, Behavioral Publications, New York, 1972.
6. Krant, M. J. The doctor, fatal illness, and the family. In *Concerning Death,* p. 55, Beacon Press, Boston, 1974.
7. Kubler-Ross, E. *On Death and Dying,* p. 29, MacMillan, New York, 1969.
8. Cobb, B. Cancer. in Garrett, J., and Levine, E. (eds.): *Psychological Practices with the Physically disabled,* p. 232, Columbia University Press, New York, 1962.
9. Kubler-Ross, E. *On Death and Dying,* p. 157, MacMillan, New York, 1969.
10. Krant, M. J. *Concerning Death,* p. 51, Beacon Press, Boston, 1974.
11. Bowers, M. K. *Counseling the Dying,* p. 60, Nelson, New York, 1964.
12. Jackson, E. N. *Understanding Grief,* p. 18, Abington, Nashville, 1957.
13. Holland, J. C. *Cancer Medicine,* p. 1005, Lea & Febiger, New York, 1973.
14. Bard, M. *Where Medicine Fails,* p. 99, Aldine Publishing Co., Boston, 1970.
15. Rusk, H. Foreword, In Garrett, J., and Levine, E. *Cancer,* pp. v–vi, Columbia University Press, New York, 1962.
16. Garrett, J., and Levine, E: *Cancer,* p. 237, Columbia University Press, New York, 1962.
17. LeShan, L. Psychotherapy and the dying patient. In Pearson, L. (ed.): *Death and Dying,* p. 40, Western Reserve University Press, Cleveland, 1969.
18. Weisman, A. D. *On Dying and Denying,* pp. 98-99, Behavioral Publications, New York, 1972.
19. Krant, M. J. The doctor, fatal illness, and the family. In: *Concerning Death,* p. 51, Beacon Press, Boston, 1974.
20. Kubler-Ross, E. *On Death and Dying,* p. 159, MacMillan, New York, 1969.
21. Bard, M. *Where Medicine Fails,* p. 104, Aldine Publishing Co., Boston, 1970.
22. Manser, S. A. A credo of patient's rights...by a patient. *The Sunday News,* p. 1C, Detroit, 1974.

Cancer: The Behavioral Dimensions, edited by J. W. Cullen,
B. H. Fox, and R. N. Isom. Raven Press, New York © 1976.

Respondent

Leonard Pearson

School of Medical Science, University of Nevada, Reno, Nevada 89507

In trying to figure out how to respond to this wealth of material, I decided to compare clinical experiences with my personal experiences. I will match Sr. Vettese and I will use a data base of one—myself. I will compare what she said with my own experiences, having had renal cancer 16 months ago; if what she said makes sense and if it applies to my experiences, I will praise it. If it does not fit with my experiences, then I feel that her ideas must be expanded, modified, clarified, or rejected. I think it is reasonable to discuss clinical experiences in terms of their significance, not necessarily in terms of the absolute size of the sample. I want to applaud Dr. Antonovsky for his concern with us as citizens and for reminding us of our need to control cancer but not at the risk of controlling and dehumanizing human beings. I wanted to challenge Dr. Peacock's glib dismissal of correlational and causal studies, particularly of the Swedish DDT studies that resulted in Sweden's banning DDT about 6 or 7 years before we did. The research there was not based on "bell ringers," but on careful, sober evidence provided by scientists of the effect of DDT on the food cycle, on fish, birds, bird eggs; the whole ecological system was involved in their decision. In this country, let us not forget the "bell ringers" for the chemical industry, the agricultural industry, the food processors, etc.

Regarding Dr. Antonovsky's smooth reassurances concerning pesticides, preservatives, and insecticides, I would have liked to ask him: "Can you reassure us with sound evidence that the synergistic effect of eating 12 ounces (which is the average amount we consume) of additives, preservatives, artificial colors and flavors, etc., has absolutely no effect on our functioning?"

I have noticed a shift in emphasis on the complexity of human behavior, something which should be self-evident. Dr. Mathews alerted us to distinguish between changing behavior and offering choices regarding future behavior. Dr. Matilda Butler-Paisley vividly pointed out that we are not dealing with passive audiences waiting to be manipulated, but that audiences themselves are manipulators who have the freedom and ability to process incoming data, to distort, and to ignore. Dr. Mendelsohn pointed out the complexities of human behavior—we are not just a combustion engine, a bunch of wires, or a plumbing system based on the hydraulic concepts of Freud. There is much more involved, and I think we would be doing a disservice to our sponsoring group if we left them to think there is a simple theory concerning human behavior.

I shall now discuss personal, clinical, and research experiences in other areas relating to our work—other possible research directions. I have been teaching thanatology for about 10 years and am impressed by the change in the field. We no longer have to persuade, intrigue, or seduce the students into studying the phenomena of death. There are 1,200 courses offered this year on thanatology in this country. I was at a conference in June on death education at the University of Washington Medical Center, Seattle, where 125 educators were present. They were teaching—nursing students, medical students, social workers, psychologists, undergraduate students in philosophy, and so forth. I helped to organize a conference in Reno. For the first time in 10 years, I have received hate mail. These are signs of progress. I have been accused of participating in the "Communist conspiracy" by looking at death and making it seem more attractive, of making it appealing to the point where people might even want to commit suicide.

There is a wealth of experience in another field of human behavior—driver education. The goal has been to change the behavior, in the near future, of potential drivers. The whole method of using scare techniques is now considered ineffective and has almost been abandoned. Driver education has been mandatory in many states for many years, and I hoped someone would report on all the information on changing behavior within that field.

Another area I haven't heard discussed is that of encouraging husbands and lovers to become involved in breast examination for cancer. Maybe this topic is taboo, but I hope we won't ignore potential sources of help in achieving our goal, which is to reduce the incidence of cancer and to increase survival. The film on breast examination I have shown to students in the past has a careful disclaimer that says: "Do not show to male students." It is incredible to me, in this era, that male college students don't know about female breasts, so I have always ignored that disclaimer and shown the film. I haven't noticed any striking increase in pregnancy, but don't really know what has happened as a result. I don't think the idea of involving husbands and lovers in the problems of breast examination is that unconventional and see no reason for NCI to consider it so. It occurs at a nonscientific level, anyway.

The last area I shall comment on concerns biofeedback and relaxation and meditation techniques. The pioneer in this field, Dr. Carl Symington, was present at the conference that produced this volume. He is a radiotherapist who has innovated the use of imagery and meditation with radiation therapy and has reported extremely successful results with those who can learn to meditate. What he has done essentially is to marshal the self-healing processes. If we can control a number of autonomic systems, can we also increase the way in which the white cells flow to a certain area? That's the implication, as I understand it, of his research. Regarding the models of human behavior, I think we have seen that the psychodynamic focus, which most of us are familiar with, concentrated a great deal on the past and to a lesser extent on the present. As to behavior modification or operant conditioning, or experimental analysis of behavior, there is a great deal of emphasis on these at present, but this will lessen in the near future. The humanistic and existential psychologies, the so-called third force, with their emphasis on value, choices, decision-making, etc., focus a great deal on the future and also on the present. I hope that research will not be limited to any single theory that explains multicausal behavior.

Dr. Holland's chapter included a number of key points. I found her emphasis on distinguishing different types of depression particularly helpful. What is normal depression? We are so used to thinking that a patient who is depressed, sad, or crying is not entitled to be that way, and that we must modify that mood somewhat, usually so that we, or the nursing staff, will feel more comfortable. Dr. Holland's distinction is spelled out in greater detail in her chapter. I think we as professionals find it difficult to allow a normal period for anticipatory grief, for mourning for the lost function or part, and for extending the limits of what we might consider normal and appropriate depression. Dr. Holland makes another point, namely, the need for trust between the patient and the healing physician. These are all extremely important points and they are part of the human aspect that Sr. Vettese was talking about.

In Dr. Krant's chapter I was impressed with several things, including the poetic as well as philosophic aspects of it. Some of the phrases are really impressive, for instance, "the withering away of the life's essential elements," "feelings of dirtiness," "hopeless irrevocability," and so on. One point had to do with the bearer of bad tidings being executed, and Dr. Krant phrased the question that is often asked by the physician reluctant to commit himself: "Should I as a physician condemn a human being by giving him the diagnosis?" I think as long as the question is phrased that way, the answer must be no. Why should anyone want to condemn another human being to an early death? My medical students often ask, "What is the point of trying to talk very much to a cancer patient? What have I got to offer him since all of my skills lie in the areas of healing and curing?" My answer is that the most powerful tool you have to offer is a relationship and that is what most dying patients want and need so desperately.

A number of studies in various age groups have shown that dying patients have two concerns. One is: "Will death hurt? Will I be in pain as I die?" We can assure these patients that there are sophisticated medications available to alleviate their pain. The second question is: "Will I be alone when I die?" We can assure them they will. In our society people die alone, in the corner bed, the dying room, the curtains drawn. Several speakers have pointed out that this is an extremely sensitive area, that is, the fear of being alone and neglected, and yet this is what often occurs. Dr. Krant also noted a certain irony in the fact that the doctor is at the center of patient care and therefore often at the center of the problem. It always reminds me of the Pogo statement: "We have met the enemy and he is us." He also spoke of the psychiatrists, psychologists, social workers, and nurses wishing to indict the heroes out of malevolence—the heroes usually being the surgeons.

I shall now discuss the diagnosis of cancer and the meaning of time to the patient—time to reassess himself, his future, his values, and his goals. Often we don't provide enough time; we don't provide enough help. In my own case, I had a nephrectomy about 16 months ago and was lucky because the cancer had not come through the capsule at all nor were there any other signs at that time. Since then, I have learned that I have a coin-sized lesion in my right lung, which was there at the time of surgery but hasn't changed in 16 months. In a conversation with the chest surgeon 3 months ago, he said, "Well, 50-50 it's malignant or benign. Now if I go in there, I am not sure that I can find it, but I can always take out a lobe or two and you are healthy enough to have a whole lung taken out. However, if you want surgery I'll schedule it on Monday." And I replied, "Wait a minute. What kind of choice are you giving me?" He said, "If you don't want surgery, I won't schedule it on Monday." I really did appreciate the fact that I was involved in the decision-making process. He was frank enough to say that he just wasn't sure; if it was soft he might not find it. I said, "What if you find out it's an old TB, because I did part of my dissertation in a TB sanatorium?" The surgeon's reply was, "Well if there is nothing there I have just wasted an operation." I thought, well, so would I have wasted that operation. So we agreed to review the situation in 3 months. Whatever that lesion is, it has not changed; it may be 1 mm smaller, which may be an artifact of the X-ray, but I am content to wait another 6 months, and another, and another.

Anyway, I thought the decision-making aspect was critical, and also the reexamination of my goals. I have decided to leave the medical school where I am teaching. I have enjoyed the teaching experience in some ways; but I've hated the interminable committee meetings and the politics. Not only do we have factions, but we have caucus meetings before faculty meetings. Therefore, our factions know what to do during our faculty meetings, and I have had it. I have also decided to return to film-making. I have made about six educational films that are dramatic films and have received a number of awards. One film, called "The Inner World of Aphasia," depicts the patient's perspective concerning what it feels like to have communication blocked off if you have a stroke or a head injury.

Discussion

Swartzes: I am a pediatric oncologist so I have a slightly different viewpoint from that of Dr. Krant. Regarding the comment that medical school education is inadequate in teaching doctors how to deal with patients, my own reaction is a more violent one. I not only think it inadequate in teaching them, I also think it destroys any feeling that students may have for human beings when they enter medical school, and, in fact, it teaches them to respond not to human beings but only to things that they have learned in school. This process begins in medical school but it gets worse during internship and training. Take for example a physician (and I am going to speak about pediatrics because that is my field) who has completed school and who then goes into pediatric internship and works in a nursery where, for instance, he should be very concerned about the feelings of parents of a critically ill infant. The doctor should at this point learn something about dealing with a person's feelings, but he is so overworked, working 36 hours or more as the system demands, that he is not taught this. Instead, he has been taught to ask about the electrolytes, the blood pressure, and the white cell count. Meanwhile, he is also in a situation where he should be inquiring about the nature of human needs and cares. I would like to challenge the behaviorists to look at this problem and to consider it an important area of research in which something can be done to promote concern for human beings. To me, the most important question is how do you instill concern, perception, patience, and all those other little things that produce a sensitive physician? I think it can all be summed up in one simple word: *love*. People seem to want to get away from that, but I think that this human element is one that the old-fashioned physicians respected. They took time to go out and see their patients, to put down their instruments and to listen, and they were able to say: "I understand what you are feeling and I want to share it with you." How can we go about instilling this kind of attitude in individuals who have been so pressured by an educational process that they seem devoid of all human emotions?

I would like to respond to one comment that I heard—that truth-telling can be "barbaric." I think it can be barbaric, but I think it is essential to be truthful in talking with the cancer patient. But truth must be tempered by concern, by perception of what the truth means to the patient, and with this goes the responsibility to follow-up on the truth, to answer all questions concerning it, and to deal with the patient's emotions.

My last comment relates to my own area, pediatrics. I have heard no mention of it and I think it is another critical area of research in the behavioral sciences. What about the child who gets cancer? What about the person who is too young to talk about what is happening to him, who doesn't know how to say, "I am afraid of dying, I am afraid of what is happening to me." How do we handle these people? I think this is a very important area for all of us to examine.

Holland: It seems to me that the attitudinal changes in the health professional in this general area is something to which we could address ourselves as a group. The behavioral scientists should look at this.

Fox: Dr. Krant, if you will look at the way in which people are made, you will notice that just as intelligence varies all the way from idiocy to genius, so too do skills vary, and in any individual you will have peaks and valleys of capabilities. Now there is a critical capability that I think you have selected as an important item. This can either be taught or it may be an innate characteristic of the individual. Aside from this capability that could be developed in the medical school—the measure of sensitivity, the ability to relate, the empathic quality that one hopes will be in the physician—what do you do about the idiot savants who are savants in medicine but idiots in sensitivity?

Krant: Last year at Tufts Medical School there were 8,000 applications for entry to 140 spots, which is typical of most medical schools. There are about 45,000 people seeking entrance to medical schools each year and, although I don't know how many thousands of them are actually admitted, the ratio is small. Clearly then, the chief concern is to select those individuals you want to enter the health-care system. This choice has already been made, of course, because most faculties have been responsible for the entry requirements of instruction to the grand sciences, the hardcore sciences. Most students who go to undergraduate school, and they are extremely competitive, plan their activities with medical school in mind. "A" averages in biochemistry seem to be required and the recipients of these and other high grades are the ones who are selected. You therefore have an opportunity to choose the kinds of students you want to see in medical schools.

Also, I think once you are in with the medical school, the question you pose seems to be something like, "Since we aren't all talented pianists, can't we all play the piano?" The answer is that there are transmittable skills that can be taught. You can help people to "see" in areas where they have never "seen" before by changing the kind of curriculum. A large part of what physicians don't do is not because they are insensitive; it is because they just don't "see". What education seems to have done is to narrow rather than broaden their vision. It is up to teachers; a faculty is influential in the expansion as well as in the contraction of vision. It is the total educational design, the goal of education, that you want to impart to the student before he leaves. The schools do have some designs, but these are submerged in the need to produce 25% primary practitioners, now that the law requires it. To produce physicians who will do 30,000 different things, however, we need 30,000 different tracks, and to me this is not educating; this is simply losing control of a process. To address these issues properly, there should be some minimal standards of educational behavioral science. I think that the schools could establish these standards and expand their educational design.

Buckley: I have a number of things to say that are relevant to this particular point. Dr. Holland talked about the problem of when and how to intervene and the question was raised of who should be doing counseling. Our agency, Cancer Care, Inc., is the regional service arm of the National Cancer Foundation. The board of directors has staked out a particular territory of concern. The first concern is the advanced-cancer patient, medically speaking. Second, and equally important, is concern for the family of that patient. The third area is the hardest-hit economic group, that is, middle-income, self-supporting people. That's the population that benefits from our direct in-person services delivered in the tri-state area of New York City—Greater New York, New Jersey, and lower Connecticut. It's a very expensive program and our board of directors picked social workers to offer counseling, professional, expert guidance, and personal services. One of our main jobs, along with providing expert counseling, however, is the coordination of services on behalf of, and as an advocate for, patients and families so that they may have the services that they need. The most distinctive aspect of our particular program as a social agency in a community is that of helping people be cared for at home whenever it is medically appropriate and sound. Getting the right people together to do this job is certainly difficult. In 1975 we reached almost 23,000 people in the tri-state area, over 7,000 of whom were advanced-cancer patients. One of the facts that emerged from this effort is that doctors are dodging the issue of diagnosis. Professionals and doctors still tend to ignore the people around the patient and the impact of these people on the patient's life. To ignore, at whatever stage, the fact that the cancer patient lives in a social unit—the family—is like taking care of a blood clot and not realizing the implications for the rest of the body; no sound physician would do that. Naturally, physicians concentrate on the disease itself. I think it is equally important that we work together for the patient as a whole person. I don't think many people know what the team approach really is, much less put it into effect. When we do achieve this approach, it's thrilling and it provides effective, comprehensive medical care.

Pearson: It's almost a truism that there are no cancer patients; there are people who have cancer. I wish there was some way we could hyphenate that word "cancer" and make it a person with "cancer-family," and bring it to the attention of all the health professionals very early. The impact of cancer is so severe that unless one considers the family as part of the sufferer, or the victim, then there is a huge gap in what we are trying to do in terms of changing the ones most directly involved—the physicians. One way of promoting change is, of course, through education in the medical schools. The other way, I fear, may have to be through legal action, either through more sophisticated bills of patient rights or through actual litigation. Patients and/or families often feel they haven't received the full story or the total truth or that they were not cared for properly, depending on how "care" is defined.

Unidentified speaker: I would like to take issue with that. There are two words that are creeping into the vocabulary of the medical system that don't belong there, but which are penetrating in a vicious way: "client" and "consumer." We have heard both of them and to me they both belittle the phenomenon of suffering. The very nature of law does the same kind of thing. If what Dr. Holland was talking about is true, if establishing relationships of trust is essential to the ability to walk through the valley of shadow—whatever it may be—then the more we talk about litigation as a means of serving rights, the more we are becoming clients. Obviously one must be careful because we are not talking about—at least I am not talking about—gross malpractice procedures. What we are talking about is that today cancer does not seem to be an equalizer; that is, the patient and his family and the ones who give care do not seem to be on equal terms. The relationship can be one of human interaction with mutual need and trust, or it can develop into a doctor-client relationship.

Pearson: Let me respond to you by using the example of the study done by the California Medical Association on malpractice suits. The association was looking at high and low suits. It found that in hospitals having a high number of claims, the physicians were indeed guilty of psychological malpractice; but there is no basis in law for psychological malpractice suits. Patients were waiting for a chance to sue their doctors because they felt that the doctors didn't care, were not sensitive, and were not spending enough time on their case. The same episode, whether it is leaving a sponge in a patient's body or falling on a mop in the hallway, would end with a million-dollar suit in one hospital and with a sincere apology from the physician in another.

Whyman: As a more recent victim of a different kind of process—that of medical education—there are a couple of points I would like to make. I notice that whenever someone here makes a statement to the effect that what we need in medicine is more sensitive, empathic, caring physicians who know how to listen as well as to talk to their patients, there is usually a smattering of applause in the audience. This is because most physicians have the right attitude. The problems go much deeper; they are not simply attitudinal but economic, social, and somewhat historical. It seems that what we are sowing now are the seeds of a 20-year historical process of inculcating the values of acute-care medicine. The medical school professors, our models as students, inculcate selected virtues in their students. The image they portray is the image of the physician as life saver, as the person who deals expertly with diagnosis. Very few of these professor models are found in chronic-care clinics; very few of the professors spend time there at all. Their time is better spent either in the laboratory or at the bedside providing acute care. The model for a medical student, therefore, is, as always, his mentor, his professor. Until that changes, I don't think that a very good behavioral science curriculum in the first or second year is going to make a difference. As someone said, as soon as the medical student reaches the clinics, that's when it really matters to him and he does not have the models at that point.

Holland: This is the same point that Dr. Peacock made about smoking—children learn from their parents. We are seeing this same learning process at the professional level between students and their professors, so I think there is a valuable principle to be drawn from both sessions.

Haley: I think some of us who are products of the established medical system and the processing have managed to break out of it. Dr. Holland asked us in this discussion to talk about support systems. I just finished one of the world's great boondoggles, a postgraduate medical course on a cruise ship. In one of my 14 teaching sessions, I discussed the management of the patient with advanced disease. That session was supposed to last an hour: it lasted an hour and a half. The students didn't want to stop. In another session I asked them to fill out a rather threatening cancer attitude survey that our group had developed. Dr. Paiva wanted some more standards, so I obtained a few for her with a captive audience (I had 41 physicians on the cruise ship). Interest was again sustained and I heard about the survey for the next week. I think, therefore, that this is my first endeavor in continuing medical education. I have been doing undergraduate and residency education, but certainly this is one place that the support system ought to be working, and at least I found a positive response to it.

At least twice during this meeting, people have talked about the isolation of patients. Cancer patients are isolated all the way through. I think the reason I wanted to bring this up is that my response to the family issue is quite different from what we have just heard. I have been impressed by the number of times that the family itself is responsible for isolating the patient. I have had to deal frequently with the difficult problem of getting the family interested, involved, and communicating with the patient. I was once chief of surgery in a state mental hospital. Again, the isolation of patients by family in that environment was frightening. What happens is that there is stress and isolation in the family before the illness. After the onset of the illness itself, fantastic guilt feelings develop that can complicate the management of the patient. I think there is another side to the family picture, therefòre, than that which has been presented.

In describing the cancer patient in the preterminal phase of his illness, there is another aspect of his state in life that has not been referred to and that is the loss of his future. We are living in a terribly future-oriented society. When you remove the future, you are going to die; you no longer need to plan. It is one aspect of isolation and one that requires a therapeutic approach. You must define the future for patients. For instance you might say "Tomorrow morning I am going somewhere else before I come to the hospital, so I'm going to be late. I won't be around at 8 or 8:30 as usual. I won't be along until noon." That is saying a couple of things to the patient. It is saying we've got a future; but it is also saying we've got a future together.

Schmale: My area is behavioral medicine and I am cross-trained in internal medicine and in psychiatry. At Rochester, we are at least trying to do the right thing by introducing behavioral concepts in the first year and keeping this as a part of training in medicine and medical skills throughout the 4 years. This morning we were introduced to the idea of the all-purpose summary by Dr. Haskins. We have heard many all-purpose reviews by many experts. I am glad that we are not going to have an all-purpose conference here. I think, however, that the problem is that we don't have all-purpose patients. We can't yet reduce psychosocial concerns to simple generalities. There is a great distance between the experts in the field of epidemiology, the systems people, the mass communicators, the social scientists who want to have the clean, neat criteria to work with, and those of us who have been working at the bedside. We have been trying to put together in operational terms, as Dr. Antonovsky said, what some of the models are, some of the generalities, some of the categories so that we can begin to reduce different kinds of responses and look at patterns and then indeed talk about principles. We do have some general principles concerning the psychology of health and disease. I don't think it has to be left to the "do-good" humanitarian aspects of us as physicians. We do have certain principles and skills with which to transmit knowledge. What are the specific elements of knowledge that we need in treating the various diseases? Cancer is the disease that we are looking at here; it is a model that can be used in many other fields.

Hayes: All of us here are concerned with and somewhat critical of the practices of some physicians in regard to cancer. What I infer from some of the comments is that we all believe those practices are related to the attitudes held by those physicians and that the attitudes could be improved in some way. We all probably subscribe to the idea that attitudes arise to some degree from the training and educational background of physicians. On the other hand, some of the data that I included in my chapter indicate that students may bring some of the attitudes with them to the medical school. Another problem relates to Dr. Krant's reference to the models, and that is that many of the people serving on admissions committees of the medical schools are physicians who possess the same qualities we find to be unsatisfactory. In choosing students for medical school, they will choose people like themselves. Therefore, we must be able, as behavioral scientists, to tell the people on admissions committees that these are the traits that will allow you to produce physicians with desirable attitudes. I do not anticipate that anything much will change until we are able to do that. Otherwise, the admissions committees of the medical schools (that is where the problem lies if there is a single focus) will continue to operate with the same biases they now hold. It is our obligation as behaviorists to supply them with a new set of standards based on some other data.

Rimer: Part of the problem may lie in the fact that all of us have grown up in a culture that discourages us from talking about extreme trauma in our lives. The only time that the patient can talk about severe pain or about facing death is when he is faced with it for the first time. I was very pleased to hear that there are over 1,800 courses on thanatology in this country. It seems to me, in the open society that we have today, with its proliferation of X-rated films, that perhaps the time has come when we can also face the extremes of life. If someone grows up in a culture in which there is understanding and open discussion of pain and the fear of dying, and this same individual then becomes a patient, the chances are that he will be able to confront the whole experience of illness, including the trauma of treatment and therapy, with better understanding and endurance. The expectation that doctors alone are going to change the attitudes toward pain and death is an unrealistic one; the general population itself must help promote the change, and open discussion of these subjects at all levels of society must take place.

Abrams: The only observation that I can make at this point is that we don't have general practitioners anymore. Most of us don't have family doctors. In addition, I don't think that the doctor who is taking care of the dying patient can—much as he would like to—help the dying patient in the areas in which the patient wants help. I believe strongly that we are going to have to add somebody else to the team, someone the doctor, the patient, and the family will accept as a mediator. The dying patient's greatest need is to leave behind a good image. He really doesn't want to talk to his doctor about some of the things that may be closest to his heart, that he may be ashamed to talk about. I would like it very much if doctors could acknowledge the fact that there may be some other person, such as a counselor, a chaplain, or a social worker, whom the patient needs and would accept. The doctor must give the patient and the family the opportunity to introduce this new person into the picture. I think this supplementary help is what is so sorely needed by the advanced-cancer patient today.

Pearson: Dr. Kubler-Ross has a new book that deals with this same idea. She believes that the use of drawings can be very helpful in the case of children with terminal illness. The children are allowed to express what they feel, what they expect to happen, in their drawings. Some of you may know an article that appeared in the *Journal of Pediatrics* about 5 or 6 years ago. The title was "Who's Afraid of Death on a Leukemia Service? Answer—The Staff." The children are often much more resilient and capable of dealing with reality than we think they are.

We are trying to teach our students, both medical and nursing students, that it is okay for them to cry. It is so hard for them to express feelings. I organized a conference last year on the health of the health professional, because our students were concerned about rumors to the effect that if you went into the health field, especially medicine or nursing, your own health was bound to be adversely affected. The rumors were confirmed. The life-span of the average male physician is 17 years below that of the average white male; drug addiction is 300% higher among physicians than among the inner-city blacks; each year 400 doctors lose their licenses to practice because of alcoholism. We don't know how many others continue to function although they are alcoholics or drug addicts. At our conference we concluded that one of the reasons for the high mortality figures in terms of living and divorce was that health professionals have been taught not to express their feelings. Since feelings have to go somewhere, the professional people may attempt either to alter them through the use of mood-changing chemicals, drugs, and alcohol, or there may be a psychological distress response, such as suicide. We are trying to learn from these findings and we are saying, "It is not only okay to feel, but it is okay to express those feelings openly."

Introduction

Abraham Brickner

Michigan Cancer Foundation, Detroit, Michigan

There is a real need to begin to look critically at how we, who are in cancer control, are going to systematically involve those in scientific behavioral research. Those of us who take care of such people do not have sufficient time to direct our energies toward implementing evaluation plans. Somehow the patient service operations group must get help from those who are absorbed in research and evaluation. This conference was ably planned by Drs. Cullen, Fox, and Isom. They have developed a provocative and informative meeting, which is a good first step toward developing the partnership between behavioral research and community cancer control.

My recommendation is that each participant read carefully the two documents included in the conference information pocket. The National Cancer Institute (NCI) *Five-Year Plan* and the NCI report of the *Conference Directors, Rapporteurs and Working Group Chairman, Volume I* will provide the necessary information on questions on funding and the nature of RFPs. The documents will also help develop insights into what the NCI objectives are and tell what programs they will support. Frankly, we will have to relate to these objectives if funding is to be forthcoming.

The first section of this volume dealt primarily with prevention, which is of great concern to the NCI. This is an area in which the behavioral scientists can have a field day. When we move into the screening and detection area, however, things get more difficult. We must know why people go or do not go for examinations, and why they delay in seeking medical help. I was interested in earlier statements to the effect that 78% of the women in this country have had a Pap test, whereas the remaining 22% are reported to have the highest incidence of cervical cancer and are not being involved in screening and detection programs. The Michigan Cancer Foundation, under a subcontract from the State Health Department, has an NCI contract to reach this target population. It is a difficult job to motivate this group of women and involve them in a basic preventive health-care program. Some problems have been identified, but a lot more information must be gathered. One could say that these women are not as worried about dying of cancer in 5 years as they are about having food on their tables or a roof over their heads, or possibly dying from the effects of a rat bite. There are higher priorities to be concerned with than preventive health care. We must develop an approach and message and present it in such a way that we encourage these target populations to participate in preventive medical care. This is where behavior modification becomes the primary objective of the program. Taking the Pap test and doing the laboratory work is easy. The area of diagnosis and treatment provides an even greater challenge to the behavioral scientists. What does the doctor do to handle depression and resistance? How does the patient respond to treatment? These questions and the answers to them lead to a deeper involvement with people. Cases are diagnosed and treatment is prescribed and then applied. We should then become concerned with continuing care and rehabilitation. Cancer, heart disease, stroke, multiple sclerosis, and schizophrenia are all chronic diseases. It is in the areas of continuing care and rehabilitation that research on the problems of behavior modification must be done. We are dealing with the patient and his family, and it is difficult work. There are unlimited opportunities for behavioral scientists to contribute to continuing care and rehabilitation of cancer patients. This section addresses itself to this area. As we see it, a team approach is needed.

My plea to each of you is to develop an operations research model. Although I enjoy reading about the hybridized concepts from university settings and the models developed there, vast amounts of clinical material on patients from different populations are available only through operating agencies. We in the metropolitan Detroit area have an overwhelming number of clinical problems that need the attention of behavioral scientists. We need this collaborative help because it is difficult for those of us who are in the field operating on a day-by-day gut level to become too involved in evaluative work. There is unusual opportunity for this partnership to develop, and the Division of Cancer Control and Rehabilitation should be one of the prinicpals.

There are concerns about getting more money, deciding where to direct our efforts, and so on; there is also the need to reorder our priorities. This volume has been devoted in part to developing a coping process. How are we going to cope with the behavioral problems? How are we going to get a group of scientists involved with us in a meaningful way so that our work will be more productive?

As an administrator, my job is that of allocating money. When we are talking about data, how do we know they are reliable, valid, and usable? Decisions concerning a rational method of allocating resources must be made. It is important to have a profile of the type of patient we see, and to know the results of our interventions. As I go to our Board, to Washington, and to others in search of support, it is evident that the results of our programs are very important. Therefore, the proper motivation and behavior of both patient and health practitioner become the keys to success. In addition, we must recognize that we are dealing with many different publics and that these publics cannot all be treated in the same way. We have a patient population of different racial, ethnic, and social groups and then we have our professional population with all of its own differences.

How do we get people of such different persuasions, all of whom are cancer experts, organized and working together to achieve our objectives? There is no question about the chief objective: we must do something about cancer. How are we going to do it, and how are we going to measure our results? This conference has helped reinforce my conviction concerning the need for cooperative action, the need to parlay clinical material into operational agencies with the assistance of behavioral research staff in its academic settings. To me there is a sense of excitement and urgency underwritten by the mandate of the cancer control program and I look to the Cancer Institute to provide opportunities to begin using cancer as a model for chronic disease control.

Cancer: The Behavioral Dimensions, edited by J. W. Cullen,
B. H. Fox, and R. N. Isom. Raven Press, New York © 1976.

A Team Approach to Coping with Cancer

Shirley B. Lansky, James T. Lowman, Jo-Eileen Gyulay, and Karen Briscoe

University of Kansas Medical Center, Kansas City, Kansas 66103

Modern methods of therapy have increased the chances of the survival in patients with malignant disease. This increased survival is particularly striking in pediatric patients. In a selected group of children with acute leukemia, the survival period has been extended from 2½ months to 5 years. This increased survival, although striking from a medical viewpoint, is accompanied in many cases with significant psychological disability. Indeed we have cared for children whose emotional problems were more debilitating than their physical disease (1). The recognition of some early emotional complications of the disease, as well as late-stage effects in children surviving the illness, led to our interest in studying this aspect of cancer care. Tumors in children are uncommon; therefore, the population we are studying does not represent a large number of cases. We have approximately 100 children under our care at all times. There are 25 new leukemic patients and 30 new solid tumors each year. Because of our limited population, we can provide an opportunity to study not only the child but also the family, siblings, and friends.

The goals of the team are: (a) to study in detail the behavior patterns of the sick child, the siblings, the core family, and the friends and relatives; (b) to define a behavioral model for this group; and (c) to develop intervention programs that will prevent as many of the emotionally debilitating complications of malignant diseases as possible. The team assembled for this study includes a number of subspecialists, each with a specific area of interest; however, a major emphasis is placed on group problem solving. The decision to start this program was originally made by an oncologist.

Obtaining detailed information on behavior patterns and emotional difficulties requires dealing with the disease in an open and free manner. When a patient is admitted to the pediatric oncology service at the University of Kansas Medical Center, he is given his diagnosis. The diagnosis is discussed with him in language appropriate to his age. The families are given any information they request, such as laboratory results and temperatures, by any member of the health-care team. They are encouraged to discuss the child's disease at the bedside and all personnel try not to discuss it in the hallway or in a separate room, since this increases the child's apprehension. This system has been in effect for approximately 5 years and appears to have no disadvantages. It did, however, bring to the attention of the oncologists many emotional problems they felt unable to handle adequately. The team approach evolved from this experience. The health-care team includes three pediatric hematologist-oncologists, trained in the traditional setting, a pediatric psychiatrist, a nurse clinician, a lay expediter, and two pediatric hematology-oncology fellows. The roles of each of these people is discussed in some detail. The group is actually a division of the Department of Pediatrics and, although members of the group hold joint appointments in other disciplines, their primary responsibility is in the division of pediatric hematology-oncology. The team is directed by the head of the Section of Pediatric Hematology-Oncology. He makes decisions regarding protocols and research. He is the chief coordinator between cooperative national research programs and the University of Kansas Medical Center. Although he has some patient responsibilities, he is regarded primarily as team leader, assisting the other individuals in their roles. He is directly responsible for maintaining the group, both financially as well as administratively, and becomes the final arbitrator in the rare intragroup disputes.

The pediatric hematologist-oncologists rotate responsibility for the medical care of patients. They are chiefly responsible for clinical decisions relating to drug therapy, toxic reactions, and other complications; however, they are attuned to emotional difficulties and deal effectively with many of them. They direct the training of the pediatric hematology-oncology fellows and participate in student and house staff education. If questions relating to priorities in patient care arise, it is the responsibility of these physicians to make the final decision. For the psychiatrist in the group, active participation with the cooperation of the medical team from the time of diagnosis throughout the illness and after the child's death provides a unique experience (2). From a public health standpoint, there is the opportunity of providing (a) primary prevention, such as alerting parents and their children to the possibilities of school phobia during the diagnostic period, (b) secondary prevention, such as counseling sessions with parents experiencing communication problems, and (c) tertiary prevention, which may include therapy sessions with children after the death of a brother or sister.

Group sessions are used effectively with this population. The child psychiatrist participates in all sessions and makes individual rounds on the inpatient service each week, seeing all the patients under our care. These periods are used both to get to know new patients and also to reinforce the psychiatrist's role on the team. In a less formal manner, but equally important, the psychiatrist tries to help each member not only with patient problems but also with personal difficulties professionals have when treating children with cancer.

The child psychiatrist coordinates the mental health efforts of the whole team and organizes research efforts. In addition to exploring new directions, the current program must be recalculated constantly. The psychiatrist and other members of the team teach both within the institution and outside it to various professional groups.

The role of the nurse clinician is perhaps best defined by the word "liaison:" she is the liaison between staff and family, medical staff and nursing staff, and patient and family.

This liaison role is one of reinforcing information the patient and family receive from the medical staff as well as one of relaying questions to the staff that the family is afraid to ask. The nurse clinician provides the professional team with awareness of various problems the family and patient may have.

After the patients are dismissed, she calls or writes to their families. This is a reassuring measure. She provides each patient with the home and office phone numbers of the team members so that he is able to contact any one of them if questions or problems arise. The nurse clinician sees some of the children for follow-up visits in the clinic. During these visits, she does physical exams and gives chemotherapy and intrathecal therapy. Time is spent in assessing the family situation during each of these visits. The nurse specialist also attends funerals or visits the mortuary. She maintains active contact after the death of the child, especially during the family's acute grief state. Although length of follow-up after death varies, certain occasions, such as birthdays, holidays, and the anniversary of the death itself, are important dates remembered with a call or letter. Attending weekly parent-child groups and staff meetings allows for communication of information and problems away from the units.

Teaching is also a part of the nurse clinician's role. She teaches nursing groups (staff and students within the institution, as well as members of the outside community), medical students and staff, and allied health-care team members. The material taught includes many aspects of chronic disease—its physical and emotional facets, therapy, pre- and postoperative care, and methods for evaluating problems the patient and family present.

The lay expediter is the unique member of our team. She has no professional education and her role, as defined here, has developed during the last 2 years. She is the mother of a child who died of leukemia while under the care of our team. The other team members feel this experience has helped her develop her special capabilities. She deals exclusively with the emotional impact of cancer upon families, and there are three important aspects of her work:

1. She gives as much help and support to families as possible.
2. She gathers and records information which might affect total patient care and relays that information to other team members for immediate use and for further study.
3. She provides a "sounding board" for other team members trying to validate new ideas or suspected problems.

The lay expediter provides a role model for parents, coming to them as a person who has been in a similar situation and therefore understanding all that their own experience entails. Her presence helps them in many ways, but mainly it impresses upon them that they are not alone and that, as heartbreaking and traumatic as their experience is, it need not be the end of their lives or their happiness.

The lay expediter enters the scene shortly after the family has been informed of the diagnosis. She introduces herself and gives a brief description of her background and role in the team. She stresses the team's concern, interest, and availability, as well as her own, and answers any questions the family might have at this time. When the initial shock of the diagnosis has diminished, she discusses with them problems that commonly arise and how they may be prevented. She tries to pick up hints of any existing problems and to help them recognize and deal with these concerns. The family is informed of help available to them from community resources, organizations, and other team members, and the lay expediter aids them in making contacts. The expediter tries to make the parents realize that their problems, including financial ones, are common to others in this situation and that most of them stem from the stress of the illness. One way of doing this is by getting them acquainted with other parents and involving them in the parents' discussion groups, in which she also participates. Whenever possible, the lay expediter takes the parents away from the hospitalized child. This allows them to speak more freely and on a deeper level. She sees them again during clinic visits and hospital stays.

Follow-up, which is accomplished by means of a call or letter the first week after the patient is dismissed, continues throughout the illness and up to 2 years after death. Special attention is, again, paid to birthdays, holidays, and the anniversary of the child's death. The lay expediter writes personal and detailed letters that deal with feelings and problems that are likely to exist at these particular times; here again, she expresses the concern and understanding of someone who has preceded them in this experience. Home visits are made periodically and are an excellent method of reinforcing her individual interest in each particular family. Whenever possible, the lay expediter attends the funeral of the child and follows the family closely with letters, calls, and visits for the first few months after the child's death.

The lay expediter is sometimes used by parents as a mediator in the parent-doctor relationship, and the parents talk freely to her of problems they are reluctant to take to the physician. At times they feel unsure of their emotional stability and fear the doctor's reaction should they ''break down.'' They frequently feel their problems are irrelevant to the child's illness or do not merit the doctor's consideration. These may be problems in dealing with their own emotions and frustrations, problems at home or work, or problems concerning their child's care.

The lay expediter is usually the first to hear things that parents feel are too ''bad'' to admit, such as being tired of the illness and wanting the child to die, wishing it was another child instead, or admitting that they do not love or enjoy a new baby as they had thought they would. Worries about their own feelings, marital problems, religious questions, and questions of funeral arrangements and autopsies are all subjects commonly discussed with the lay expediter.

Often the parents test the honesty and openness of the physician by asking the lay expediter questions that have previously been answered by the other team members. Many times it is necessary for her to reinforce her statement that she has no medical knowledge. In nearly every case, she is asked by the parents if they really will be informed by the physician when death is near. Parents are encouraged to take their questions directly to the physician or other appropriate team member. However, if they are hesitant to do so, they know (unless they have requested that the information be kept confidential) that the lay expediter will relay the information to the other team members.

In general, the lay expediter provides a nonthreatening yet empathic atmosphere that encourages parents to vent their feelings without fear of rejection or repercussion.

The individual team members fill their roles as described. There is obviously considerable overlap and duplication of effort. This is not considered wasteful or detrimental. It assures the patients and their families of receiving help and information from different members of the team and reinforces the team concept for them. The team meets for 1 to 2 hours each week to exchange patient information, develop family therapy plans, and discuss problems. The entire team makes inpatient hospital rounds one afternoon a week. These rounds convince the patients that we do operate as a team. They demonstrate to the patients, the attending medical students, and house staff the importance of total patient care.

In any group of people working closely together for a long period of time, conflicts occasionally develop between individual members. This certainly has been true for our team. The most obvious breaks occur between those members most clearly involved in physical care and those who attend to emotional needs. How are priorities established when the physical care, which may include protocols demanding 5 days after every 21 days in the hospital, adds to the problems of the child? We have chosen to handle these situations in the same manner as we approach family problem solving—by open discussion during team meetings. It has proved quite successful.

The house staff represents still another group in which the contribution by oncology team members is directly correlated with interest in our program, as well as with excellence of care for the child cancer patient. This same approach is true for the nursing staff. They, too, need information and support for their job of direct patient care and the other staff members try to provide this.

Many of the team members are asked to talk to community and state lay groups as well as to professional audiences. This is time well spent. Once they understand the nature of the team's work, both the lay and the professional groups alter their attitudes and become more helpful in dealing with individual families.

The information presented in this report was gathered by a number of techniques, and much of it by individual team members. Specific data for school attendance and psychological testing were generated by prospective studies described in detail in this report. Group sessions are another principal method used effectively both for gathering information and for conducting therapy. These group meetings are of different composition and structure. Two weekly meetings are held for parents. They are attended principally by mothers, but the number of fathers who come is increasing. This is a time when the participants expect to share their fears, guilt, and questions about peripheral issues and also get to know one another. Much of each session is devoted to a discussion of family interaction. Anxiety may be very high at the outset, particularly for new members, but this often gives way to relaxation and even laughter during the hour.

A children's activity group follows one of the parents' sessions each week. Both in- and outpatients, as well as siblings, participate in this group. Children are not separated on the basis of age or severity of illness. An activity that can be enjoyed by all ages is planned by the occupational therapist. The children immediately see that their own illness is not an isolated occurrence. They become aware of children who are sicker, healthier, or the same as they are. Side effects, such as baldness and weight gain, are common to the majority of children. There is also an opportunity to see other children's condition improve as well as worsen.

An adolescent group has recently been formed. This group attempts to cope with the problems so important at this particular age: isolation, regression, and the teenager's fear of death. They are more likely to talk about their special concerns in their own group, but they also participate in the children's session.

A small, weekly group for mothers who have already lost children deals with the problems of reintegration of the family following death and with the many and long enduring manifestations of grief. Many definitions of problems relating to grief have come from this group.

In general, the many emotional difficulties and behavior patterns uncovered by these group techniques seem to fit a model related to various stages of the disease. Many of the same problems recur at several stages; more often, however, reactions seem to be related to one stage. The various phases and frequently observed behavior patterns in our population are defined in the following sequence.

PHASES OF THE ILLNESS

Diagnosis

The oncology team operates on the premise that openness and honesty are the most satisfactory methods of dealing with both the parents and the children. The referring doctor is asked to tell the family that he suspects the child may have leukemia. During the initial evaluation, the word "leukemia" is used and some information about the disease is supplied. Often the patient is transferred from a small community hospital to a large medical center or cancer center. This is quite frightening for many reasons: it places financial stress on the family, separates the family physically, and confirms the seriousness of the child's condition.

A conference is held on the second day of hospitalization with both parents and as many members as possible of the hematology team. The diagnosis is given and explained as fully as the parents understanding will allow. Life expectancy in terms of statistical data and treatment protocols is discussed. The parents are told that they are free to choose whether or not their child will participate in the treatment regimen, and that treatment will be continued only as long as it is having positive results. The immediate reaction of the parents is usually one of shock and grief. Two questions frequently asked are: "How will he die?" and "Will death be painful?" Studies have shown that the parents almost always assume the child is going to die immediately. Further information given during the meeting is not assimilated.

Induction

The parents are visited twice daily by the hematologists for the next several days while the child is being treated and, it is hoped, going into remission. They are told the results of all laboratory work and given a report of the child's current status. This first, or induction, phase is a period during which most parents isolate themselves because of their intense grief. They limit their communication to the oncology team and the nurses caring for the child. They comprehend some of what is told them, but much of it has to be repeated many times.

Parents find themselves beset with numerous problems throughout the child's illness. In addition to those resulting directly from the illness, many normal daily problems are magnified by the ensuing stress. The tangible difficulties, such as finances, work, home arrangements, and transportation, are aggravated by the two most prominent emotions felt by parents during this illness: guilt and fear. They fear the return of the disease, side effects of the drugs and changes in the child's body image, and the suffering and death of the child. Guilt ensues from the feeling that they (the parents) have caused the child's illness directly or indirectly, or are selfishly prolonging the child's suffering by allowing him to receive treatment.

Remission

If the child responds well to treatment and enters a remission phase, the parents stop grieving, become elated, and sometimes deny that the child is fatally ill. The necessity of continued follow-up and therapy must be stressed, particularly with children whose remission is long. During the period of remission, the child often must adjust to a changing body image, such as gaining weight on steroids, then losing, only to gain again in a few months when the treatment protocol once again demands steroids. The pattern is the same for hair loss. These body-image changes are particularly difficult for the older child and adolescent to face, and they may become so unnerving that the child wishes to terminate therapy because of them. Parents are generally overwhelmed by the abundance of help and support showered upon them immediately following the child's diagnosis or death. Then they suffer deeply the pangs of the nearly total isolation that often occurs shortly thereafter. Close relatives often cause problems, offering unwanted advice or seeking support for themselves. Grandparents can be "the straw that breaks the camel's back" for families who are trying their best to cope with a devastating illness. They offer unwanted advice such as, "Those doctors don't know what they are doing—take the child elsewhere." They are oversolicitous and undermine the parents' discipline: "How can you punish that child when you know he won't live long?" They overindulge the sick child with gifts, and this causes two problems: it frightens the child because he knows that only people who are not expected to live get this type of attention, and it causes animosity in the siblings who feel left out.

Relapse

The first relapse is a blow almost as severe as that of the diagnosis. The denial often used by parents is no longer effective and the fear of death again becomes acute.

The child, who has been dutifully taking his daily medicine and submitting to painful intravenous and intrahecal medications because of the assurance that he will stay well if he complies, now doubts the entire process. Parents empathize with their children and worry about what the child is thinking and going through. They find it difficult to treat the child normally. They may claim to do so yet guard themselves against future regrets by giving in to his whims.

Parents are beset by questions and decisions throughout the child's illness and after his death. They wonder why or how the illness happened; how to treat the ill child; how to know what problems are and are not caused by the illness; and how to divide their time between siblings and the patient.

One of the most evident problems is the breakdown of the family unit. Mothers develop a symbiotic relationship with the ill child and devote most of their time and energies to the child's care. Both mother and child suffer from separation and anxiety. In many cases, the child sleeps with the mother. This is true even of teenage children. The mother tries to take the entire burden of the illness on herself. Fathers are slowly pushed out of the scene and withdraw, usually taking on an extra job. Mothers are torn between the needs of the siblings at home and the ill child, and feel resentful of the responsibilities placed on them. Fathers feel guilty and rejected because of their lack of involvement. The parents feel they are not receiving the kind of support they need from each other. Communication consists of little more than the mother giving second-hand reports of the child's clinical progress to the father. The parents avoid communicating on a deeper level in an effort to protect one another. Most plans and conversations revolve around the sick child. Siblings manifest behavioral problems as a result of their own fears, guilts, and resentments. Employers are often a problem, and the self-employed parent must find a way to keep things going while he is away. Financial problems become horrendous and include not only medical bills but also transportation costs, expenses of living away from home, and the effects of time lost from work.

Siblings who, prior to the illness of their brother or sister, had been getting along well both at home and at school, suddenly develop behavior problems. This appears to be a result of several factors. As mentioned earlier, the mother spends most of her time attending the sick child with little attention to the others in her family. Father is away from home working extra hours. The siblings feel resentment toward the child who is receiving all the attention but feel extremely guilty if they complain about it. The only way to expose their frustration, therefore, is by unacceptable behavior at home or at school.

Parents often seek support from the siblings, searching for someone with whom to share their sorrow, and they feel hurt when siblings do not react to the child's illness or death with the intensity of grief expected.

Terminal Illness

During the terminal phase of illness, there is vacillation between hope and the knowledge that death is near. Parents also are fearful that the child's agony will be prolonged because of their own selfish desire to see him live. They are unable to make decisions concerning continuation of medical treatment if there is no hope for meaningful life. The child often asks questions about death and this is very hard for the parents at first. Often one spouse is unable to respond to the other's needs but feels an overwhelming desire to be comforted. At the time of death, they have to make difficult decisions concerning which family members will be present, whether or not to permit an autopsy, and which funeral home to use.

After Death

The funeral is a very important event. Most of the parents find that they are the comforters rather than the comforted. At the time the child dies, many parents have passed beyond the state of acute grief and may actually be relieved. During this early stage they may become frenetically involved in many activities. The deeper effects of grief appear later on.

Grief has different time and experiential components in our population from that described in the classic work of Lindeman. Whereas time intervals are mentioned to give a reference point, there are no rules concerning periods of grief. The first several months are spent in a somewhat numb state. After the actual event of the death, the acute pain is over and the task is thought to be one of getting beyond the loss and reintegrating. There is such dramatic relief at this point that a state much like euphoria is experienced. During this period, therefore, one can talk about the child and the illness with little evidence of distress; there are no tears, there is no flooding of consciousness with the child's image.

During this same period, however, there is a feeling of the presence of the dead child. This occurs at times when the family is all assembled, such as at mealtime. There is a conspicuous gap at the dinner table. In any family setting, the child's presence is felt. For the mothers this means that whenever they are asked by new acquaintances how many children they have, they immediately respond with the total number of children before the loss.

The memory that does remain is that of the illness itself. For a long period this is all that is available, and it is very distressing when the child's face cannot be remembered at all. There is a strong desire to hold onto the memory at the same time that an active effort is being made to forget.

The mothers often report being irritable and impatient during the first year to 18 months. This is particularly true of them when they are at home with their families. The men, as perceived by their wives, go to work, then sit in front of the television and sleep when at home. Communication continues to be as limited as it was throughout the illness.

In many families there is an open desire on the part of either one or both parents to have another child. This desire is actively denied as a wish to replace the dead child. There is an ambivalent situation going on in this case. The wish for a baby is a wish to fill the void of dependency that the sick child occupied. A baby is certainly both dependent and time-consuming. On the other hand, the loss of the sick child provides a new-found freedom. Initially this freedom is painful and one is not able to enjoy it. In addition, there is guilt in the savoring of it. The recurrent need to have a new baby may last as long as 2 years. If a baby should be born during this period, the maternal attachment appears to be incomplete. Within our population, one infant was born during the grieving period and failed to thrive. The only cause found was inadequate attachment to the mother with psychological deprivation during the first year of life.

For up to 2 years there is a careful avoidance of activities in which children of the same age as the dead child are involved. At the same time there is a furtive searching in crowds for a face that is reminiscent; if this face is found, however, feelings of anxiety and depression arise. There are ambivalent feelings toward other children with the same illness—sometimes there is hope that they will survive, but more often there is resentment and a wish that they too would succumb. Because this thought is unacceptable to the parents, they disguise it by saying that they wish the child and his parents were free of the suffering.

The second period following death comes as a surprise to some parents. During the first year they worked actively on detaching themselves from the child but now in the second year they find that even little things suddenly produce tears. Although this emotion is not associated with the pain experienced during the last stages of the illness, it is extremely distressing to outsiders who think that the bereaved has all these feelings under control. There is also a period beginning between the second and third year (sometimes later) when the parent begins to recall events of the child's life prior to the illness. This is a pleasant experience. The parent then begins to wonder if he or she will envision the child as growing up. One mother visited the children's section in a cemetery and found an answer to her question on graves of children and infants who had died 25 to 30 years previously. There were toys and objects appropriate to the age at which the child died.

The feelings and observations we have been discussing are those of mothers whose children have died during the past 5 years. It is readily apparent that the loss of a child is a pervasive, long-term, slowly resolved process.

While our primary concern is patient care, we feel it is necessary to validate all our observations and continue to evaluate our program.

RESEARCH

Specific research results have been obtained in two areas: (a) school attendance as an indicator of age-appropriate behavior, and (b) projective testing as an assessment of the child's coping mechanism. These studies were accomplished with the full, informed consent of the participating patient or his family. School attendance is the main parameter of a child's social behavior outside of the family. When we began studying this behavior in detail, we found an inordinate number of cases of school phobia. This observation could be validated because of the careful attendance records kept both by the school and by the hospital.

A study was done on 11 cases of school phobia identified in our clinic (3). This phobia was recognized as occurring at an unusually high rate in the population of children with malignancies. It is one of the problems described above as affecting the quality of life for the child and his family.

School phobia in both physically healthy children and children with cancer is characterized by refusal to attend school, fear of separation from the mother, and somatic complaints. In the child with malignancy, school phobia has two unique aspects: (a) a high rate of occurrence, and (b) marked regression.

Children with malignancies may have many physical problems, but they use complaints similar to those of physically healthy counterparts to express anxiety. The phobia begins insidiously in both groups with a complaint of headache or stomach pains. The mother responds by permitting the child to stay home for a period of time. The ambivalence of a mother encountering this behavior in her child is heightened when the child has a malignancy because, in managing the malignancy, she must rely greatly upon the child's report of new or recurring symptoms. A visit to the doctor may assure her that there is no physical basis (malignant basis) for the current complaints. If they disappear when school is not in session, that is further confirmation of the phobic nature of the complaints. Treatment of school phobia is extremely difficult in children with malignancies. The course of the cancer and the uncertainty of life thwart intervention. The real answer lies in prevention. From the time of diagnosis our oncology team discusses the importance of attending school. The families are told that maintaining a normal life style, including school attendance, prevents emotional deterioration. In another study, we obtained school attendance records for a random group of children being treated for malignancy in 1970 (before our program began) and compared them with the school attendance records for a group known to have school phobia. Days in hospital or clinic were accounted for. For the random group, the mean number of days attended was 78 out of a possible total of 180. For the group known to have school phobia. the corresponding mean number of days absent was 47 (Fig. 1).

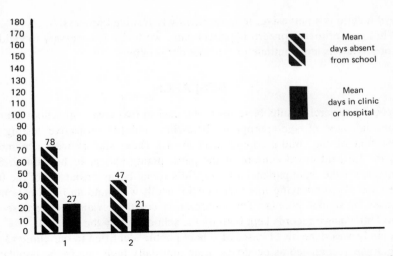

FIG. 1. Comparison of means for (1) School phobia cases (N = 6, representing 20 yrs malignancy) versus (2) Nonschool phobia cases (N = 15, representing 44 yrs).

Another study followed an observation that the sick child seemed to have a decreased wish-fulfilling fantasy (4). Is this lack of fantasy a result of having to attend to all the details of his illness? In other words, are we burdening the child with our open system? Also, how do the children experience their illness? The following questions were asked: (a) Do the older youngsters handle the stress of illness better because they have developed more mature ego functions, or do the younger children manage better because they do not understand the total situation and can use more primitive defenses, such as denial? (b) Does the sex of the child influence his functioning? The hypothesis from clinical observation was that males, who are usually more gross-motor oriented than females at the same age, suffer more because of the physical confinement and immobilization that the disease and its treatment impose on them.

Projective testing, including Rorschach, Thematic Apperception Test (TAT), and sentence completion, were used to answer the preceding questions. Eighteen children, 9 boys and 9 girls, between the ages of 5 and 15 years were tested.

The results were as follows. The younger boys displayed a significantly higher anxiety level than the young girls, but the older boys were able to view the world more realistically than the older girls. With respect to fantasy, the children's disposition to fantasy was not diminished, but the content of their imaginings showed a relative diminution of positive (pleasant, wish-fulfilling, fanciful) aspects. Unstructured situations elicited more anxiety and provided an atmosphere in which there was a tendency to distort reality.

This supports our clinical data, which indicate that children do better in an open, structured setting in which they have clear explanations of their condition and treatments. Under these circumstances they cope amazingly well.

Other soft results of our research on the program's effects are as follows:

1. Fathers are involved in the direct care of the child, including staying overnight in the hospital.
2. Families are returning to the Medical Center after the death of the child.
3. There is mutual support of families, particularly at periods of crisis.
4. Open discussion by parents of their fears of death occur prior to the terminal phase of the child's illness.
5. Parents are willing to look at their total family commitment rather than attending solely to the needs of the sick child.
6. Because of open discussion there are no dark secrets and we have no screaming, frightened children during their terminal illness. The child is composed as he nears death.

CONCLUSIONS

We have described a team approach to treatment and research in the psychosocial rehabilitation of children. A model of the emotional reactions of the child patient and involved family based on the various stages of the disease was proposed. Specific data for school attendance, as well as the results of projective tests for this patient population, were reviewed. These results demonstrate not only the problems and coping behavior experienced by these children but also the methods used to define the problems and the therapy programs designed to deal with them.

Many of the problems defined have not been studied by our group. The stresses on marriage at the time of illness are being examined using a number of parameters. The reactions and coping mechanisms of siblings are being studied Because we have concentrated on childhood malignancies, we have made only limited forays into the adult cancer patient's behavior. When family therapy has been used, however, it has been effective and shows that the experiences of these families are mirror images of those we have encountered in pediatrics. Much more intense study of this adult population is needed.

We have been intrigued by the information differential—who tells what to which team member. In our open team system for dealing with the disease, it is apparent that patients frequently give totally different answers to the same question asked by different team members. This has obvious implications for these cancer patients, and we feel it deserves systematic study.

REFERENCES

1. Ablin, A. R., Binger, C. M., Stein, R. C., et al. A conference with the family of a leukemic child. *Am. J. Dis. Child.,* 122:362 (1971).
2. Binger, C. M., et al. Childhood leukemia. *N. Engl. J. Med.,* 280:17–21 (1969).
3. Bozeman, M. F., Orbach, F. C., and Sutherland, A. M. Psychological impact of cancer and its treatment. *Cancer,* 8:1–18 (1955).
4. Easson, W. M. Management of the dying child. *J. Clin. Child Psychol,* 3:25–27 (1974).

5. Friedman, S. B., et al. Behavioral observations on parents anticipating the death of a child. *Pediatrics*, 32:610–625 (1963).
6. Futterman, E. H., Hoffman, I, and Sabshin, M. Parental anticipatory mourning. In: *Psychosocial Aspects of Terminal Care*, pp. 243–272, Columbia University Press, New York, 1972.
7. Futterman, E. H., and Hoffman, I. Shielding from awareness: An aspect of family adaptation to fatal illness of children, *Archives of the Foundation of Thanatology*, 2:23–24 (1970).
8. Goggin, E., Lansky, S. B., and Hassanein, K. Personality characteristics of children with malignancies. Submitted to *J. Acad. Child Psychiatr.*
9. Heffron, W. A., Bommelaere, K., and Masters, R. Group discussions with the parents of leukemic children. *Pediatrics*, 52:831–840 (1973).
10. Hoffman, I., and Futterman, E. H. Coping with waiting: Psychiatric intervention and study in the waiting room of a pediatric oncology clinic. *Compr. Psychiatry*, 12:67–81 (1971).
11. Howell, D. A. A child dies. *J. Pediatr. Surg.*, 1:2–7 (1966).
12. Humphrey, G. B., and Vore, D. A. Psychology and the oncology team. *J. Clin. Child Psychol.*, 3:27–29 (1974).
13. Kirkpatrick, J., Hoffman, I., and Futterman, E. H. Dilemma of trust: Relationship between medical care givers and parents of fatally ill children. *Pediatrics*, 54:169–175 (1974).
14. Lansky, S. B. Childhood leukemia: The child psychiatrist as a member of the oncology team. *J. Am. Acad. Child Psychiatry*, 13:499–508 (1974).
15. Lansky, S. B., and Lowman, J. T. Childhood malignancy: A comprehensive approach. *J. Kans. Med. Soc.* (1974).
16. Lansky, S. B., and Lowman, J. T., Vats, T. S., and Gyulay, J. School phobia in children with malignancies. *Am. J. Dis. Child.*, 129:42–46 (1975).
17. Lascari, A. D., and Stehbens, J. A. The reactions of families to childhood leukemia. *Clin. Pediatrics*, 12:210–214 (1973).
18. McIntire, M. S., Angle, C. R., and Struempler, L. J. The concept of death in mid-western children and youth. *Am. J. Dis. Child.*, 123:527–532 (1972).
19. Morrissey, J. R. Death anxiety in children with a fatal illness. *Am. J. Psychother.*, 606–615.
20. Nagy, M. A child's view of death. In Feifel, H. (ed.): *The Meaning of Death*, McGraw-Hill, New York, 1959.
21. Orbach, C. F., Sutherland, A. M., and Bozeman, M. D. Psychological impact of cancer and its treatment. *Cancer*, 8:20;33 (1955).
22. Smith, A. G., and Schneider, L. T. The dying child. *Clin. Pediatr.*, 8:131–134 (1969).
23. Solnit, A. J., and Green, M. Psychologic considerations in the management of deaths on pediatric hospital services. *Pediatrics*, 24:106–112 (1959).
24. Spinetta, J. J., Rigler, D., and Karon, M. Anxiety in the dying child. *Pediatrics*, 52:841–845 (1973).
25. Sutow, W., Vietti, T., and Fernbach, D. *Clinical Pediatric Oncology*, pp. 4–5, C. V. Mosby, St. Louis, 1973.
26. Waechter, E. H. Children's awareness of fatal illness. *Am. J. Nursing* 71:1168–1172 (1971).

Cancer: The Behavioral Dimensions, edited by J. W. Cullen, B. H. Fox, and R. N. Isom. Raven Press, New York © 1976.

Respondent

Jacob Schonfield

University of Maryland Hospital, Baltimore, Maryland 21201

Twenty years ago in one of the earliest reports on leukemic children and their parents, Bozeman et al. stated: "Although the mothers were aware of the hierarchy of the doctors, acceptability depended more on a physician's ability to establish warm emotional rapport than on his hospital rank. The physician's ability to form a good relationship with *the child* was above all else basic to the parents' acceptance of him as a physician for their child." One gets a feeling very early, therefore, in the study of leukemic children and their families of how important a feeling of caring and warmth is in the treatment of these children.

The most convincing aspect of your program, Dr. Lansky, is the impression one gets that your group really cares for the leukemic child and his parents. You are not just taking care of the child's medical needs, but also attending to the emotional needs of both the patient and his family. This comes through in your effort to maintain contact with the family after the death of the child. Simple things such as remembering the anniversary of the child's dealth or his birthday, are, I am sure, deeply appreciated by the parents. I know of no other program in this country that maintains contact with the family of the leukemic child for 2 years after his death. Such actions by your team must come through to the parents as the genuine concern of one human being for another, and this may be more important to the child's welfare than the best medical care in the world.

Several other important matters came to my attention in the early article by Bozeman et al. One of them is the continuity of care by professional personnel. Bozemen states that examination by different doctors and unsatisfactory information gave many of the parents the feeling of lack of continuity and unintelligent planning in treatment. By presenting the team as a unit and allowing the parents to talk to any member of the team, as well as by pooling all information among team members, you avoid this lack of continuity.

Finally, Bozeman et al. report the parents' resentment of clinic management that is characterized by regimentation, bossiness, lack of consideration, impersonality, or inefficiency. I certainly don't get the feeling from your report that your team had any of these attributed to its operation, vis-a-vis the parents or the leukemic child.

I also want to applaud your decision to speak openly in front of the child about the diagnosis. I have found in working with adult cancer patients that over 90% of them know that they have cancer although nobody has ever mentioned the word to them. We are beginning to realize that although very young children, even as young as 4 years of age, may not have an intellectual grasp of what death means, they still react emotionally to the fact that they have a dreadful illness that no one wants to talk about. They pick up subtle clues from the way adults react to them that something awful has happened. It is much better to talk about this openly than to pretend the child isn't capable of comprehending the meaning of a fatal illness when emotionally he clearly is.

I would also like to commend Dr. Lansky and her colleagues on the excellent idea of using as a lay expediter a mother who has lost a leukemic child. One often hears parents of leukemic children express doubts concerning the ability of the professional staff to put themselves in the position of parents of a child with a fatal illness. The fact that you have such a parent on the team means that there *is* someone who has gone through this same frightening experience, who has survived, and to whom one can express one's deepest fears and most unacceptable wishes because presumably she has felt the same things at one time.

I do have a few questions to address to Dr. Lansky and her team. Several authors have described the almost symbiotic relationship between the mother and her leukemic child, symbiotic to the point where even teenage children are allowed to sleep in the mother's bed. How do you handle the separation between mother and child when the child is hospitalized? Do you allow the mother to feed, dress, and otherwise take care of the child in the hospital or do you insist that these duties be carried out by hospital personnel? If the nurse or some other professional takes care of the child's needs in the hospital, there is bound to be some conflict with the mother over this in view of the unusual closeness between mother and child outside the hospital. How does your team cope with this problem? In addition, it might be interesting to look at school phobia from the point of view of separation fears on the part of the child as a result of actual separation from the mother. For instance, have the children who evince school phobia experienced greater separation from their mothers during hospitalization? Or is it the child whose mother is allowed to perform the usual mothering tasks in the hospital, and who consequently is never totally separated from her, the one who shows up more frequently with school phobia? Or is the significant factor in school phobia the mother's personality and how this meshes with her child's needs, regardless of the kind of separation experience the ill child has had?

I would like to ask a second set of questions, Dr. Lansky. You state that you are available to the team members if they want to ventilate their feelings and, presumably, their frustrations. I wonder to what degree being a team member reduces this need for "external" support. Is it easier as a member of a team to cope with the inevitable hostility that parents of a dying child express toward the medical personnel who are unable to save their child's life? Are these angry feelings somewhat diffused because they are now directed toward not just one or two people but toward the entire team? Do your team members find it easier to cope with parental hostility because they act as a team and have the support of other team members in whatever intervention, if any, is used?

Finally, I would like to ask Dr. Lansky about her work in counseling the siblings of the leukemic child. Binges et al. recently reported that 50% of the siblings whose brother or sister had died from leukemia had difficulties in coping. This was signaled by severe enuresis, headaches, school phobia, depression, abdominal pains, and severe separation anxiety. Dr. Kubler-Ross reports meeting with a group of such siblings after one of them complained that Dr. Kubler-Ross had plenty of time for their parents and for their sick brother or sister but no time for them. She says that this meeting was one of the most rewarding ones she has had, and that it provided her with all kinds of insights into family problems she was not aware existed. What has your experience been with siblings of the leukemic child? Do you think it is best to counsel them individually or have you tried any group sessions, either with or without the parents? Just as the parents seem to gain support from other parents facing the same situation, don't you think the siblings might benefit also if they met brothers and sisters of other leukemic children and shared their experiences and problems with them?

Response to Dr. Schonfield

Shirley Lansky

The problem of a symbiotic relationship developing between the mother and the sick child is one that we have been concerned about for some time because of its far-reaching effect on the mother, the child, and the other family members. The question is: How do we handle this matter when the child is hospitalized? We encourage parents to stay with their sick children because most of our patients come from out of town. It is very helpful to the little children to have their mothers available to support them and assist in the treatments. This is also true for the older children. In both instances, however, we must weigh the effects of the support and constantly be aware that overinvolvement may occur.

With older children we encourage the mother and the child to separate frequently. The mothers often go out for meals together. This is mutually supporting for them and at the same time they exert a subtle peer pressure on the mother who may be reluctant to leave her child for any length of time. We also encourage children to perform as many self-care activities as they can. Their mothers may assist them with those that they cannot perform. Fathers have been participating more in the child's care—staying overnight and bringing the patient to a clinic. This is probably the most effective method of preventing a symbiotic relationship.

We are fortunate in having a nursing staff that is very attentive to the needs of both child and mother. Because their efforts receive support, nurses have been able to discuss their frustrations in trying to care for a child whose mother will not permit him any independence. It has been some time since a mother and a nurse have become embroiled in a conflict over the question of who would care for the child.

School phobia does not seem to occur more frequently in the children of mothers who assume an exclusive care-taking role. The statements made by Dr. Schonfield regarding the mother's personality and how this meshes with the child's needs are more of an expression of what we have observed with this entity. The prevention of school phobia also depends on how well we succeed during the first hospitalization in convincing the family that they need to return to their usual activities. When we are successful in getting this message through to them, school phobia does not develop.

With regard to the questions concerning the team, what we have described is the sharing of responsibility in our work. However, we also share the hostility of parents; we share the grief of the loss of the child. Often the anger is not directed at the team but at an individual. This individual may hear about it from another team member rather than directly from the child or parent. Here again, we look at this openly and see if there is a basis for it. We attempt to correct the situation if this is possible, or we tolerate the parents' anger knowing it is associated with their grief over the child's death or approaching death.

As I mentioned earlier, siblings are recognized as having very special needs. We have begun to study them and their problems. At present we see them in our children's group, in family conferences, and on an individual basis. Because most of our families come from out of town it has not seemed practical to get them together on a regular basis, although we hope it will be possible to do this in the future.

Respondent

Ruth McCorkle

University of Iowa, Iowa City, Iowa 52240

Dr. Lansky's chapter describes a treatment and research program, using a team approach, for the psychosocial rehabilitation of children with leukemia. My comments will be directed at two major areas of her report. First, I will raise some questions relating to the research program and methodology outlined in the chapter, and, second, I will comment on several of the treatment and substantive areas of the study that include the team members' findings.

THE RESEARCH APPROACH

Research is the vehicle or process used by the scientist to develop and test knowledge. The body of accumulated knowledge that purports to describe some selected aspects of the universe is known as science;[1] therefore the researcher seeks to discover scientific knowledge. In other words, the researcher's discoveries must be capable of being proved or disproved by anyone with the necessary intelligence to use the technical devices of observation and experimentation (2). The study reported by Lansky and her team seems designed to construct a theory about progressive illness and coping rather than to rigorously test hypotheses.

The Lansky study is exciting because the authors attempt to go beyond the scope of the present literature describing psychological responses to cancer in general (3–9) to concentrate on the response to one specific disease in one population, i.e., leukemia in children. There have been some previous attempts to describe this group and their needs in the literature (10–12); however, this study is unique because it uses the team approach to effect a favorable behavioral response to coping with a progressive illness within the family unit.

One difficulty I had in viewing this chapter as a scientific endeavor was my own inability to understand exactly what was done by the team on a day-to-day basis. In other words, could the study be described in such a way that other teams could be formed across the country to achieve similar effects? If the team approach were used in caring for other types of cancer patients, it also would be helpful to have answers to the following questions: If you were to repeat the study, what things would you do again, and what changes and recommendations would you make? How were you able to predict certain difficulties or benefits for the patients and their families in coping with all aspects of leukemia? Were the interventions of groups, such as a children's activity group, an adolescent group, and a group of mothers who had already lost children, used in a systematic fashion? What effects, in fact, did these interventions have on the behavior of patients, families, and staff? Were there any situations in which specific interventions were not used and a comparative analysis of groups was done? Were the children and families observed at regular intervals

---

[1]Richard Rudner makes the distinction between science as a process and science as a product: "On the one hand (as process term), it is used to refer to the activities or workshops of scientists or scientific institutions, i.e., to experimenting, observing, reasoning, reading, organizing research projects, etc. But on the other hand, the same term is employed to refer to a result of these activities or processes, to the product of scientific activities, i.e., to a corpus of statements purporting to describe one or another aspect of the universe and embodying what counts as our scientific knowledge" (1).

throughout their illness? Were the same data collected on all children and family members? Was each team member reliable in observing similar behaviors and in recording the observations? And what, in each of your own observations and experiences, were the most difficult times?

These questions are raised not to criticize the work of these individuals but, in fact, to support their endeavors. It seems imperative that these questions be considered in planning future interventions and that the data in our reports be analyzed explicitly so that others can utilize our findings effectively for the patient's benefit and for the further development of knowledge.

THE HUMAN APPROACH

My remaining remarks will focus on various interventions discussed in the chapter. Dr. Lansky and her team are obviously dedicated to the caring of human beings (13). They work in an area that requires a great deal of time and personal devotion. There is no question in my mind that their patients benefited from their care.

The team members have focused their collective efforts on attempting to enhance the quality of life for the child and his family. They have gone beyond the issue of whether or not to tell an individual he has cancer and have tried to help the child feel less sick. There is general agreement among those who argue against telling that giving the diagnosis anticipates profoundly disturbing psychological effects (14). This team not only anticipates certain effects but also ameliorates them by joining forces to help the patient, his family, and the medical staff. They are dealing with the certainties of leukemia. They are willing to take what knowledge they have of the illness and its treatment to plan and implement a *support system* for the child and his family.

They have learned that individuals with a progressive illness need contact with one key person on whom they can rely when the going gets rough; that the emotional commitment associated with this type of health care is exhausting and that it is essential to have their own support system built into the team. No individual alone can help a child and his family deal with these devastating events. Support must come from many people administering to various needs throughout the illness. The use of a lay expediter is a good example of a special kind of support. I know of only one place where volunteers are used in a similar way and this is at Saint Christopher's Hospice in England. The volunteers are supervised by Mrs. Hanna, the administrative director of volunteer services.

It is apparent from the study that communication among team members is essential. The medical therapies must be planned and shared so that individual members can answer questions from patients and their families in a consistent manner. The finding that patients or family members or both choose one team member with whom to communicate is extremely important for the practitioners to know. How many of us have stopped to consider how many times a patient may have to discuss his physical condition in order to keep the individuals involved in his care informed. The entire team approach is concerned with identifying appropriate communication strategies needed to assist the child, family, and staff in dealing with the consequences of illness. Dr. Lansky and her team were able to identify many behaviors. Two of the most prominent and difficult ones to cope with are the feelings of guilt and fear. It would be helpful if the specific communication strategies used to cope with guilt and fear could be put into effect so that health-care personnel in other institutions could assist individuals in dealing with these feelings. In addition, it would be helpful to know if Dr. Lansky and her co-workers were able to recognize those factors that made the program successful for some families and not for others.

My final comments focus on two areas that are indirectly related to the chapter. One is the patient's increased awareness that people with similar diseases receive different types of treatment. Recently I attended the Cancer Treatment and Rehabilitation Conference in New York City. I was overwhelmed by the number of different protocols used in the medical management of cancer. My concern is not whether different programs of medical research should or should not be used in the treatment of individuals with cancer, but that we as behavioral scientists address ourselves to this issue. We need to identify communication strategies to help these individuals make informed decisions and to offer them continued support.

Finally, I must comment on the concept of pain control in the individual with progressive cancer. Dr. Lansky's team reports that patients and their families often fear that death will be painful. Pain is certainly not experienced by all children with leukemia; but for those individuals in which it does occur, it can be devastating. To me, it is inconceivable that a patient with progressive cancer, no matter what type, has to experience pain longer than necessary to assess it and to determine a control. Yet, I consider this one of the major nursing-care problems encountered in our hospitals today. It seems to me that pain control should be one of our main priorities. This session is entitled "Living with Cancer" and pain relief is a prerequisite for living. One possible solution might be to compare individuals with progressive cancer to those with other chronic illnesses, such as diabetes or heart disease. For example, a physician or nurse would not think of withholding insulin from a diabetic patient. The diabetic patient needs insulin to live and the physician would be charged with malpractice if he ordered insulin to be given only when a diabetic coma occurred. The person with cancer may need his pain medication as regularly as the diabetic patient needs insulin or as the cardiac patient needs heart pills. Individuals should be allowed to be free of pain and not be reminded of their symptoms simply because the physician is not skilled in prescribing adequate and sustained relief. It is a very rewarding experience to help an individual determine the adequate dosage of his pain medication and the time interval needed between administrations of it. In addition, it allows the individual some control over what is happening to him.

In conclusion, I want to commend Dr. Lansky and her team for their achievements. It is never easy to condense and solidify 5 years of work into an hour presentation. My responses to this chapter have been directed to its research approach and to the elements of human compassion evident throughout. No matter what direction research takes as a result of this conference, I hope that we will always be guided by compassion.

REFERENCES

1. Rudner, R. *Philosophy of Social Science,* p. 8. Prentice-Hall, Englewood Cliffs, N.J., 1966.
2. Feigel H. The scientific outlook: Naturalism and humanism. In Feigel, H., and Brodbeck, M. (eds): *Readings in the Philosophy of Science,* pp. 8–18, Appleton-Century-Crofts, New York, 1953.
3. Finesinger, J. E., Shands, H. C., and Abrams, R. P. Managing emotional problems of cancer patients. *Cancer Bull. Cancer Prog.,* 3:19–31 (1953).
4. Bard, M., and Sutherland, M. Psychological impact of cancer and its treatment. *Cancer,* 8:656–672 (1955).
5. LeShan, L. Psychological states as factors in the development of malignant disease. *J. Natl. Cancer Inst.,* 22:1–18 (1959).
6. Rothenberg, A. Psychological problems in terminal cancer management. *Cancer,* 14:1063–1073 (1961).
7. Hinton, J. The physical and mental distress of the dying. *Q.J. Med.,* 32:1–21 (1963).
8. Senescu, R. A. The development of emotional complications in the patient with cancer. *J. Chronic Dis.,* 16:812–832 (1963).
9. Feder, S. Psychological considerations in the care of patients with cancer. *Ann N.Y. Acad. Sci.* 125:1020–1027.
10. Bozeman, M. F. et al. Psychological impact of cancer and its treatment-III. The adaptation of mothers to the threatened loss of their children through leukemia: Parts I and II. *Cancer,* 8:1–19; 20–33 (1955).
11. Binger, C. M., et al. Childhood leukemia—emotional impact on patient and family. *N. Engl. J. Med.,* 280:414–418 (1969).

12. Waechter, E. H. Children's awareness of fatal illness. *Am. J. Nurs.*, 1168–1172 (1971).
13. Benoliel, J. Q. Discussion of the concept of care in contrast to the concept of cure. The concept of care for a child with leukemia. *Nurs. Forum.* XI:194–204 (1972).
14. Donald, O. What to tell cancer patients. *J.A.M.A.*, 175:51–53 (1961).

Response to Ms. McCorkle

Shirley Lansky

We hope that our work can be translated to other groups. We want to quickly reemphasize, however, that the evolution of this group was important to the final structure of it. At different centers around the country there may be different types of people available. It is the interest, the ability to cooperate as a team, that makes a group viable.

The one member that appears to be the pivotal person is the lay expediter. This person, having had the experience of losing a child, can provide a great deal of empathy, but must clearly know his or her own emotional status. Goodwill alone and having had the experience is not enough. This person also must have a period of time away from the illness to put her own grief and mourning into perspective.

Miss McCorkle asks if we observe families throughout the illness. Yes, we do from the time of the diagnosis until at least 2 years after the death. The question is: What makes the program successful for some but not for others? We have a fairly high participation rate in the many activities mentioned; however, there are some who refuse to participate in anything other than the essential medical program. Many of these people say that they have never been comfortable in groups of people and are afraid of losing their composure in uncontrolled expression of their fear and grief. Sometimes people who are reluctant initially will begin to participate later on. The people who do participate maintain contact with us for a long time, those who do not participate sever contact with us soon after the death of the child.

A question was asked regarding interrater reliability. Although this has not been done in a formal way, we do spend much time at our team meetings discussing our observations and why we have made them.

Discussion

Louis Fink: Dr. Lowman, is each pediatric cancer patient in your hospital managed by a multidisciplinary group from the onset? If so, are the multidisciplinary members of the group all in-house professionals? Does your present team function with each member of the multidisciplinary group?

J. Lowman: To answer the first part of your question, we are all in-house members of the staff. We have tried to expand our numbers and have been moderately successful in several cases. We are in a fairly low physician-population state and our basic premise is that the child treated near his home is the happiest child. Unfortunately, we really don't have that option in some cases because of the low population base of physicians in the state of Kansas, so we are in-house basically. As I said, we have expanded on a few occasions to include physicians out of the university system. I don't see any particular reason why this should not be done. Most children receiving treatment today require reevaluation at a large center during periods of their care, so in nearly all cases they would be going back and forth for some of their treatment. I didn't understand your last question.

Louis Fink: The last question relates to the various phases of patient management in the hands of different professionals and different disciplines. Does the present team apply themselves at each stage of the management?

J. Lowman: Yes, if the child is, for example, primarily receiving radiotherapy, the emotional support team will continue with that child through that course of therapy. The same is true for surgery. Once we are associated with the child, we essentially never leave him and his family until at least 2 years after the death.

Louis Fink: Then you would say that throughout the management of the patient at the various stages of each discipline there is total communication via your present team.

J. Lowman: There are obviously occasions when communication breaks down between patient and team and it creates a very difficult problem.

D. Hayes: Our institution has also subscribed to this approach, and we are also a member of the Acute Leukemia Group B so that we probably deal with some of the same protocols. In our case, we have found that the addition of a specially trained chaplain to our team has been helpful. We, of course, are the buckle on the Bible Belt and the social significance of religion in North Carolina, Tennessee, Virginia, and South Carolina, the states that constitute our referral area, is such that we have found the chaplain to be a particularly valuable adjunct to the team. I would like to ask you if you have, in assessing the value of the team approach, considered the possibility of measuring it in terms of cost benefits. This is what we have attempted to do. Leukemia, of course, is a costly disease in both adults and children and we have found that in measuring the number of hours saved on the part of the family in babysitting time, travel time, and in hours spent away from the hospital because the team is giving them adequate support, we have saved them approximately 50% in time and an equivalent amount of money. In adult leukemia, we found that the cost to the family ranges from about $8,000 to $32,000, with an average of about $16,000. We have not been able to achieve the same sort of cost saving in the treatment of adult acute leukemia, probably because the outcome is so much poorer, but I would be interested in your reaction to this cost-saving approach.

J. Lowman: Well, I think that's exciting; it's one of the areas that interests us. We have not used this sort of approach. Because of the population size we serve, our program is a moderately expensive one. We feel that the number of health professionals involved is quite high for the number of patients served. However, one of our objectives is to show that much of what professionals do in this realm of health care may be done poorly, and second, that this area does not really require the degrees and education that most professionals possess. The work of Karen Briscoe, our own lay expediter, is a good example of what the nonprofessional can accomplish. One of our proposals, therefore, is to estimate the cost of using good nonprofessionals in our health care and then see how we come out. We're just beginning to feel that we're hampered by professionals in achieving our goals.

Zwartjes: I think your approach to the total care of the patient is superb. How can you afford having a full-time psychiatrist on your team? Where do you obtain financial support for a patient advocate (lay expediter)? These are two of our biggest problems. What about the problems of the child who has survived his disease and is now faced with the backward attitudes of society toward it? What about the teenager whose parents have a hard time committing themselves to sending him to college? What about the boy who has had leukemia for 5 years, and who tries to get a job, and is turned down because of his disease? I'd also like to respond to your thoughts about expanding the number of physicians on your team. We're in a similar situation in Denver in having to cover largely rural areas, and we have found that a good way to do this is to bring the physicians in from various communities on a 3-month basis to acquaint them with our programs and then to set up one physician within about a 50-mile radius of any particular area for referral. Considering your situation in Kansas, this might be an approach that would work for you also.

J. Lowman: We've been fortunate to have begged and borrowed money from several sources. Karen Briscoe, for example, has been supported by the Kansas Division of the American Cancer Society for 3 years. Part of Dr. Lansky's work was supported by small research grants; some of our programs have been supported by private donations. We are fortunate in having a group of angels, I suppose that is an appropriate term, that have been interested in this program for some time and have supported it. Ours is also an institution in which the physician's income reverts to the department and, in some cases, divisions, so that the treatment of many of our patients has been paid for in this way. Many of our patients are covered by very good catastrophe clauses. I think Dr. Lansky is the one to answer your question concerning the children who survive.

S. Lansky: We don't have a large population, but we certainly are seeing the same things that you mentioned. We are just beginning to study them analytically. One of our cases of school phobia, for instance, was that of a child who is in his eighth year after primary diagnosis. He's had no relapses and yet he did not go to school for 5 of those 8 years. I agree with you, therefore, that this kind of problem must be attended to and our concern with it will become a more important part of our program as time goes on.

A. Brickner: I'd like to close with two comments. One of the papers that I want to write some day is called "Everybody Talks to the Executive, but to Whom Does He Talk?" and I think I am going to substitute the doctor for the executive. I think that insufficient support for the physician himself is one of the really critical problems to be examined. The other comment is that during my days as a militant-acting citizen, I was on the Board of Commissioners in the county I live in and on one particular issue I was approached by a constituent who came up to me and said, "Abe, that was a great thing you did, a beautiful compromise." Then a group of constituents approached me on the same issue and said, "You sold out."

Cancer: The Behavioral Dimensions, edited by J. W. Cullen,
B. H. Fox, and R. N. Isom. Raven Press, New York © 1976.

Decision Making for the Terminally Ill Patient

Norman K. Brown, Maria A. Brown, and Donovan Thompson

*School of Public Health and Community Medicine, University of Washington,
Seattle, Washington 98105*

DEFINITIONS

Decision making has become as much a part of our behavioral science vocabulary as problem solving was 5 years ago. The word *decision* comes from Latin, "de-" meaning "of," or "from," and "caedere" meaning "to cut." Hence, when a decision is made, one cuts off the question or the dilemma. When decisions are made concerning the medical treatment of terminal patients, cutting off debate may also mean cutting off the life of the patient.

Until recently the term euthanasia connoted mercy killing. When medicine became capable of prolonging life, the modifiers positive (active or direct) and negative (passive or indirect) were prefixed to euthanasia to distinguish mercy killing first from mere withdrawal or withholding of life-prolonging treatments in the second (1). Unfortunately, the expression *negative euthanasia* still carries the original emotional connotation of mercy killing, which will probably prevent its becoming a colloquial phrase in our society. Recently the Euthanasia Society of America changed its name to the Society for a Humane Death for this reason. Nevertheless, negative euthanasia will be used in this chapter because of lack of a better substitute at this time.

WHO MAKES THE DECISIONS?

Decisions about health are made many times in the life of an individual. We face minor illness often and frequently make our own decisions about diet, work, and medications. However, when faced with a major or terminal illness, most of us voluntarily enter the health-care system in which our role in decision making varies.

As depicted in Table 1, the health-care professionals generally assume an increasingly active role in making technical decisions about steps to be taken as the illness becomes more serious. As the health-care professional becomes more aggressive in decision making, the patient tends to become more passive. There are at least 10 reasons for this shift of responsibility in health-care decisions from

TABLE 1. *Role of patient and professional in technical health-care decisions*

Severity of illness	Relative aggression of decision makers		Examples	
	Self-family	Professional	Condition	Action taken for
Minor	++++	0	Headache	Aspirin
Minor	+++	+	Cough	Antibiotic
Moderate	++	++	Appendicitis	Operation
			Ulcer	Medications, diet
Major	+	+++	Heart attack	Coronary care
			Auto accident injuries	Intensive care
Terminal	0 ◄►++++	++++◄►0	Terminal cancer	Intensive care Withdrawal of treatment; Dying at home

the patient to the health-care professionals themselves. These reasons may be divided as follows:

1. Patient reasons
    a. Lack of knowledge and experience with illness and the complex machinery used to treat it
    b. Weakness and passivity created by disease, drugs, or treatment procedures
    c. Increased isolation as a result of being in intensive- or coronary-care units
    d. Substitution of trust in the health-care professionals for "informed consent," which becomes nearly impossible to achieve in technically complex situations
2. Health-care professional reasons
    a. Increased specialization of health-care professionals, who tend to have more rigid treatment methods—and alternatives—with very sick patients
    b. Increased numbers of consultants who have difficulty meshing decisions with one another let alone with the patient
    c. Errors of omission that, unlike errors of commission in prolonging life, have led to malpractice suits
    d. Apparently endless availability of society's resources—i.e., dollars—for technological treatments
    e. The Hippocratic Oath which forswears the use of a deadly drug
    f. A lack of awareness on the part of both health-care professionals and patients of the moral dimension in making technical decisions (2).

The passive role of the patient with a major illness has so far been reasonably well "accepted" by patients and their families provided a relative recovery ensues. Hackett and Cassem (3) found, however, that 18 of 19 patients placed on a cardiac monitor in an intensive-care ward used partial or major denial of fear "to allay anxiety and to minimize emotional stress." When the patient with major illness either suddenly or gradually becomes terminal, patients, families, and many others in society suddenly turn into "activists." The health-care profession-al battling with a severely deranged physiology by means of an increasingly aggressive technology may find himself with a terminally ill patient who now asks to be part of the decision making process.

We therefore see the health-care system paradoxically deployed for the battle to preserve life at the brink of terminal illness when, and at this moment, the patient or his family suddenly calls a halt to the proceedings. Two important questions are immediately apparent in this crisis situation: (a) What decisions are being made? and (b) Who is making the decisions? If these questions can be answered, then the impact of decisions and whether what "is happening" as opposed to what "ought to be happening" become the next logical queries. Answers to these last questions help us alter or adjust current terminal care so that it is consistent with society's needs.

CURRENT ATTITUDES: SOME DATA

Let us examine the data we now have on the attitudes of both physicians and society. Table 2 summarizes surveys in the literature of attitudes toward euthana-sia, both negative and positive, in several moderate-sized populations. Without dwelling on every reference, I shall note a few points:

1. Endorsement of negative euthanasia ranges from 61–97% in all populations except those of nursing home nurses and Iowa physicians.

2. Although the nursing home study hardly fits with the others cited because of its small population, I have included it because the analysis was done in detail for 10 patients. You will note that the response range in favor of allowing death was consistent with our "average," except for those nurses who wanted to prolong life in 9 out of 10 of these patients.

3. The percentage of respondents in favor of positive euthanasia was lower in every study than that for negative euthanasia.

4. Americans polled by Gallup were among those most in favor of positive euthanasia. Fifty-three percent of them were in favor of it as opposed to only 36% in favor in 1950.

5. Religion made a consistent difference in six populations surveyed in that Protestants were more in favor of euthanasia (both types) than Catholics. One investigator went so far as to say, "When physicians debate the morality of infanticide, they do not speak as medical men, their opinions are not informed by peculiarly medical concerns. Rather, they speak as Catholics, Protestants, Jews and agnostics...their opinions are based on the same (religious) factors as those which form the opinions of laymen." (4)

TABLE 2. *Surveys of attitudes toward euthanasia*

Ref.	Population studied	Date	Geographic area	Number surveyed	Number respondents	Replies (%)	Negative euthanasia (% in favor)	Positive euthanasia (% in favor)	Some characteristics of respondents	
									More in favor	Less in favor
7.	Internists and surgeons	1961	Chicago	250	146	58		63	Prot., Jew., no religion	Catholic
8.	Physicians	1962	US	?	?	?	81	31	Prot., Jew.	Catholic
9.	British MDs	1965	Britain	1,000	?	?	76			
10.	Professors of medicine	1969	US	344	333	97	86	18	Other, Prot.	Catholic, Jew.
10a.	Univ. of Wash. grads.	1970	Wash. (State)	1,179	632	56	75	35	Other, Prot.	Catholic
4.	Faculty: med. and ped.	1970	US	627	454	72	67		More scientific orientation, Jew., Prot.	Less scientific orientation, Catholic
11.	Attend. MDs Univ. and comm. hospitals	1970	Seattle	460	418	92	59	31	30–39 yr anesth., path., rad., psych.	>60 yr surg. special.
12.	Nurses univ. and comm. hosp.	1971	Seattle	744	677	91	85	36	Surg. special., E.R.–O.R. pediatrics	
13.	4th yr med.	1971	Wash. (State)	84	82	97	90	50		

	Year	Location						Notes
students ('69)			83	81	98	69	50	
1st yr med. students ('72)	1971	Wash. (State)	10	7	70	70		
14. Nursing home patients	1971	N.Y.	10	10	100	70		
their families			10	10	100	60		
their physicians			10	10	100	10		
their nurses			?	?	?	—		
15. Americans	1973	US	?	?	?		53 (36 in 1950) 11	
16. MDs & DOs	1974	US	3,000	933	31	71		Psychiatrists, internists, Prot., Jew., >30 yr / Ob-gyn pediatric. Catholic <30 yr
17. American Soc. of Abdom. Surg.	1974	US	?	ca.1,000	?	97		
18. Physicians	1974	Iowa	2,290	1,145	50	47	26	Respondents (27%) / Nonrespondents (16%)
Interns and residents			322	177	55	52	37	Infrequent contact with term. patients / Frequent contact with term. patients
Univ. faculty			267	147	55	34	25	<30 yr / 30–60 yr
1st and 4th yr med. students	289		133	46	70	50		>60 yr <30 yr Rural / Urban

6. Physicians in certain specialties were more in favor of euthanasia—ironically those physicians who are the least likely to be responsible for making such a decision.

7. Obstetrician-gynecologists, surgical specialists, and pediatricians were those least in favor of euthanasia. Yet the nurses in two of these areas were among those most in favor, suggesting that coordination of emotional goals on this topic may not be optimal on these services.

8. Although the surveys in which the response was less than 90% show excellent general agreement with surveys above 90% response, it should be noted that surveys with lower percentage responses may be less representative. For example, Travis et al. (5) pursued 82 nonrespondents and found them much less in favor of positive euthanasia than respondents (16% versus 26%).

DECISIONS FOR NEGATIVE EUTHANASIA IN A CONVALESCENT CENTER: SOME DATA

If the majority of our society is in favor of negative euthanasia, what is occurring in actual practice? From the findings (reviewed in Table 2) it seems likely that decisions for negative euthanasia were being made. Travis et al. (5) found that their respondents performed negative euthanasia about as often as they favored it. We believed that identifying and quantifying such decisions would be of value if we are to improve terminal care and make the role of the health-care professional in these decisions one that is more compatible with society's needs.

Wishing to find a place where a number of such decisions might be made, we turned to a metropolitan extended-care facility. Our study included all admissions during a 1-year period. I shall concentrate on the patients admitted with a cancer diagnosis to demonstrate the details of our method of identifying decisions for negative euthanasia. Then I shall summarize factors that are related to negative euthanasia for all patients.

Of 728 admissions in 1973 by 284 community physicians, 99 had an admission of cancer. Although 14% (99 of 728) of the admissions were for cancer, 33% (40 of 123) of the deaths among all admissions were those of cancer patients (Table 3). Fifty-eight of these 99 cancer patients developed a "poor" condition or a significant fever ($>101°$ on two occasions in 24 hours), with outcomes as shown in Table 4.

TABLE 3. *Occurrence of poor/febrile episodes and death among 728 admissions to an extended-care facility*

Diagnosis	Number	Number of poor/ febrile episodes	Percent with episodes	Number of deaths	Percent dying
All other	629	143	23	83	13
Cancer	99	58	58	40	40
Total	728	201		123	

TABLE 4. *Outcome of 58 poor/febrile episodes in 99 cancer patients*

Hospitalized	10
Resolved "poor"/fever	7
Died in facility	40
Died at home	1
Total	58

Those who became "poor" or febrile, but were not hospitalized, were defined as subjects for potential negative euthanasia (i.e., the physician was likely to have withdrawn or not instituted therapy that would otherwise have prolonged life). Further study of the medical records of these 40 deaths showed strong evidence of the physician's decision for negative euthanasia in 28 patients (Table 5).

Twenty-eight of the 40 (70%) of the cancer deaths in an extended-care facility were judged to have been those associated with negative euthanasia. Those deaths with negative euthanasia represented about one-fourth of the cancer patients admitted (28 of 99).

Although this study demonstrates an impressive frequency of decisions for negative euthanasia in cancer patients, the small number of patients studied and the possible bias of one facility limit further interpretations. A partial correction for the small numbers may be found through examination of all 201 patients who developed a febrile or poor/critical episode. In addition, we have sufficient numbers to examine some of the factors that may be related to these decisions. (See Tables 6-9.) Again without citing reference numbers, several points are worth noting.

1. Men were more likely to suffer a crisis, yet less likely to be "treated with" negative euthanasia than women.
2. Patients with cancer were more likely to suffer crises and to be "treated with" negative euthanasia than were patients with other diagnoses.
3. Whereas crises occurred in patients of all payment classes (private, Medicare, welfare), there was a direct relationship between frequency of decisions for negative euthanasia and responsibility for paying the bill.
4. Single or married individuals were more likely to be "treated with" negative euthanasia than widows.

TABLE 5. *Physician's decision for negative euthanasia among 40 cancer deaths*

Progress note with direct statement of intention	16	
No antibiotic for fever	7	28
No life-prolonging orders after hopeless prognosis statement	5	
No evidence of decision for negative euthanasia		12

TABLE 6. *Examples in medical records of entries indicating definite negative euthanasia (NE)*

Age and Sex		Diagnoses	Progress note/order
79	M	Cancer	Discontinue all medications; Demerol and Phenegran PRN (as needed).
79	F	Cancer	Keep patient comfortable. Patient is terminal.
79	F	Cancer, CVA	Patient appears terminal—no effort to be made to maintain her.
71	M	Cancer	Family requested IV to be discontinued. Complied.
72	M	Cancer, fever	Condition is deteriorating—do not believe artificial support (IV's, nasogastric feeding, etc.) is warranted here.

5. With respect to religion, Catholic physicians and patients alike consistently avoided negative euthanasia decisions.

Since many of these factors are themselves interrelated, a final analysis will have to take these interrelationships into account. For example, most welfare patients were less than 65 years of age, so decisions in favor of negative euthanasia might have been less frequent because of age as much as because of inability to pay. Methods of analyzing possibly interrelated factors are available, but have not yet been applied to these data.

In conclusion, our study has shown.

1. Decisions are being made for negative euthanasia in at least one metropolitan convalescent center.
2. Data in preliminary form have been presented demonstrating that 28 of 99 patients dying with cancer in an extended-care facility in 1 year had decisions made for them that could be labeled as negative euthanasia. The effects of such a decision upon the surviving family, the patient, and the health-care professionals have not been evaluated but merit better definition.
3. The small numbers and the restricted population in this study are too

TABLE 7. *Factors associated with negative euthanasia decisions*

Factor	Patient more likely to be/have
Sex	Female
Admitting diagnosis	Cancer
Payment class	Private > Medicare > welfare
Marital status	Single or married > widow
Religion	No preference or Protestant > Catholic

TABLE 8. *Negative euthanasia decisions in 201 patients with poor/febrile episodes*

Patients	No	Yes	Decisions (total)
Male	77	24	101
Female	60	40	100
Total	137	64	201

inadequate for extrapolating data applicable to our society. Rather, these results should be viewed as a stimulus to further broad-based investigations with greater potential validity.

RECOMMENDATIONS

1. The construction of a new morality of decision making for patients who are terminally ill, particularly with cancer, appears warranted. The data presented indicate, in a preliminary way, the ethics or norms of such decision making in one setting for cancer patients in our society. Such ethics of decision making are not necessarily moral, i.e., right as opposed to wrong. However, the availability of more representative data and knowledge concerning these decisions, coupled with intensive analysis of individual attitudes toward dying, should provide a strong

TABLE 9. *Factors associated with negative euthanasia decisions in patients with febrile "poor"/"critical" episodes: Seattle, 1973*

Admitting diagnosis	Percent negative euthanasia decisions during a crisis
CVA	21
ASHD	20
Fracture	36
Cancer	45
Other	30
Payment class	
Private	38
Medicare	31
Welfare	27
Marital Status	
Single	38
Married	37
Widowed	27
Divorced or separated	20
Religion	
Catholic	18
Protestant	34
Jewish	None among 4
Other	35
None or not stated	36

foundation for an exchange of ideas among health-care professionals seeking to improve the care of the terminally ill patients.

2. Some suggested questions to answer in improving decision making for terminal patients are:

   a. Can we improve communication between health-care professionals and patients on the moral as opposed to the technical aspects of the decisions (2)?

   b. Negative euthanasia is an upsetting expression to many; can we find a more acceptable yet accurate expression for this action that would facilitate open discussion of the subject (6)?

   c. Patients seeking a particular range of moral options in their care may be better off if they enter the health-care system capable of providing these options. Can we assist patients with cancer in choosing physicians, even changing to physicians whose value systems are more compatible with their own? The studies reviewed here indicate that a Catholic patient with cancer and a Catholic physician might work much better together during a terminal illness than, for example, a Protestant or Jewish patient and a Catholic physician.

   d. What is the impact of a decision in favor of negative euthanasia on the surviving family members? Did the survivors or the patient or both participate in the decision?

REFERENCES

1. Rachaels, J. Active and passive euthanasia. *N. Engl. J. Med.*, 292:78–80 (1975).
2. Cassell, E. J. Making and escaping moral decisions. *Hastings Cent. Stud.*, 1:53–62 (1973).
3. Hackett, T. P., and Cassem, N. H. Patients facing sudden cardiac death. In Schoenberg et al. (eds): *Psychosocial Aspects of Terminal Care*, pp. 47–56, Columbia University Press, New York, 1972.
4. Babbie, E. R. *Science and Morality in Medicine: A Survey of Medical Educators*, pp. 157–170, University of California Press, Berkeley, 1970.
5. Travis, T. A., Noyes, R., and Brightwell, D. R. The attitudes of physicians toward prolonging life. *Int. J. Psychiatr. Med.*, 5:17–26 (1974).
6. Biorck, G. Thoughts on life and death. *Perspect. Biol. Med.*, 11:527–543 (1968).
7. Levisohn, A. A. Voluntary mercy deaths. Sociolegal aspects of euthanasia, *J. Forensic Med.*, 8:57–79 (1961).
8. Editorial: Euthanasia is justified (in the opinion of 31% of U.S. doctors) when..., *New Med. Materia*, pp. 31–40, 1969.
9. Platt, Lord. Euthanasia. Meeting October 13, 1969. *Proc. R. Soc. Med.*, 63: 659–661 (1970).
10. Williams, R. H. Number, types and duration of human lives. *Northwest Med.*, 69:493–496 (1970).
10a. Williams, R. H. Qualitative and quantitative problems in generation. *Northwest Med.*, 69:497–502 (1970).
11. Brown, N. K., et al. How do nurses feel about euthanasia and abortion? *Am. J. Nurs.*, 71:1413–1416 (1971).
13. Laws, E. H., et al. Views on euthanasia. *J. Med. Educ.* 46:540–542 (1971).
14. Miller, M. Decision-making: The death process of the ill aged. *Geriatrics* 26:105–116 (1971).
15. Gallup Poll. Euthanasia poll, news in the world of medicine. *Reader's Digest*, p. 113, February, 1974.

16. Scott, J. T. Physicians' attitude survey: Doctors and dying: Is euthanasia now becoming accepted? *Med. Opinion,* 3:31–34 (1974).
17. Lagone, J. M. Surgeons and the dying patient. *Abdom. Surg.,* 16:283–286 (1974).
18. Noyes, R., Jr., and Travis, T. The care of terminal patients: A statewide survey. *J. Iowa Med. Soc.,* 63:527–530 (1973).

Cancer: The Behavioral Dimensions, edited by J. W. Cullen, B. H. Fox, and R. N. Isom. Raven Press, New York © 1976.

Coping Behavior and Suicide in Cancer

Avery D. Weisman

Harvard Medical School, and Massachusetts General Hospital, Boston, Massachusetts 02114

There is something vaguely disquieting about appearing near the end of a program. Time itself has almost run out. The resemblance to a fatal outcome is too close, as if only consideration of death remains. But this is not my purpose.

Like war, cancer is a kind of ultimate disorder that few people want, but no one is fully capable of preventing. Declarations testifying to its undesirability are deplorably ineffectual. Some of this may be due to man's violence and self-destructiveness, a kind of social suicide. But cancer is like war in another respect, too. Fatal outcomes are still more frequent than solutions or cures, despite our most valiant efforts. Until mankind finds a final biological solution to cancer, every rational means to identify the illness, contain its spread, and alleviate distress will be required.

The diagnosis of cancer may itself terrorize people, evoking the image of invalidism, incapacity, and death, regardless of the actual prognosis and available treatment. Nevertheless, without minimizing the gains and dedication of people engaged in efforts to control cancer, death is common, and the catastrophic effects on people cannot be adequately measured by statistics alone. In a word, cancer is far too serious to be left to physicians.

How any cancer patient copes or fails to cope with psychosocial problems at different stages of illness will be our concern for many years to come. We should also consider the destructiveness and death rate of suicide in our population. It is now the tenth leading cause of death, rising in incidence as people grow older. Cancer and suicide are, literally, urgent matters of life and death. It is the combination of both with which I am concerned today, because suicide and vulnerability, one aspect of suicide, may offer still another avenue to improve our management of psychosocial problems related to cancer.

Regardless of personal attitudes toward suicide—whether it is an inherent right or an unforgivable offense—it is clear that some cancer patients, facing a grim or uncertain future, will opt to terminate their lives. Self-destruction may be thought of as both an ultimate dissolution and a form of coping with problems. In any event, just as cancer is regarded as. the prototype of a fatal illness, suicide represents the paradigm of social and emotional vulnerability.

INCIDENCE OF SUICIDE IN CANCER

Danto (1) has pointed out how little information we have about the actual incidence of suicidal behavior among cancer patients. Isolated reports show a higher frequency of suicides among older males with cancer than in comparable age- and sex-corrected general populations, a finding which is true to a lesser extent for females with cancer. Campbell (2) simply compared the prevalence of cancer with suicide by cross-checking names in public health registries. Although she found only a small number of completed suicides, she excluded patients with highly curable skin cancers, implying that a person with a curable cancer would not commit suicide. Moreover, she listed no examples of suicide by ingestion. Since most suicide attempts are effected by overdoses of medication, it is reasonable to assume that Campbell merely alluded to the incidence of cancer and suicide, without giving a full account of it. Achte and Vauhkonen (3) found that slightly more than one-half of suicides in general and in medical hospitals in Finland in particular suffered from terminal cancer. However, Farberow et al. (4), working with Veterans Administration statistics, discovered that about 25% of general medical and surgical hospital suicides occurred among patients with neoplasms; an overrepresentation by 12% of hospital populations. They found that the tendency to suicide was not associated with any one type of cancer; all cancer patients were vulnerable. Most importantly, suicides took place when patients were outside of the hospitals. The lethal methods were those using firearms, hanging, and jumping—tactics that could hardly be overlooked by medical examiners. Once again, ingestion was not reported as a common method of attempting suicide.

Dorpat et al (5) noted that among older men and women who commit suicide, physical illnesses, including cancer, were common, although the correlation between suicide attempts and cancer was not statistically significant. It is estimated that attempted suicides exceed completed suicides by as many as 15 to 1, but no one is really sure because of discrepancies in reporting, equivocation among suicide attempters, denial of intention after the fact, and failure to recognize life-threatening behavior.

LETHALITY AND VULNERABILITY

My thesis is not that suicide and suicide attempts may be more frequent than is reported or diagnosed, but that lethality is simply an extreme example of how vulnerable many cancer patients are. Suicide attempts are but tragic symptoms of the psychosocial distress that some cancer patients are forced to endure. Abrams (6) has eloquently described many crises with which cancer patients contend and has shown how effective psychosocial interventions might be for patients with distressing emotional plights.

Lethality may be defined as the disposition to take one's own life, although experts are divided about the range of lethal behavior (7). As yet, there is no successful instrument to predict suicide (8), nor even agreement on why suicide occurs (9). We can, however, divide lethal behavior into: (a) overt attempts, (b) thoughts, threats, and impulses, i.e., suicidal ideation, (c) life-threatening behavior, in which a person jeopardizes physical survival through a potentially destructive act, and (d) vulnerability, a set of distressingly ominous traits and symptoms frequently found among people regarded as suicidal risks.

It is the diagnosis and management of *vulnerability,* even in the absence of the other three forms of lethal behavior, that challenges cancer professionals. Obviously, profound dejection, inability to establish lasting relationships, intense and extended anxiety, poorly controlled frustration and anger, failures in coping with previous problems, destructive methods of neutralizing tension, and regressive interactions with reality are often sufficient to establish a suicide alert (10). From many reports concerning high suicide risks, we, at Project Omega, have selected 13 traits, called "vulnerability variables" (Table 1), that can readily be recognized, rated, and compared with their opposites. Intermediate states, not listed in Table 1, can also be scored and coded for computer analysis.

COPING AND VULNERABILITY

Identifying the cancer patient with high vulnerability is not primarily intended as a means of finding the suicidal risk. It also helps to discover ways in which coping behavior is impaired, so that psychosocial interventions can be initiated for those people most in need. However, there are patients who may be judged emotionally unstable or vulnerable by most clinical criteria, and who still accept the diagnosis of cancer, follow through with treatment, and do not undergo psychosocial relapse.

Coping is a problem-solving process which, if effective, brings relief, reward, quiescence, and equilibrium. As is true of motivated behavior in general, coping consists of active measures to master and aversive efforts to avoid or minimize specific threats. If a person cannot cope effectively, then varying degrees of turmoil, anguish, frustration, despair, and suffering result. The common aim, therefore, of all coping strategies is to contain a *recognized problem.* Unless a patient identifies a threatening problem and can inform us about how he or she managed the ensuing conflict, no clinician can be sure that what is observed constitutes coping behavior. In other words, we must first focus on a specific problem, then find out what a patient is now doing or has done about it. Lacking

TABLE 1. *Vulnerability variables*

Hopelessness	Worthlessness/self-rebuke
Turmoil	Isolation/abandonment
Frustration	Denial/avoidance
Despondence/depression	Truculence/bitterness
Helplessness/powerlessness	Repudiation of others
Anxiety/fearfulness	Closed time perspective
Exhaustion/apathy	

this kind of information, the most that a clinician can do is to observe behavior, which may be defensive, and to discriminate traits and symptoms of vulnerability.

The literature of coping and adaptation is so enormous that I may be forgiven for not attempting even a capsule summary. Because there are already several excellent summaries on the subject (11), my very disinclination is an illustration of coping, which might be called "Avoidance by rationalization." If I had more time and space available, I could, however, cope with this problem by "selecting relevant and important research and sharing information" with you. Please note that the "-ing" in coping signifies that coping is an on-going process, not a fixed set of responses.

Every individual, whether a patient or not, has distinctive personality characteristics that help to determine coping behavior. Information processing, judgments about priorities among problems, perceptions of values and necessities, and effective readjustments for differences between old and new problems are probably inherent in every instance of coping behavior. However, in everyday coping, there is a melange of selection and suppression, confrontation and avoidance, acceptance and denial, recognition and redefinition that constitute an exceedingly complex situation for clinicians and clinical investigators.

The reference to the intricacies of coping behavior should not be construed as recommending surrender. After all, regardless of our conceptual difficulties, we do manage to cope with a host of problems every day, despite oscillation between effective resolution and significant vulnerability. It is both possible and practical to cope by "compromising with complexity" and settling upon observations of what patients commonly do or fail to do in the course of dealing with problems relating to cancer. Table 2 shows 15 different coping strategies that are neither too general for practical application nor too specific for cross-patient comparison. Although these strategies can and do overlap to some extent, they are distinctive enough to be useful.

TABLE 2. *Common coping strategies*

1.	Seek more information
2.	Talk with others to relieve distress
3.	Laugh it off
4.	Don't worry, try to forget
5.	Put mind on other things
6.	Positive constructive action based on present understanding
7.	Accept, but rise above it; find something favorable
8.	Stoic acceptance of the inevitable
9.	Do something, anything, however reckless, impractical, etc.
10.	Do what worked in other situations
11.	Reduce tension by drinking, drugs, etc.
12.	Get away by yourself
13.	Blame someone or something for your condition
14.	Seek direction and do what you're told
15.	Blame yourself, atone, sacrifice

CASES OF CANCER AND SUICIDE

Although cancer and suicide do occur together, individual case studies are rarely reported in depth. Project Omega, named after the Greek letter symbolizing the end of life, has studied hospitalized patients who are preterminal, suicidal in the recent past, or both. Initially, our emphasis was on developing the "psychological autopsy" for better understanding of these patients. Some of our subjects in the preterminal phase were, of course, cancer patients. How they coped with incipient death was useful in reconstructing the psychosocial context of dying (12).

Our current aims emerged from understanding that death styles are determined by life styles. Even though terminal cancer is only one possible outcome of the chronic illness called cancer, our belief is that measurable and practical data can be found comparing patients with recently diagnosed cancer with more advanced cancer patients according to their coping strategies and vulnerability to various concerns.

During the first phase of our work, about seven patients were admitted with the combination of cancer and a recent suicide attempt. Each patient was examined using clinical interviews, psychological testing, social case work assessment, and psychological autopsy. It is not necessary for death to occur to conduct a psychological autopsy. Several other patients were simply seen in consultation or accidentally encountered during other work.

One man with terminal Hodgkin's disease jumped or fell from a hospital window without giving any previous warning. The other six patients attempted suicide (one woman threatened another attempt while hospitalized) before admission. Three suicidal patients were in an early or controlled stage of cancer: a 67-year-old man with a recent resection for annular carcinoma of the colon, a 50-year-old woman with a radical mastectomy who overdosed with sleeping medicine as she neared completion of radiation therapy, and a 31-year-old woman with long-standing psychiatric problems, including preoccupation with suicide, who made a low-lethality attempt with sedatives. Her Hodgkin's disease was inactive and not being treated at the time.

The remaining three patients were preterminal. A 37-year-old woman with brain and lung metastases was told she needed total brain radiation. Six days later, suffering both confusion and anxiety, as well as pain, she swallowed a small amount of meperidine (Demerol®) and phenobarbital. A 75-year-old man with severe pain and advanced pancreatic carcinoma tried ineffectively to hang himself, and several days later, to drown himself, before being hospitalized. A 34-year-old woman with an extensive gastric cancer made two attempts with alcohol and medication, and a third attempt by jumping ineffectively in front of an oncoming automobile.

Detailed analyses of these and other patients who had attempted suicide only in the distant past are beyond the scope of this presentation. However, leaving aside the question of the man who was found dead below a hospital window, only two of these patients explicitly wanted to die. Even in these patients, as well as in others whom psychiatrists thought to be depressed, the dejection was not clearly unadulterated: rage, feelings of worthlessness, confusion, apathy, and painful isolation were easily recognized. Two patients disclosed life-threatening behavior. Five patients showed prominent themes of denial, death, loneliness, and anger in the Thematic Apperception Test (TAT), regardless of what they may have said during psychiatric or case work interviews. Only one patient had previously attempted suicide; four patients were very sick at the time of their attempts, despite the overall prognoses in their cases. According to an *ex post facto* vulnerability rating, done after the psychological autopsy, six patients were in the high to high moderate range. Only one patient was considered low moderate, and this patient showed much denial.

What can be said about these cancer patients who attempted suicide? The series was, of course, too small for far-reaching conclusions. Moreover, other patients who had contemplated suicide in the past did not attempt it, even in the depths of terminality. Despite their physical incapacity, there was no obvious connection between the diagnosis of cancer and the attempt at suicide, except through the intervening variables of family problems, unresolved anger, abuse of alcohol (three cases), confusion, and pain. We noted the prevalence on the TAT of denial, depression, loneliness, and anger. Previous psychiatric symptoms were not significantly correlated with higher vulnerability in these patients, but denial in an extreme degree seemed to be more typical of suicidal patients than were symptoms of earlier depression. A female patient who was not in this series reported that when she first discovered that her symptoms, including pain, were due to kidney cancer she tried to kill herself by ingesting a handful of sleeping medicine, but had fallen asleep after being given an injection of a narcotic. When she awakened the following morning, the sleeping medicine was still clutched in her hand. Was this suicide "attempt" or suicide "intent" only?

CANCER AND VULNERABILITY

Investigation of highly distressed suicidal or cancer patients who have, at the most, only fleetingly considered suicide has led us to think of lethality as subordinate to the general concept of vulnerability, not the reverse as we thought originally. In other words, suicide is an aberrant coping strategy that is used only by a very small number of cancer patients, whereas high vulnerability cancer patients may be not at all suicidal in thought or action. Therefore, our present focus is on how readily the vulnerable patient can be recognized so that appropriate psychosocial interventions, not suicide alerts, can be instituted.

Worden et al. (13) developed regression equations that permit comparison of observed with expected survival times for cancer deaths, when corrected for age, sex, site, staging, and treatment. These equations can be used in measuring survival quotients alone, and survival quotients used for appraising the effect of psychosocial factors on the length or quality of the terminal stage of life. Weisman and Worden (14) found, for example, that terminal patients who kept or developed cooperative and responsive relationships toward the end of life tended not only to survive longer, but also to have better deaths, using the criteria for the appropriate death (15). In contrast, patients showing apathy, depression, death wishes, and long-standing mutually destructive relationships over the years survived for shorter periods than expected.

The factor of denial is difficult to assess in isolation, apart from other considerations. Most cancer patients are aware of their diagnoses, especially in the terminal phase, whether or not they have been expressly informed earlier. Those few militant and unyielding deniers in the preterminal period also had long-standing fears of doctors, and came to the hospital at advanced stages of illness. They were antagonistic or paradoxically lighthearted in talking about their sickness. Several expressed only the fear of protracted pain, as, indeed, it is difficult for anyone not to do.

Let us imagine your feelings if, tomorrow, you were found to have any form of malignancy, ranging from the most trivial epithelioma to the gravest lesion. What would your immediate response be? If the known statistics were favorable and the treatment said to be successful in a rather large percentage of cases, would this be sufficient reassurance, or might there be a thought that, just possibly, you were the exception?

In an effort to explore the existential plight of patients recently given the diagnosis of cancer, at five different sites (cancer of the lung, breast, colon, Hodgkin's disease, and malignant melanoma), Worden and Weisman found that vulnerability scores were moderately high in practically every new patient, but that most managed to adapt quite well during the first 3 months. Moreover, existential concerns were sources of more trouble than even worries about health complaints (local, pain, systemic) except among men with severe symptoms relating to cancer of the lung. Women with breast cancer were vulnerable in proportion to the treatments required. On the surface, therefore, the treatment given corresponds to the prognosis because the more serious the prognosis in certain breast cancers, the more intensive is the treatment. When a woman is considered "inoperable," she gets chemotherapy and radiation, both of which are apt to produce longer lasting side effects than surgery alone. Nevertheless, the phrase, "on the surface," must be used because existential concerns can be more intense among patients in whom the likelihood of survival is reduced.

About 10% of patients with newly diagnosed cancer in our series of consecutive admissions report having been desperate enough in the past to have thought that life wasn't worth living and that suicide was a possibility, even before the diagnosis of cancer. We must insert a caveat, however, that in the first phase after cancer diagnosis, the therapeutic atmosphere is usually optimistic and the treatment conditions are the most favorable. Patients who considered themselves habitual pessimists showed more vulnerability traits when they became cancer patients. The fate of vulnerability when recurrences, relapses, or refractory responses occur later is a problem still to be systematically studied.

Using multivariate analyses of vulnerability scores for 189 patients with newly diagnosed cancer followed for 3 to 4 months after the diagnosis, initial treatment, and primary assessment of personal and psychosocial factors, it was found that the

13 variables of vulnerability clustered into 4 factors covered by the terms, *denial, annihilation, alienation,* and *destructive dysphoria.* Details of this analysis will be published separately. However, the coping strategies used by patients with the highest vulnerability scores tended to be those of repudiation, avoidance, suppression, defiance, or just plain apathy, which itself is a sign of futility and exhaustion. Denial was a common strategy for coping and a form of vulnerability. The suggested explanation is that denial is often useful for brief periods provided that it does not contradict reality too flagrantly. On the other hand, patients who initially denied the seriousness of the diagnosis, if, indeed, they accepted it at all, were also those who had higher alienation scores, which meant repudiation by and of others, as well as painful isolation.

DISCUSSION

As is true for the use and abuse of alcohol, vulnerability and coping effectiveness can fall within normal limits or be the forerunner of cumulative incapacity. For example, who among us has never felt depressed, angry, alienated, or dysphoric? Denial is not only useful at times, but also probably necessary to muster other strategies and resources for taking positive actions. We need no longer debate, however, whether denial should or should not be fostered in every patient for the duration of illness. It is a strongly independent vulnerability factor even in the first few months of cancer.

An informed patient is a better patient. One who understands uncertainty and can share concern, selecting, and readjusting is better able to cope effectively than someone who simply avoids, distracts, and discharges the tension built up by the facts and complications of illness and related psychosocial problems.

No one has an unlimited repertoire of coping strategies for all occasions. Obviously, some people are more vulnerable and less resourceful than others. No form of coping is ever infallible, nor can it be understood without knowing the problem or context in which it is activated. Nevertheless, there would be no sense whatsoever in instituting psychosocial rehabilitation and in planning behavioral contributions to the continuing care of cancer unless we felt able to fortify some coping strategies and to discourage others.

Patients who have the most trouble coping effectively are often those who feel most powerless, frustrated, painfully isolated, and who lean heavily upon suppression, denial, and avoidance. Other patients who cope poorly are apprehensive about abandonment while, at the same time, repudiating efforts to help. They expect little of themselves, less of the world, and practically nothing of the future.

There is no doubt that successful and prompt cancer treatment is a great tonic for vulnerability. Until the utopian vision of universally available help becomes a reality, our task is to refine methods of recognizing high vulnerability and low capacity to cope. We do have indications that psychosocial factors influence the length of survival, but any conscientious cancer worker believes that length of survival is by no means the only or sufficient aim of management.

The best copers are patients who avoid avoidance, openly confront problems of highest priority, seek out competent help, and use it effectively. If this sounds like a platitude or redundancy, it is only because the effective encouragement of coping strategies requires that we call upon strategies that are likely to be effective. Although we seek support systems that reduce suffering and disability in any chronic illness, somehow it is more imperative to do this for cancer patients.

PRACTICAL APPLICATION

It is easy to take care of patients who need very little care. The most effective physician or other health professional is one who treats patients who are not very sick and who suffer only from self-limited illnesses. The opposite is true for everyone engaged, however distantly, in any aspect of the continuing care of the cancer patient.

Suicide research is not irrelevant to the study of cancer because we must learn to detect signs of vulnerability among cancer patients even if actual suicide attempts are infrequent. And it is just possible that by appropriate intervention attempts that might occur are prevented. Social alienation, self-destructiveness, and demoralization are threats that afflict not only patients, but even cancer workers themselves. Informed collaboration between behavioralists (please do not expect a succinct definition of what rehabilitation, continuing care, and psychosocial professionals do) and oncologists is fully as important as informed consent between physician and patient.

Present aims and future prospects indicate a belief that our purpose is to be a psychosocial counterforce for improving the quality as much as the length of life for cancer patients. Denial, alienation, annihilation, and destructive dysphoria are apt to differ from person to person at different stages of cancer and with various kinds of treatment. For example, when do we decide that any patient should expect only palliation, not cure? Surely, if results from any treatment are problematic, at best, then some patients are receiving only palliative treatment from the outset. Others who have more reason to be optimistic are discouraged by the professionals who decide that treatment of cancer is likely to be futile unless the disease itself can be extirpated with finality.

I recommend an enlightened realization of uncertainty, but one that calls upon every available resource. Practical alleviation includes psychosocial enhancement of coping and reduction of vulnerability. Few terminal patients ask for cure, only for a sense of relief and a feeling that someone cares. We professionals should cope also by meeting defiance and negation with trustful preparation in settling for a little gain and not expecting absolute cure, lest we fall into abandoning the patient who cannot fully cope.

CLOSING THE CIRCLE

Support systems in the field of cancer are necessary both for patients and for health professionals. We cannot overestimate the toll exacted from workers and patients in emotional and psychosocial strain. Some cancer patients will attempt suicide, but not because of cancer. Secondary suffering, a concept partially covered by what we call "vulnerability," is an existential condition that can compromise our best strategies. Outright pessimism may be misguided because to be a cancer patient does not necessarily imply a bleak future. Even a bleak future does not justify capitulation to the inevitable, but only an acceptance that challenges our competence in coping.

There is no doubt but that it is compassion for humanity that has aroused our interest in an autonomous choice concerning death and dying. Sustained efforts to better the lot of cancer patients at every stage of illness, including the preterminal phase, means only that each of us works within finite time and is unable to do all that he might wish. Had we knowledge, skill, and leverage enough to come in at the opportune moment, to be called upon and to implement what is already recognized, it would help map out the vast ignorance still before us.

The Living Will (16) is a gesture toward a humane treatment of patients who are beyond the reach of palliation or at least a return to partial function. It is intended to rebuke and restrain those who would substitute technical triumphs for realistic rehabilitation efforts and psychosocial care. Better trained rehabilitation experts who are grounded in the facts and factors relevant to comprehensive treatment of individuals, not tumors alone, who are prepared and permitted to share in decisions with physicians and patients, will do much to alleviate the fears of cancer patients. The Living Will is not a fully legal document. But the wide interest shown by the lay public in its objectives implies that because of the inherent vulnerability that many people feel with respect to cancer and other serious illnesses, they are willing to sign a lethal document or what amounts to a suicide note.

Our best coping strategy for dealing with all forms of cancer is not denial, surrender, or grandiose statements. Rather it is a realistic appreciation of psychosocial as well as physical problems in cancer. Succeeding generations will confront, redefine, and negotiate with available strategies. In this way, we come nearer to closing the circle on cancer.

SUMMARY

1. Suicide is a small but statistically significant strategy for coping with cancer. As is true of many suicidal data, it is underreported and underinvestigated.

2. Aside from actual suicide attempts, there are other forms of lethality shown in thoughts, impulses, life-threatening behavior and in emotional and psychosocial signs known as vulnerability.

3. From the viewpoint of cancer management, it is more important to recognize signs of vulnerability than of lethality. Vulnerability can be understood as a combination of traits or as a product of four factors: denial, annihilation, alienation, and destructive dysphoria.

4. Cancer patients who are measurably more vulnerable, and not necessarily suicidal, tend to use strategies of avoidance and repudiation, withdrawing into

painful isolation and fearing destruction from some external source. In contrast, patients who cope more effectively with cancer are found to accept the diagnosis, seek more information, share concern with significant others, actively voice their needs, and to redefine and rise above the threats they find in their plight.

5. Until the final biological solution to cancer is found, behavioral factors deserve careful investigation and intelligent application. The distress of being a cancer patient is not necessarily a catastrophe. Failure to cope with psychosocial problems in cancer may, however, seriously reduce the survival time and value of treatment.

6. Comprehension of psychosocial factors in suicide as well as the terminal stages of cancer may help clarify and improve strategies for coping with cancer at any stage.

REFERENCES

1. Danto, B. The cancer patient and suicide. *J. Thanatol.*, 2:596–600 (1972).
2. Campbell, P. Suicide among cancer patients. *Conn. Health Bull.*, 80:207–212 (1966).
3. Achte, K., and Vauhkonen, M. Suicides committed in general hospitals. Psychiatria Fennica (Finnish Psychiatry). In *Yearbook of the Psychiatric Clinic*, pp. 221–228, Helsinki, 1971.
4. Farberow, N., Ganzler, S., Cutter, F., and Renolds, D. An eight-year survey of hospital suicides. *Life-Threatening Behavior*, 1:184–202 (1971).
5. Dorpat, T., Anderson, W., and Ripley, H. The relationship of physical illness to suicide. In Resnik, H. (ed.): *Suicide Behaviors*, pp. 209–219, Little Brown, Boston, 1968.
6. Abrams, R. *Not Alone with Cancer*, Charles C. Thomas Co., Springfield, Ill., 1974.
7. Shneidman, E. *Deaths of Man*, Quadrangle/New York Times Book Co., New York, 1973.
8. Beck, A., Resnik, H., and Lettieri, D. (eds.): *The Prediction of Suicide*, Charles Press Publishers, Bowie, Md., 1974.
9. Lester, D. *Why People Kill Themselves: A Summary of Research Findings*, Charles C Thomas, Springfield, Ill., 1972.
10. Schuyler, D. *The Depressive Spectrum*, Jason Aronson, New York, 1974.
11. Coelho, G., Hamburg, D., and Adams, J. (eds.): *Coping and Adaptation*, Basic Books, New York, 1974.
12. Weisman, A. *The Realization of Death: A Guide for the Psychological Autopsy*, Jason Aronson, New York, 1974.
13. Worden, J., Johnston, L., and Harrison, R. Survival quotient method for investigating psychosocial aspects of cancer survival. *Psychol. Rep.*, 35:719–726 (1974).
14. Weisman, A., and Worden, J. *Psychosocial Analysis of Cancer Deaths*, Omega *(in press)*.
15. Weisman, A. *On Dying and Denying: A Psychiatric Study of Terminality*, Behavioral Publications, New York, 1972.
16. Mannes, M. *Last Rights*, William Morrow & Co., New York, 1974.

Cancer: The Behavioral Dimensions, edited by J. W. Cullen,
B. H. Fox, and R. N. Isom. Raven Press, New York © 1976.

Respondent

Ruth D. Abrams

*Patient and Family Counselor Consultant,
Chestnut Hill, Massachusetts 02167*

I share Dr. Weisman's uneasiness in appearing at the Omega stage of this conference. Keeping this in mind, I shall not overburden you with all my interpretations but instead elaborate on some significant statements made by Drs. Weisman and Brown.

I shall first focus on remarks of Dr. Weisman. He suggests, and I strongly agree with him, that crisis intervention should be available to these patients. The form it takes depends, as he so well states, on the positive and negative qualities that the individual embodies. Obviously, most of the people that could and should be helpful in the area of intervention do not possess the qualifications and capacities of Dr. Weisman. We appreciate, however, the distillation of his thoughts and his efforts to broaden the quality and the extent of patient care.

I am pleased that denial on the part of the patient for shorter or longer periods of time is endorsed by him, as long as it is not continued indefinitely or, as I would add, to the detriment of the patient's own self-image. The patient even without disease is in such a complex situation that to superimpose a positive threat increases the necessity for broad spectrum care conjoined to more specific areas of medical care. In other words, Dr. Weisman succinctly expresses this thought when he says that "cancer is far too serious to be left to physicians."

Discussion

M. Krant: I would like to ask whether it would be possible for us to take a dialectical look at three different values. I wonder, in fact, how we can integrate them to make sense out of some of the propositions that human beings face.

Let me suggest that these three values are operational or functional for us. One value is that of the sanctity of life—that life is pure, good, and must be maintained. The second value, I think, is self-control, and by this I mean being in control of your own life. Nobody should take this control away from you. The third value, I think, is an ethic that is around a great deal: One should not suffer. This ethic was manifest in the traditional Westerns in which if a horse broke its leg, it was mandatory that his owner take a gun out and shoot him. Similarly, if a man found a friend of his dying from torture at the hands of hostile Indians, he felt obliged to shoot his friend and put him out of his misery.

What is suffering, and how do we relieve it? Does a human being have control over relieving it in his own way? The other point, of course, is can he relieve suffering in his own way if this way conflicts with the sanctity-of-life principle? In not confronting the value structures and trying to reexamine them, we often take a passive position. We prolong agony mercilessly. We make people stay alive in ways that are unacceptable to them by taking the passive position that we'll do nothing more. On the other hand, we hesitate to do something positive because this seems to violate the sanctity-of-life principle. I think we need much more discussion of the three values I have mentioned here to understand what our position really should be. This discussion should take place at all levels of society.

Hayes: I am afraid I fail to share Dr. Krant's optimism or high expectations of humanity, but I think that perhaps it might be more realistic for society to approach this particular set of problems on a basis that everybody in society understands. There are only a few levels on which this can be done, one of which happens to be the financial level. I can think of an example from our own experiences to illustrate my point. In a section of North Carolina we supplied a series of mobile units with personnel and equipment to handle coronary cases to resuscitate people before they got to the hospital. We found that previously they were dying on their way to the hospital. On cost-accounting this procedure, we found that every resuscitation (i.e., somebody who survived 6 months after the procedure was done) cost $19,000. We submitted a proposition to the voters in the form of a bond issue asking if they were willing to pay for this kind of an effort to maintain life. The answer was an overwhelming NO; none of the voters had any difficulty in understanding the question when it was put to them in monetary terms. I think if you approached people in Dr. Krant's way, with which I certainly agree, many of them would simply not invest enough of themselves in the discussion to arrive at any answer.

Brown: I like the three values Dr. Krant mentioned. I was wondering if I could add one more—in the form of a question: what would be the greatest good for the greatest number? In addition, I would like to amplify a little on the sanctity-of-life. It seems to me that the second two values that you gave—self-control and the ethic that one should not suffer— both tend to favor negative euthanasia decisions, whereas the sanctity of life principle would tend to oppose them. The only way that I can see of integrating the life-principle with negative euthanasia at this point is through the development of ethometrics, which is a matter of measuring life, how much life there is in an individual and what type of life would have more value than another. When I say the greatest good for the greatest number, I am implying that the dollars we have here are the result of taking resources from one situation and putting them into another.

Holland: Is this a way of measuring the quality of life—survival? Ethometrics? That's a new one. Dr. Weisman.

Weisman: Well, Dr. Krant, the values that you mentioned are only the beginning. I think we should add another one—that one person's values are not necessarily those of another person. To impose our particular values on someone else is a risky business. I love getting into philosophical discussions, and I have also learned to resist them. Let me just cite a recent example. I got a call one Sunday morning from a woman who used to work with us. When she became pregnant, she resigned. She is married to a lawyer. Her father, a banker and an alcoholic, had been brought into Massachusetts General Hospital and was in the intensive-care unit. To complicate matters even more, he had a rare blood type and in a few hours had already gone through 12 units. The father had said specifically to his doctor that he preferred to die drinking rather than to give it up for the sake of a few extra years of life. Nevertheless, with a very able surgical resident in charge of the intensive-care unit, the father was treated for bleeding esophageal varices. The daughter told the surgeon she didn't want her father treated any more and that he should not be in the intensive-care unit. The father had already indicated when he was reasonably well that he didn't want extreme measures taken. The blood ammonia was too high however, at this point; the patient's earlier statement was disregarded. The surgeon quite rightly said that when anyone comes in the door of the hospital, there is a tacit expectation that he is there for treatment. The statistics at Massachusetts General Hospital, regardless of blood ammonia levels or other medical data, is that about 10% of patients with bleeding esophageal varices can be pulled through. The surgical resident had ethical obligations. We had some fun, then, for the next 48 hours; we summoned a hospital lawyer and a director. The father died within 48 hours, but the issue remains. Can we solve it by settling on the kind of values that any of us might advocate for ourselves? If I were terminally or irreversibly ill, I am not sure who should make a decision for me. The Living Will, as you know, has been recommended, but it has no legal significance. I was going to say lethal significance, I meant legal but I also mean lethal—my unconscious as always is a couple of steps ahead of me. You may have full confidence today in what you would like to have done when you are sick. When your life is on the line, the Living Will may become a suicide note. I guess that is what my unconscious meant.

Antonovsky: I was very pleased when Dr. Krant made his comment and when Dr. Weisman pointed out that different people have different values. When Dr. Hayes got up, however, and said that Dr. Krant was optimistic, I was amazed. I thought that Dr. Krant had made a profoundly pessimistic statement. Then I found the answers to why Dr. Hayes thought he was optimistic. Dr. Brown, being particularly American, used the word *integration.* I guess I became non-American during the many years spent away from this country, and the reason I regarded what Dr. Krant said as being profoundly pessimistic is because of the impossibility of reconciling his three values. No matter what an individual decides he will be thought "wrong"; nevertheless he makes that decision and then must go on living with being "wrong."

Krant: I would only reiterate that I was indeed being pessimistic, but not too much so. I think there is another phenomenon, however, that I find over and over again; can you live with a bad decision? This is the sort of thing you were talking about before, Dr. Weisman, namely, if I know what's right, do I have to accept your bad decision? In this case, what you seem to be saying is: "That man is making a bad decision to terminate his life in a certain way, to do what he wants to do, and there is a surgeon saying, but I know what is right, because I do what I do. I cannot tolerate his bad decision."

I think there are others who have criticized psychiatry as being an instrument of bad decision erosion, that is, if the person is at odds with society and doesn't make a decision, somebody in power says, "Yes, I agree with that decision." The psychiatrist frequently becomes the agent of conviction in one way or another and says that the person has no right to hold to that decision. The psychiatrist manipulates him into abiding by our medical decision which is "right", and I would like to raise that as another necessary debate point.

Holland: I think if we have any particular rule by which we operate, it is that we try to help a person find what he wants for himself, perhaps sometimes in a way that leads to criticism of psychiatry for the opposite reasons. I do not think the psychiatrist is as much an "agent of society" as he is someone who tries to help an individual find his own way.

Lowman: I think decision making is even more complicated in children, and I couldn't let this pass by without bringing it up. We don't give them the legal right to make their own decisions until they are 18. I think they have that capability, however, by the time they are 7 or 8 and maybe even younger. It becomes a very difficult task, because we give two people—the mother and father—that right if both of them are legally responsible. They rarely agree, the child may disagree with both of them, and this whole area becomes more and more complicated. In fact, frequently we have the sad experience of recommending that therapy be stopped (we mean that in an active sense), whereas the parents insist that it be continued, even though it is against the child's own wishes. We're really caught in a tremendous legal dilemma to say nothing of the philosophical and ethical one.

Holland: The decision making becomes more and more complex, the more we discuss it and become aware of the various facets.

Fox: I feel a little distressed because I think your response to Dr. Krant reflects the point of view of your own profession, namely, psychiatry. What you said is certainly correct. Your objective is to try to ascertain the intentions of the patient. But I believe that Dr. Krant's point was not restricted to psychiatry, however, and, in fact, it is my impression that the direct opposite obtains for the other disciplines in medicine; namely, that the other doctors do not hold the view that the patient's intention is the most desirable one. Dr. Krant's tenet is entirely correct for some of the subspecialties.

Whyman: As I listen to the discussion, it gets more and more parodoxical in a way. To talk about psychiatry for just a moment, I think both of you may be correct. It depends on the work you are doing, and on your professional background. One of the parodoxes as Dr. Fox just mentioned is that, on the one hand, we in the mental health profession in our desire to help people make their own decisions are willing to involuntarily commit them. On the other hand, the surgeon will say to the patient, "You don't want this operation." Therefore, he doesn't get himself into our predicament.

Brown: I want to talk to Dr. Antonovsky a minute about my "integration." I think you might find that if you went to some of the physicians in Israel who are delivering care that they would have a somewhat similar integrative attitude. I don't see that I can practice medicine myself without disintegrating unless you either "clone" my own germ plasm so that my patients are just like me or send me all the patients that fit my bias. I've got to sleep nights too, and it is hard for me not to take the conflicting values that Dr. Krant mentioned and to try and pull them together in a way that permits me to give care. Maybe this is part of the conflict in this conference that we've talked about.

Unknown: This changes the subject a little but, but Dr. Weisman, I wonder if you have any statistics or information on the people we have heard about recently, relatives who in some way cause the immediate death of the suffering patient. How many people actually do this? Is there any follow-up, and what becomes of these people after they perform these acts?

Weisman: You mean that the relatives actually cause the death of the patient?

Unknown: Yes, we have heard of several situations of this kind recently. For example, there was a case in which a brother shot a suffering brother. I wonder how frequent such cases are. Then, what happens to people after they've committed these acts? Is there any follow-up, any support?

Brown: I don't think there is. In fact, one of my recommendations was that we should try to find out who is in fact making the decision, who is dominating, and who is merely participating in the decision. What are the effects on the people who participated and on those who didn't? Obviously some people are pretty angry because they didn't participate, and that is how we get the editorials in *The New York Times*. But what about those who did take an active part and I assume there must be some. I think from my own experience that there are not, perhaps, in terms of shooting somebody, but in terms of proposing a plan or agreeing with one such as the daughter did in Dr. Weisman's case.

Weisman: I would like to supplement Dr. Brown's comment, and I am sure Ruth Abrams would, too, because you've emphasized an extreme, aberrant example of the suffering that the "significant others" undergo. We referred to the bereavement of the family and there are statistics and information (I don't think the two are necessarily mutually exclusive) about the higher incidence of physical and emotional disorders in bereaved families for the first couple of years after the loss of the "significant other." We haven't really talked about the best way to manage bereavement. Is anticipatory grieving therapeutic? How long should the normal grief response go on? I think shooting your brother is just one form of grieving, but it should remind us that much less flamboyant types of bereavement exist and deserve management.

Goldstein: I don't usually defend physicians, but the surgeons are receiving excessive criticism from everybody, and that distresses me. It seems to me that there is a dual meaning in many things said, "Let's be absolutely honest, let's provide our patients with a lot of data about what we think, what we do, and what we don't do." But the surgeons take abuse because they throw somebody out for not going along with what they want to do. That is a very honest, if blunt, response. Here is what I do, here are my reasons for doing it, if you don't want it find another doctor. I do that, too. I tell the patient to go to someone else if he wishes to remain the way he is. My data tend to confirm that, but my data are self-serving, self-fulfilling too, which is one of the most significant findings in our field. More important, there is a feeling that people make decisions, and that there is a known true self here. I find that a somewhat invisible commodity that has intrigued me for many years, just as religious ideas do. There may be a true self, and people may make a decision at a very young age. I think two of my children were born at age 5; they don't act very young. In any event, people make decisions, and it seems to me that they change their decisions at intervals. Decisions are ambiguous, complex things, and the more complex the issue, the more complex, difficult, and subject to change the decision is. The notion, therefore, that people at any given age make the decision, that we have an understanding of that decision, and that it has its own wisdom and its own sense, seems to me to be a reaffirmation of an invisible process about which we have little data. The notion that psychiatrists are the high priests of conformity to their own decisions or other people's decisions is again an understatement and shows a lack of understanding of the complexity of the decision process. Now, I am not exalting psychiatrists either; I don't do that. What I am suggesting is that people ought to talk to their patients about what they do or plan to do. If psychiatrists are ambivalent or open, or understanding about changing decisions, they ought to declare themselves so. If surgeons feel they do not want to deal with the patient who doesn't listen to them, they ought to say so. Any physician ought to explain his procedures to his patients. To say that he has no biases concerning his patient or his patient's decision has to be either self-distortion or a lie.

Holland: The necessity of open communication on both sides is in a way what you are advocating. I don't think there would be any disagreement with that.

Cullen: Thank you, Dr. Holland, for keeping us on schedule. I have taken a lot of notes after listening to the foregoing erudition. Yet, I am not going to say very much. Everyone knows that government people are bureaucrats, that they really don't have any ideas, that they sit in Washington on a big pile of money and write papers about unimportant things. Actually it's really not that way at all, and I think this conference is a demonstration of the fact that we are truly searching for ideas. We don't have the best solutions, I will admit that. When Gertrude Stein was dying, she mumbled several times, "What's the answer? What's the answer?" and people kept asking her, "Gertrude, what do you mean, 'what's the answer?'" Finally, she said, "What is the question?" And she died, Maybe that is what this is all about—what are the questions? Indeed when we set out to have this conference, our first thought was to ask: what are the questions to which we in Washington must address ourselves?

I have heard some excellent ideas. I have met some exceptional people; and I congratulate you for your critical thinking, your expertise, for the insight, and for all the heuristic, valuable information with which you provided us.

On this note, I'm going to introduce the next three people, who will attack some of these questions. As I said in the very beginning of this conference, I have given them an impossible task. I have asked not just for a summary, but for an integration of what has been said, implied, or created.

Cancer: The Behavioral Dimensions, edited by J. W. Cullen,
B. H. Fox, and R. N. Isom. Raven Press, New York © 1976.

Summary

Inferences and Synthesis of Significant Results

Ruby N. Isom *

JRB Associates, Inc., McLean, Virginia 22101

Dr. Pearson mentioned that the role of the respondent was not defined, but our role was clearly defined. Dr. Cullen said we were to listen to the somewhat disconnected topics and speakers from various fields (these fields all imperfectly balanced and somewhat fragmented) and then select and describe in 15 minutes the salient ideas we thought worth submitting to a second conference of practitioners and behaviorists. The practitioners and behaviorists would then translate these into the cancer control programs to be used by the Division of Cancer Control Rehabilitation (DCCR) and eventually by the whole world of cancer control. I suspected this task would be difficult and then I met with Drs. Leone and Schonfield, and they reassured me that the task was impossible. The data base for that conclusion is very small, however, and the methodology very imperfect in determining that fact. I am, therefore, only one-third certain that it is accurate. I have thrown out the 32 pages of conference material that I worked on last night. I will concentrate instead on the things that seem a little more certain to me, based on my perspective as a community health educator. I'm like Abe Brickner, in that my concern is with the community right now. The mandate from Congress to the DCCR is to rapidly disseminate new and existing knowledge about cancer to the professional and lay community, and that is what I must do as a community educator trying to understand and use these imperfect fields we have been discussing. It seems that the field of behavior change is at least no more uncertain and incomplete than it was when I was in school, and this is reassuring. It hasn't gotten worse, but there are things I thought we needed to know more about, such as delay. I agree with Dr. Hulka that the methodology is inconsistent and imperfect, and I'd like to see it improved, I'd like to see more work done on delay. This is the most important thing we have been discussing. Why are we losing hundreds of thousands of people annually to cancer because of delay? I'd like to find the answer to this, using the right methodology in a consistent fashion. Then I could improve my community program. I like the word *credibility*.

*Present address: Community Resources Development Branch, Division of Cancer Control and Rehabilitation, National Cancer Institute, Bethesda, Maryland 20014.

Trustworthiness and expertness were discussed by Drs. Bohlen and Klonglan and I think health professionals have to face the issue of increasing their credibility. A favorite hymn that I sing regularly concerns changing our behavior. We must all change our behavior so that we can provide a model in the community. If we don't do this, then we shall have to face the fact that our impact as communicators will be reduced accordingly. By the way, don't you think being an expert, as well as being a model, will make you also the communicator for the community? We have to realize that there are very few of us here that could communicate well in certain high-risk neighborhoods. Even the patients we have here that are communicating, could not really talk to all these other patients from troubled areas. High-risk patients are very different from the verbal, educated, and motivated patients that we have seen at this and other conferences. I'd like to know more, therefore, about the credibility issue and how we can reassess ourselves.

We have to be a little cautious in our statements and recognize there are limits to our truth. I am saying this because I am thinking about the breast self-examination (BSE) program and how religiously we are using that program. We must recognize that, for instance, there are limits to the BSE and the people should not be so sure of it that they will then ignore other facts from other parts of the program. Right now, for example, I am doing a survey to try and find a gynecologist who does not regard the seven danger signals as a sign of my old age. The doctors know the information very well and I know it very well, and so far, the last four physicians I have seen have assured me that my condition is nothing more than the result of my advancing years. I have mimeographed chapters from cancer medicine and distributed them to these same doctors because even though I might have a problem, they would not know it. I don't think I have a problem, but this issue has become a challenge to me.

Another topic discussed here is not one of my favorite subjects; it is something called "school health education." I dislike it because I have spent a number of years trying to get school health education into local schools. As was pointed out here, it is expensive, it is time consuming, and the teachers don't particularly like it. If you recall what health education was like in your school, you probably remember that you didn't like it either. The school system, including the medical school system, is so crowded with knowledge, we have to do something to make room for school health education. I think we should be talking about pilot programs, to evaluate it and its cost effectiveness. We should try it, and if it works, let's change our present system and see if we can demonstrate the value of this kind of education to our school children.

I enjoyed the presentation on diffusion theory, although I realize it is offensive to a group of professionals to use any education methodology except the lecture, which is the least effective method. It is all right to go out into the community and use the flannel boards and audiovisuals, but it is terrible to use these with professionals because they might get the idea that that is an exciting way to impart information. What I like about diffusion theory is the possibility of applying it in our conference and cancer centers. I'd like to see us use it, test it, and evaluate it to see if we really can have an outreach program. You will note that we are using the term *outreach,* and I suspect that many people don't know what this means.

One useful comment that I heard was that we should be more precise in using words such as information, education, awareness, and behavior change. I am tired of hearing health education called a failure, when actually it is an information program and it may yet succeed at that. We must base our cancer education programs on objectives. I like the handout we got from Dr. Antonovsky, and I think it will be very useful, but I think the objectives also have to be realistic, functional, and measurable. They have to relate to the goals and objectives of cancer control programs—not to some aim that I have as a health educator or to some purpose Dr. Leone has in his hospital work, but to the objectives of the overall program. These objectives have to fit together, and if the aim is more information, let's acquire it. Let's not apologize because our objective is to tell a woman where the Pap clinic is. Let's succeed at that because to increase her awareness is to perform a very useful service. If the objective, on the other hand, is behavioral change, let's state the aim that way and evaluate it accordingly. We should choose the methods most likely to achieve our goals.

We haven't talked much about methods here. Someone did say to leave education to the educators. We tend to do that. If we were more active, our methodology in this respect would probably be a great deal better. What I got out of this conference superficially are things I already knew but of which I needed reminding. Because it is impossible to do what I am supposed to do, I thought I would have a little fun with word association. I selected the term *social pressure* and I immediately thought of *community organization.* I hope this means that we are going to really do something about the system and do some organizing of the community.

As I continued my association game, I remembered that they talked about the live demonstration of the BSE on television and I thought of Mrs. Ford. I remembered that the surgery she had was developed in 1897. They talked about the American Cancer Society's use of recovered patients and I remember the last page of the fact book in which they list all the people who have died from cancer. I then thought about someone who said it may be more effective to put the message in ongoing television shows, and I wished the person had said it "should be" or "is not," rather than it "may be." Then I thought of Dr. Mark Goldstein and Dr. Richard Evans. These two names seem to belong together and I couldn't decide which was more significant. One of these men keeps defending behavior modification and the other one seems to be trying not to attack it. Theirs was a good program. Someone mentioned that we have no data to show that health education is cost effective, and I thought of social casework, public health nursing and psychiatry.

Louis Leone

Rhode Island Hospital, Providence, Rhode Island 02902

I present my thoughts on the conference from the viewpoint of a clinician in oncology. I have a rather simplistic approach to this matter. As the conference begin, all of us had certain concepts of what we call cancer, particularly its medical and biological significance, and as the conference ends, this aspect of cancer remains the same in our minds. It has changed considerably for me, however, and probably for many others here, in that now it has become something that causes a life-changing occurrence in patients and a psychosocial change of magnitude. We are not really dealing with a simple cell phenomenon, but something that affects many lives, both within the patient population and within the population as a whole. We determined this in the early part of the conference. Its affect on physicians was clearly defined: "cancer" as a biological entity affects physicians in one way but, as we have seen today, the connotations of the word *cancer* affect behavior of physicians in still another way. The chapter writers and respondents accepted the proposition that cancer affects all of us in certain ways. Some of them described this affect on behavior, some of them attempted to produce evidence of it, others attacked this evidence. In general, the discussions on the first day suggested that we didn't have a data base, and we had some conflicts. As a final gesture to the conference I don't think that one should start attacking the attackers of those attacked. However, the first morning sounded more like a biological scientific meeting. People were simply attacking each others' data and the respondents seemed to be saying that there was no real data anyway and that everyone should start all over again. It occurred to me as the meeting progressed that it doesn't matter very much whether we have the kind of data or theoretical propositions being discussed. This is a recurrent theme in discussions of cancer that I think is very important from the standpoint of the clinical group. When I talk about clinicians, I am not talking about physicians alone. Much of the progress in cancer has been based on empiricism, and there is nothing in the world the matter with accepting a great deal of what has been said as more or less self-evident. Delay does occur. There is evidence, it is self-evident almost. The patient or the individual who refuses to go into prevention or screening systems does not want to be involved in this for some reason; that is a fact. The remarkable psychological and social traumas that are associated with cancer in the individual affect treatment, rehabilitation programs, continuing care, and follow-up planning. If we could have a data base that was totally reliable, we probably would be told to try and identify the problems, subject these to the usual scientific approach, and then determine the etiology and pathogenesis. Then, almost before these data reach the journals, therapists would propose remedies for the problems consistent with the data presented, and sooner or later a cure would result. In medicine there are many examples of this. This is not true in cancer; there is no rational treatment for cancer. I cannot really see a great conflict. I think this simplistic approach may be offensive to some of you, but there are many examples in cancer management and ideas pertaining to cancer that are purely empiric. The most exciting one, that all of us understand, is the effect of an empiric approach on acute lymphoblastic leukemia in children. There is no doubt that the patient with acute lymphoblastic leukemia statistically has a better prognosis for survival, and good wholesome survival, than the patient with premetastatic lymph nodes in the axilla after a radical mastectomy. This is a fact. Whether it will be borne out as leukemia treatment evolves, we are not yet certain.

We do have some material, then, with which we can work. I think delay factors in high-risk populations do exist. The impact of the system itself, the care system, on behavior in physicians, patients, and other personnel is important. Most of the emphasis has been on physicians, but I imagine that nurses, clinical psychologists, and social service people could put themselves in the physician's place. He is attacked heartily because he is insensitive, he's cynical, and he doesn't communicate. I think those are facts; I think we've observed them.

Concerning the matter of communication, I react in a somewhat subjective or crusader-like fashion to the effect of the mass media. I think the American Cancer Society has a crusader-like method of communicating; it is not totally successful. On the other hand, I sense the approach to the public through communication channels is so empiric that we have essentially no data base. Some of the interpretations, however, are very suggestive. The Pap smear was advertised early in the 1940s through this kind of informational immersion, and we now see much less advanced carcinoma of the cervix. Maybe a fuller analysis of how this came to pass would give us more confidence in this type of approach. There are more sophisticated presentations. Dr. Mendelsohn and others tried to explain how we can theorize and how we can make models; this is certainly a path that we should follow. To the crusader, the approach of Drs. Klonglan and Bohlen is very attractive. I am not able to evaluate its usefulness, as was recommended, or to select specific groups from the population, identify their needs, and approach them. These are bases for clinical investigation through cancer control programs.

Throughout the conference the matter of coping with cancer was presented very colorfully at times and concentrated on the physician's role. At one point, I think I concluded from the discussions that the physician probably should no longer bear the whole burden of communication with the patient and, at this same point, the team concept of coping was introduced. The systems that have been presented as clinical programs usually apply to an extremely small segment of the population of cancer patients. They are good models and we hope that they will receive support through cancer control programs. Many patients are taken care of, throughout most of their illness, by doctors still practicing medicine on their own. The possibility that physicians will respond favorably to this group concept really seems remote, but this approach should be investigated. I noticed that examination of the physician's behavior in an experimental setting was not described in any great detail at this meeting. I think Dr. Hayes mentioned some studies that probably included some physician attitudes and performance. But the actual objective interviewing, questioning, and the filling out of a planned protocol on physician behavior and patient concepts of physician behavior, have not been done, and it may be that such a study would help us in altering the attitudes of physicians. Remember, the physician still uses the term "my patient." In the team concept presented, the ultimate word was that of the physician. If there is a matter pertaining to chemotherapy, only the physician can give the answer. He leads the team and therefore he gives the answer. He maintains his image of a leader with his patient. I am not criticizing that, I am just saying that is the situation. Clinical investigation into these matters may lead us to a better understanding of what makes the physician and his colleagues function in their characteristic way.

The plight of the terminal patient also absorbs my attention. I don't like that term *terminal* and I am sure this is one of my defenses. We use the word *preterminal* and this certainly doesn't change the situation any, but *terminal* still connotes to most people a decision made either passively or indifferently that the patient will indeed die. The demonstration today helps show us that this decision can be a positive act reflective of real understanding and direction. The patient's own coping with this matter from the time one considers him irreversibly ill is still a very difficult area. I think physicians tend to reject the patient at this moment more than at any other time in the illness. Investigation into this area is important for the sake of helping the whole team cope with the patient's needs before it has been decided that he should have either passive or active euthanasia or before the patient himself makes a decision. Sometimes the patient maintains this irreversibly ill status for 6 months before the decision of death is accepted by physician, family, or patient. My overall reaction then is that we need some investigative approach, but this should be undertaken with a real aggregation of the research elements in the psychological area, and in those of the clinical people. I don't think we need be concerned that this will produce a dichotomy. I think in cancer, of all the areas of medicine, the integrated or interrelated independent activity of pertinent medical and scientific groups has resulted in tremendous advance. I cite the chemotherapy area again. The vision of people like Rhodes, Burchena, and Karnoffsky, who directed and fostered the concept of almost forced integration of their interests with those of the basic science people, resulted in a concept that persists today in treatment areas. I think the next discussion between the groups represented here should highlight their beginnings and build on them with examinations of the material that I believe many of you feel is highly empiric, possibly not without a solid scientific base, but material which nevertheless has great pertinence to survival, to cure, and to worthwhile and high-quality survival in patients with cancer.

William N. Schoenfeld

Queens College, Flushing, New York 11367

My fellow discussants and others on this program have said that they wished they had more time to speak; as for myself, I wish I had less!

On the hotel elevator, a young man carrying a baby and accompanied by the child's mother looked at me and asked, "You are going to be summarizing the sessions?" "Well," I replied, "I don't have much to say." "I am sure it will be interesting," he said. "I am particularly interested in what you have to say about the outcropping of Indiana limestone up in the panhandle.'' My eyes must have rolled a bit, because he looked startled, and asked, "Aren't you in the Texas Agricultural Limestone Convention?'' "No, I am not,'' I answered with some relief, "but I don't mind summarizing for you, if you wait until after 2:00 tomorrow when I will have had a bit of practice.''

As my friends have said, summarizing a meeting like this is really an impossible task. Everyone here has been experiencing the same kind of self-examination that the physicians and patients who have spoken have described in connection with cancer control, detection, and treatment. They have reported their reactions, both personal and professional, to a wide range of related situations. Now I must tell you about my reactions to those reactions, and to this conference generally. When I leave here, I will be going back to an environment in which my students and I spend some of our time tearing into one another's intellecutual creations without any quarter, and my first impulse is to do the same here. But in truth that would help no one in this case. So I tried to look at this conference from the vantage point of an outsider assigned to listen to your presentations and to extract that which seemed most meaningful. That task has not been easy. For example, I have been asking myself, "How hard-nosed ought I be?'' In 3 days of talk, there are bound to be questionable statements, such as the one that a statistical test has proved that some observation is "beyond chance expectation,'' when that is just not true and would never be asserted by a responsible statistician.

Such points are proper reservations about particular studies and conclusions, but they are not important to the function of this conference. I have some other reactions that I think may be important. One of them is that many of the researches reported here have involved groups of people distinguished by some criterion, or set of criteria, which are of little or no relevance in dealing with the individual patient. Figures and correlations from a group study do not readily permit predictions about any individual within the group. It has long been recognized that inferences from group data cannot be made about an individual with satisfactory reliability unless those correlations run in the .90s, and, of course, such values are rarely, if ever, achieved.

For example, women who come for a Pap test may be categorized into groups on the basis of race, or age, or whatever. But when a physician in a clinic is confronted by one female, and wonders why *she* hasn't come in for a Pap test before, the physician isn't helped much by observing that she is white, 35 years of age, and that other statistical considerations regarding her criterion group affiliations are such and such. It seems to me that a conference like this should be raising the question, "How do we move realistically from the research level to health application?'' The same problem also arises in behavior research laboratories. Both behavior theorists and laboratory workers today dispute the relative merits of experimental designs which employ groups of subjects as against individual organisms: The problem for them is what can validly be learned from an individual organism, and what can be learned from a group. It is the same problem as that faced by the community health researcher and the clinical worker, except that in laboratory circles the problem is not one of life and death. In medicine, of course, it is just such a problem, and bridging the gap between the group and the individual becomes truly important.

I find also that I have, on occasion, been listening to people who share the same view, but argue about it as if they didn't. I have observed that the same thing can occur in all sciences: People can insist on disagreeing, often rationalizing their supposed differences by using different words for the same things. On the other hand, it seems to me that, in any science, the search for areas of agreement is much more important than an emphasis on areas of difference, whether supposed or real. I do not find it very interesting when one researcher reports his findings, only to have another one arise to declare, "I have contrary findings." I hear, I register, and I decide that I probably have nothing to learn from either one of them. I am looking for persons who agree, and I try to teach my students to do the same. To my mind, in science it is more important to demonstrate that somebody is right, to confirm the work, than it is to show that the person was wrong. It may not be as glamorous, and you may not get the credit for a scoop, but that is how science progresses in the long run. At this conference, for example, the term *behavior-mod* has proved to be emotionally charged. Someone defends it, then someone attacks it, then a third speaker ignores both while proceeding to agree with the one or the other. One such case is the equivalence (I am speaking for myself, of course) between a "behavior modifier" and a "social communications engineer." As I heard the two parties described, and allowing for the brevity of the descriptions, they seemed to operate the same and to have the same goals. Yet the similarity was ignored, while the latter term appeared to be acceptable to some conferees who were attacking the former.

I am going to avoid the more philosphical questions to which some of the conferees have addressed themselves. Questions, and a doctor's decisions about who shall live and who shall die, and what the criteria should be for assigning life or death, are indeed important, but, if you are going to become involved in them, I think you must be prepared to become more than amateur philosophers. It may prove to be as full time a preoccupation as medicine or clinical psychology. Philosophers have been considering such problems for several thousands of years; their discussions and solutions can be read any time, and anyone venturing into this area will find there is much to be learned and mulled over. The word *religion,* for example, has been mentioned here very sparingly. Yesterday, I counted only six times that it was used, and today only a few additional times. God has been mentioned, I think, twice. Many speakers here have emphasized how important they deem the patient's own point of view about his disease and his fate. Yet, the patient's religious views have been largely discounted. At this conference, religion has not been a prominent theme. I am not saying it ought to have been; medicine and psychology do not often find religion a congenial companion. But an investigator's attitude and knowledge of religion can seriously influence research in such a field as this conference deals with. They can affect, for example, how he samples a population in community medicine studies and what he regards as a proper sample. Suppose he aims to compare Catholics and Jews in their reactions to disease, or to cancer detection programs. Jews are as different from one another in their religious outlooks as Catholics are from Unitarians. There is no "Jewish" attitude toward euthanasia or birth control, while practicing Catholics vary from traditionalists to those who play guitars and sing folk music at holy communion. There are more important religious considerations than these, of course, and I am saying only that an ignorance of them, or a deliberate neglect of them, can only obscure an understanding of a patient's reactions to his disease, his treatment, and his fate.

I don't have many more things to say. One of them may offend you, but I hope not because it is not so intended. Most of what I have heard about death and fear, about the cancer patient who is afraid to die, the patient who can look forward only to a future that is no future, who can expect only the loss of his happiness, who is afraid of pain and suffering—most of such talk is culture-bound. That does not necessarily mean it is bad; after all, your patients are culture-bound, too. But the notion that a person necessarily fears death is not true in all cultures, nor is it always true even in our own culture. What a person believes about death depends upon how he has been raised. It is not necessarily true that everyone is afraid of not having a future. If you approach such problems from a medical or psychologic conviction that the ultimate good for terminal patients is not to be afraid of death, or that your job at the end is to relieve his anxiety over a futureless future, you are likely to miss things that are more important to him. Among them, if I may return to religion for my example, is the patient's religious solutions to his problems. If you approach him on a secular level alone, as medicine and psychology are apt to do in our heavily secular and scientific culture, you will fail to see much that that patient who has had a religious background is doing. Moreover, a prejudicial secular approach may deny to a religious patient the best solutions available to him, that is to say, religious solutions. Social psychologists have long known that a patient will respond to a question partly in terms of what he thinks a listener expects from him. If I were a behavior modifier, or a social communications engineer, concerned with a patient's attitudes about death, mortality, and the future, I would ask myself, "What does this patient *need*?" not only "What does he want?", but "What does he need?," and need in an objective sense, not merely in a predilective sense. His real need may be for religious counseling. One of our conferees mentioned that he joins forces with a chaplain occasionally; actually, I think he said that he "uses" a chaplain occasionally. There is nothing wrong with using a chaplain, unless you don't like chaplains. The patient might benefit much from it, and if you are going to meet your patient's needs on his own terms, and not your own culture-bound ones, maybe you ought to make your peace with the chaplain. He might have more to offer than a secular culture cares to admit. That is what I mean when I say we are often culture-bound; in this case, perhaps I should say "subculture bound," because medicine and psychology sometimes behave as if they were a culture within a culture.

I have two recommendations for future conferences of the National Cancer Institute, and perhaps for all conferences such as this. I speak partly from my own experience in arranging conferences, and partly from what I have gathered from others who have done so. One recommendation is that some time be allowed for small, self-selected groups of conferees to meet in different rooms so they can talk about specific problems of mutual interest, or where they can meet someone they have long looked forward to meeting. I tested that idea once at an international conference of ethologists and experimental psychologists for which I had responsibility, and it was a notably successful and popular arrangement. My second recommendation is that when people are asked to summarize, and urged to make the kinds of unguarded statements that I have been making, that time be allowed for the audience to react. Not only would that be fair, but I suspect it would enhance whatever value that remarks such as mine may have.

Addendum

The following papers were not presented at the Conference; the authors, however, were part of the invited audience. Because what is contained in these papers is of substantial interest to the Division of Cancer Control and Rehabilitation, the editors agreed that these ideas should be included as addenda.

Cancer: The Behavioral Dimensions, edited by J. W. Cullen,
B. H. Fox, and R. N. Isom. Raven Press, New York © 1976.

Remote Medical-Behavioral Monitoring: An Alternative for Ambulatory Health Assessment

Gerald H. Stein, Mark Kane Goldstein, and David M. Smolen

Medical and Psychology Services, Veterans Administration Hospital, and Center for Ambulatory Studies, University of Florida, Gainesville, Florida 32602

Ambulatory health care has the major goal of comprehensive rehabilitation of the patient and his family, that is, the restoration of the patient to the highest and fullest level of functioning within the family, at the job, and at recreation within the limits of the medical status (1). A recent study demonstrated the problems in assessment of both the process of ambulatory care and in the measurement of outcomes (2). Brook and Appel reported the surprising results of a careful assessment of the quality of health care, suggesting that in ambulatory settings little or no relationship exists between the physician's judgment of appropriate treatment and the actual patient outcomes (3). Moreover, a study of posthospital ambulatory care for inner-city patients reported that a significant number of patients suffered increased morbidity or decreased function related to inadequate follow-up care (4).

It is difficult to assess the conditions affecting patient deterioration and gain outside the hospital; only intermittent samples of medical and behavioral data are ordinarily available from ambulatory patients during the brief bimonthly clinic visit. These data typically are subjective patient comments or are confounded by the limitations of clinic evaluation and thus may offer little reliable information for appropriate intervention (5-10). Fries recognized this problem and suggested an electronic data-processing format for collecting objective clinical-status data from ambulatory patients *during* visits to the clinic. In the attempt to develop an adequate functional relationship between treatment process, delayed outcome, and patient rehabilitation, new data-gathering procedures must be evolved.

Thus, this report describes a method whereby ambulatory patients collect and transmit systematic medical and behavioral information about their daily functioning. This process offers a format for continuous flow of data directly from the patient's home environment to the practitioner.

METHOD

Subjects

We selected the patients in this study from the General Medical Clinic, Veterans Administration Hospital, Gainesville, Florida, between January and April 1973. The clinic serves posthospital-care patients and is staffed by 20 medical residents (rotating between the Veterans Administration Hospital and the Department of Medicine, College of Medicine, University of Florida, Gainesville), a staff physician, and a staff psychologist. Based on personnel time and patient availability, 28 patients (see Table 1 for diagnoses) were asked to record daily frequency of events associated with regimen compliance and to transmit these data at 2-week intervals to our laboratory. The mean age of the study patients was 46.1 years. Of the study patients, 25 were white and 3 were black; all were males.

Specification of Regimen

Particular behavioral aspects of each patient's regimen were precisely specified so that the patient could record the frequency of these events daily at home, for example, total ounces of fluid consumed, minutes worked (see Table 2). These pinpointed problems or behaviors were placed into four generic aspects—activities, appetitive behaviors, medical indicators, and social behaviors. Each patient's medical history was reviewed to clarify prior medical instructions offered to the patient in the management of his disease. The subsequent regimen was selected to maximize the patient's ability to record clinically relevant information in a precise manner. Table 2 presents the behavioral targets for self-recording of each aspect together with the direction of desired change. Suggestions and instructions were given to increase, decrease, maintain, or simply to measure and report the frequency of these regimen items (see Table 2).

For example: Patient A had a 5-year history of chronic chest pain, obesity, inactivity, and frequent general medical clinic visits. Physical examination and laboratory and angiographic studies were consistent with moderate coronary artery

TABLE 1. *Primary presenting diagnosis of study patients*

Musculoskeletal (rheumatoid arthritis, low-back pain, others)	13
Coronary artery disease and hypertension (myocardial infarction, angina)	5
Psychophysiologic reaction	5
Alcoholism	3
Others (e.g., diabetes)	2
	28

TABLE 2. *Regimen Aspects*

Behavioral targets	Direction of desired change[a]
Activities	
Number of minutes of work in house	↑
Number of minutes of work out of house	↑
Number of minutes spent walking	↑
Number of repetitions of exercise	→
Number of games played	↑
Number of minutes spent outside house	↑
Number of minutes spent watching TV	r.f.
Number of minutes resting	↓
Number of minutes sleeping	↑
Appetitive behaviors	
Number of ounces of liquid consumed (pint used for liquid measure)	r.f.
Number of new foods eaten	↑
Number of occasions salt added	↓
Number of bites of food	r.f.
Number of cups of coffee	↓
Medical indicators	
Number of chest pains reported	r.f.
Blood pressures taken by patient	r.f.
Number of vomiting episodes	r.f.
Urine sugar test results	r.f.
Number of minutes breathing in bag[b]	r.f.
Number of total medications taken	→
Number of trinitroglycerins taken	r.f.
Social behaviors	
Number of church contacts	↑
Number of persons visited	↑
Number of visits received	r.f.
Number of minutes of family interaction	↑
Number of personal contacts[c]	↑
Number of pleasant spouse episodes	↑
Number of job-seeking contacts	r.f.

a ↑ = increase; → = maintain; ↓ = decrease; r.f. = report frequency of occurrence and results where tested.
b Patient with hyperventilation syndrome.
c All contacts, including telephone.

disease. The number of clinic visits and the patient's frequency of complaint regarding chest pains were increasing disproportionately to the clinical course. The cardiologist advised the patient to increase his physical activity, to reduce his weight, and to self-regulate his medication (trinitroglycerin). The cardiologist also instructed the patient to follow the treatment plan carefully, and 1 month later no change was noted in the frequency of chest pain, in weight, or in stated activity level. A study-group assistant then provided the patient with a self-monitoring "time line" (Fig. 1) to record the daily weight, the number of minutes per day spent walking, and the number of trinitroglycerin tablets ingested. The original advice given to the patient by the cardiologist was then repeated, and the patient was now asked to record these events at home as they occurred. The data (returned in preaddressed stamped envelopes) suggested increases in activity and regulation of trinitroglycerin and a slight reduction in weight during the 3-month interval of self-monitoring. Self-initiated clinic visits did not occur during this period, and physical examinations at monthly intervals revealed no change in the patient's cardiac status.

Some patients were given only one regimen aspect to follow, and several patients kept track of three aspects concurrently. Charts and stamped return envelopes were supplied to each patient with standardized instructions for recording and returning the data. Patients were instructed to keep continuous records of their regimens—on a time line for each prescribed aspect—for at least 1 month. Thus, the time of occurrence and duration of each regimen event were recorded daily and transmitted to the hospital. All data returned were computer analyzed in a time-series design to establish the cumulative daily frequencies reported for each regimen aspect and to determine the amount of change or trend. To establish the trend direction, we employed the method of least squares to determine best linear fits to the logs of the reported daily frequencies (11). A sign test was employed to

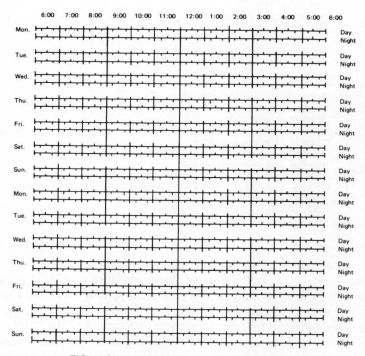

FIG. 1. Chart for continuous record of a regimen.

determine probabilities associated with observed trends in the reported data (12).

RESULTS

The 28 study patients returned continuous data on a total of 52 regimen aspects (Table 2). We initially requested 4 weeks of data, but in certain categories the data were transmitted for considerably longer periods. Reported activity regimens followed the direction of desired change (increased activity) in 19 records, were contrary in 5, and were unchanged in 3 (P = .003). Appetitive data suggested a compliance trend in 8 reports and noncompliance in 2 (P = .05). Reports of medical indicators suggested no change in rate in any of the categories monitored for baseline frequencies. Social-behavior data suggested increased interpersonal contacts in 3 reports, no change in 2, and decreased interaction or contacts in 3 (P > .05). The average number of "data days" (consecutive daily reports received) for each trend are reported, along with the trend outcomes for each monitoring category in Figure 2.

DISCUSSION

Whereas the results suggest the potential usefulness of this procedure for

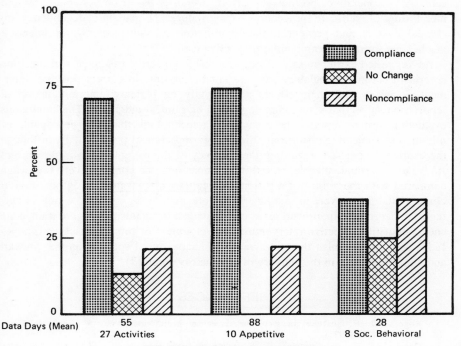

FIG. 2. Trends by monitoring category.

assessment and control of variables associated with chronic illness, the reported trends must be viewed conservatively and with interpretative caution. The data are rudimentary and only represent patient behavior in recording and transmitting information to the medical monitoring laboratory. Clearly, the relationship to clinical outcome and to health-related measures needs to be established, notwithstanding frequent implicit association with desired clinical trends. Moreover, no basis currently exists to assume that the reported rates of behavior are valid, that is, the data could be distorted or biased by the patients. This procedure thus represents a restricted attempt to elicit from ambulatory patients continuous reporting on their daily medical compliance and disease-related behaviors that have well-documented clinical concomitants. A wider normative base of information is also needed to determine the effective limits of remote ambulatory monitoring and of the types of clinical problems most amenable to this technique.

In particular, the vast increase in the number of ambulatory cancer patients necessitates an improved contact technology. Increasingly large numbers of ambulant leukemia and lymphoma patients using potent and effective chemotherapeutic agents require continuous surveillance from overtaxed health resources. The minute daily adjustments required after massive reconstructive cancer surgery (e.g., colostomy) are overwhelming for some patients and may be eased through a remote daily contact system. These patients often require interaction with a clinician because of post-operative adjustments which represent failures of self-care. A postoperative, posthospital effort, which is based on systematic remote monitoring of self-care procedures, may reduce the patient's dependency on clinical contact and prevent further debilitating consequences by serving as a mechanism for reinforcing regular preventive care.

As suggested earlier in this report, acceptable objective treatment and outcome criteria in chronic ambulatory care are notably absent. In current practice, treatment decisions and their effects rely heavily on patients' intermittent verbal reports, on subjective symptomatology, and on clinical judgment. The continuous evaluation system reported here suggests a technology that may be capable of minimizing subjective distortions, thus increasing clinical precision. Even though the cautions expressed, regarding the accuracy of the patients' data in the current study, are essential, the biases and inaccuracies may be comparatively few when compared with the ability of a patient to recall significant medical information at clinic visits. Moreover, an automated remote monitoring system, which is currently undergoing experimentl tests, can provide a mechanism for more immediate and systematic corrective intervention. Development of this approach can, hopefully, serve to diminish the prevalence of chance and of speculation that Stewart and Cluff document in the delivery of ambulatory care (13).

REFERENCES

1. Rogers, D. E. Shattuck Lecture—the American health-care-scene. *N. Engl. J. Med.*, 288:1377–1383 (1973).
2. Donabedian, A., and Rosenfeld, L. S. Follow-up study of chronically ill patients discharged

from hospital. *J. Chronic Dis.*, 17:847–862 (1964).

3. Brook, R. H., and Appel, F. A. Quality-of-care assessment *N. Engl. J. Med.*, 288:1323–1329 (1973).
4. Brook, R. H., Appel, F. A., Avery, C., Orman, M., and Stevenson, R. L. Effectiveness of inpatient follow-up care. *N. Engl. J. Med.*, 285:1509–1514 (1971).
5. Fordyce, W. E., Fowler, R. S., Jr., Lehmann, J. F., and Delateur, B. J. Some implications of learning in problems of chronic pain. *J. Chronic Dis.*, 21:179–190 (1968).
6. McWhinney, I. R. Beyond diagnosis. *N. Engl. J. Med.*, 287:384–387 (1972).
7. Mechanic, D., and Volkart, E. H. Stress, illness, behavior, and the sick role. *Am. Sociol. Rev.*, 26:51–58 (1961).
8. Silver, G. A. *Family Medical Care*, Harvard University Press, Cambridge, 1963.
9. Felix, R. H. Helping to meet the health care needs of the nation. *JAMA*, 220:1334–1337 (1972).
10. Fries, J. F. Time-oriented patient records and a computer data-bank. *JAMA*, 222:1536–1542 (1972).
11. Penneypacker, H. S., Koenig, C. H., and Lindsley, O. R. *Handbook of the Standard Behavior Chart*, Precision Media, Kansas City, 1972.
12. Siegal, S. *Nonparametric Statistics*, McGraw-Hill, New York, 1956.
13. Stewart, R. B., and Cluff, L. E. A review of medication errors and compliance in ambulant patients. *Clin. Pharmacol. Ther.*, 13:463–468 (1972).

Cancer: The Behavioral Dimensions, edited by J. W. Cullen,
B. H. Fox, and R. N. Isom. Raven Press, New York © 1976.

Antismoking Project

Louis U. Fink

Midland Industries, Inc., P.O. Box 5685, Orlando, Florida 32805

Smoking is currently the most serious of cause-connected health factors facing the human race, and is responsible for one-third of the deaths of men between the ages of 35 and 50.

An exhaustive list of projects directed at smoking cessation indicates no measure of success to date, with statistics noting regular annual increases in the number of smokers. Although currently adult males show a decrease in the number of smokers, teenagers and adult females more than balance the male ex-smokers via steady increases in new smokers.

Educational means of disseminating the hazards of smoking are vastly overshadowed by the promotional impact continuously provided by the tobacco industry. Despite the obviously slanted deleterious format of this daily promotion in national newspapers, government has done nothing to control it.

The formidable hold of the tobacco industry on legislators has been successful in totally counteracting attempts to limit or restrict this promotional impact, constantly delivered to the smoker and ex-smoker by the tobacco industry, a promotion that appears to be entirely motivated by economic goals. Accordingly, antismoking education has been unable, for the most part, to affect the ongoing conditioning of the public by the tobacco industry, notwithstanding the obvious health hazards involved.

Because smoking begins with behavior involving the social environment and becomes a sustained part of the smoker's daily existence, it would be well to examine the relationship of the present smoking environment to one's image.

Currently, smoking is socially accepted at all levels. Parents freely smoke in the presence of their infant and adolescent children. Adults smoke in public places, including eating establishments, with no regard to the discomfort of neighbors, and actually discard their tobacco garbage into the dishes at their tables and on the floors, with no concern about the pollution they generate thereby. Smokers in public places, common carriers, and even in private residences of others are surprised and sometimes even angry when asked to restrict their smoking for the benefit of others nearby. Most of this social acceptance for smoking is generated and augmented by the psychological impact of the tobacco industry's advertising format, and causes the average smoker to feel that he has the "right" to do as he pleases in smoking wherever, whenever, and however he decides. In the face of health statistics relative to the certain health conditions he will bring into his life expectancy by continued smoking, the smoker rebels by asserting his right to do unto himself as he wills it. He feels he is part of the smoking environment, as an "organized" part of society, and looks upon the nonsmoker as an "outsider" or as one loosely connected with society, or possibly as a "square" or "health freak." The smoker enjoys an image reinforced by constantly repeated tobacco-industry urgings and approbation. This, I believe, is the Achilles' heel of the tobacco industry, if recognized and exploited as such.

Smoking is obviously, to both smokers and nonsmokers, an activity that is costly, is the greatest fire hazard, and affords no beneficial residue as compared to other consumer commodities. Smoking admittedly is a dirty, smelly activity, resented often quite openly by intimates. Smoking is known by the majority to be a health hazard. One the economic side, increased tobacco prices, by virtue of increased taxation or sales prices in many states, only temporarily diminished sales in such areas. When the smoker surrendered his antagonisms to higher costs, tobacco sales swung upward again.

The tobacco industry thus is able to demonstrate that it can, at will, compete with any other consumer commodity industry most successfully for the consumer dollar.

Despite the fact that most smokers readily admit to a desire to quit smoking, and even look to the distant future when they will quit, the smoker will require far more than persuasion or dictatorial edicts if he is to give up smoking.

Industry has repeatedly demonstrated that it is fully capable of consumer persuasion toward fads or styles by image creation. The consumer can be conditioned to apparel trends, driving speeds, eating habits, and so on, simply by the creation of "the image of the masses" as being the norm. This regardless, in some cases, of the jeopardy or even discomfort of the consumer in so doing. The taking up of a current fad or even a way of life being promoted is a sure way for one to reinforce his image as others see him and, thus, feelings of inferiority or insecurity as related to his social environment are replaced by self-assurance and confidence.

Why not use the converse of this concept to solve the smoking problem? If smoking is begun by social environment and is reinforced by social acceptance and industry acclamation, why then should it not be possible to reverse the procedure and damage the image of the smoker as a smoker?

Many built-in "tools" are presently available to accomplish this reversal. As there are different patterns of behavior for different individuals, so are there different behavior patterns for smokers. For but one example, antismoking educational efforts have enjoyed some progress relative to adult males, but practically zero effect when directed at persons under 25 years of age. Still, persons under 25 react more conclusively to promotional efforts involving their wearing apparel than do older adult males. This same behavior pattern seems to hold in the marketing of automobile styles and types (Ford/Mustang promotion to "the lively set").

These facts indicate that whereas people under 25 place a priority on those industry PR efforts enhancing their image, these same people pay little heed to educational efforts directed at their health jeopardy. This leads to the conclusion that image in this age bracket is most important and that the social environment of smoking enhances their image and therefore reinforces their decision to continue smoking.

Recent formats in newspaper advertisements by cigarette makers show a defensive philosophy new to the tobacco industry in that the formats now appeal to the smokers' "rights to their own decisions" in the face of increasing data concerning health jeopardy from smoking. The industry is telling the smoker that he has the right to continue getting "pleasure" and "taste" from smoking, regardless of what others may advise.

Society's attitude toward smoking at the turn of the century required the smoker to give heed to where he smoked, and demanded that he seek permission before smoking in the presence of others, whether they were smokers or nonsmokers. Society cast aspersions upon females who smoked, even surreptitiously, so that they smoked at the risk of total destruction of their social image. It was not until Lucky Strike cigarettes reinforced woman's image with a successful promotion of "Don't reach for a sweet, reach for a Lucky instead (and you won't get fat)" that women began smoking in force, and continued in increasing numbers in the face of health hazard warnings.

Obviously, if the smoker were held as a social outcast by the majority (the nonsmokers), the smoker's image would be damaged beyond rapair or defense, and this would begin a steep downward trend in the number of smokers. The most "image-conscious" (adult females and those below 25 years of age) would be the first to quit smoking, and would be most vulnerable to health education related to smoking.

By identification of new techniques, field testing via community funded programs, evaluation of the results of such programs, and their demonstration in large-scale community environments, means can be found to reverse the current social acceptance of the smoker.

This would serve to cancel for the long-term future increasing numbers of cases of lung cancer and other smoking-related diseases in adult women and teenagers.

Cancer: The Behavioral Dimensions, edited by J. W. Cullen,
B. H. Fox, and R. N. Isom. Raven Press, New York © 1976.

Can-Dial:
Cancer Public Information Through the Telephone

Edwin A. Mirand

Roswell Park Memorial Institute, Buffalo, New York 14203

In recent years, the problem of cancer has become a topic of increased concern. Unfortunately, with the exception of the American Cancer Society's efforts at smoking dissuasion, little has been accomplished in the area of public education and cancer. Roswell Park Memorial Institute, as a comprehensive cancer center, is interested in promoting better health behavior, especially regarding the prevention, early diagnosis, and management of cancer. In an attempt to facilitate this task, a system of easily accessible tape recordings containing information about cancer was developed.

CAN-DIAL

The principal objective of the Can-Dial Public Information System is to provide immediate information on a variety of cancer-related topics to the general public. A second, but still very important, objective is to evaluate the effectiveness of such an effort as far as increasing public knowledge about cancer and influencing preventive health behavior.

Interested individuals are able to listen to prerecorded tapes on a variety of topics over the telephone. An operator takes incoming requests, answers questions, collects initial information about callers, and plays the tapes selected. The system, which is toll-free, operates 16 hours a day, 7 days a week. The current Can-Dial tape library contains 32 taped messages, recorded in easily understood, nontechnical language. A set of Spanish translations is available for use by the 30,000 Spanish-speaking residents of Erie County, New York.

Since inception of the program in April 1974, response has been excellent, indicating acceptance and use by the public, as well as a measure of initial success. Although response was relatively light during the beginning stages, it has consistently increased until utilization now approximates the maximum capacity of the system. This is no doubt due, at least in part, to an intensive advertising campaign using public service time on television and radio, announcements in newspapers and other forms of printed media, and distribution of large quantities of brochures containing information about the program.

EVALUATION

Because evaluation is a major aspect of this program, a large part of this report describes the evaluation effort to date. Two types of evalution are being conducted. The first involves a constant monitoring of the system in which respondents are asked at time of contact to voluntarily provide certain descriptive information about themselves. Response in general is also monitored and analyzed. This stage of evaluation provides descriptive data about users and use of the system. It allows us to keep track of the system and to implement any changes that might be indicated which would provide better service. The second type of evaluation entails interviewing a sample of respondents and comparison with a random sample of nonusers in the Erie County area.

In this manner, we hope to ascertain user motivation, knowledge and information gained, action taken, and user benefits attributable to the system. Since we are just beginning the second phase of our evaluation efforts, comments will be limited to the information that has been obtained from our monitoring efforts.

PATTERNS OF RESPONSE

As of January 26, 1975, a total of 25,267 calls had been received since operations began in April 1974. During this same period, a total of 22,347 tapes were played. The discrepancy between calls received and tapes played is due to calls for information, wrong number, and hang-up and/or crank calls.

Since inception of the program, the daily average (mean) number of calls received has been increasing steadily. For instance, during the first three months of operation, an average of 52 calls per day were received. This rose to a mean response of 91 calls per day in July and August, 109 calls per day in September, and 114 calls per day in October. Average daily response has more than doubled since the program began. Daily fluctuation has been considerable during this time, with response ranging from a low of 13 calls to a high of 206 calls per day. There seems to have been a tendency for response to increase as public awareness about the program's existence increased.

PROMOTION AND RESPONSE

A major interest is to evaluate the effectiveness of various types of promotion. Our preliminary analyses for the first 6 months of operation show brochures to be the most effective as far as total response received disregarding cost-effectiveness. When respondents were asked to cite their source of information about Can-Dial, 3,597 mentioned brochures, the White Directory (Yellow Pages) was second with 3,004, followed by television and radio—1,239; schools—1,096; friends and relatives—1,041; and printed sources—221.

IMPACT ON CANCER CONTROL

Although it is difficult to evaluate the impact of this system on cancer control at this time, we are able to glean some clues as to its possible effectiveness. For instance, if we examine the subjects requested, it becomes evident that some of the most prevalent types of cancer are also areas of concern to the general populace (Table 1). For instance, the tape most frequently requested is "If You Want To Give Up Cigarettes," with "The Effect of Cigarette Smoking on the Non-Smoker" ranking third, and "Lung Cancer" ranking sixth. Given the well-documented deleterious effect of smoking on health in general and especially its etiologic role in lung cancer, the popularity of these topics seems well justified. Other areas where high interest coincides with relatively high incidence or mortality include breast cancer, cancer of the colon and rectum, and uterine and cervical cancer. However, high incidence sites that do not seem to be receiving enough public interest include prostate, pancreas, and perhaps bladder cancer. The tape on pancreas cancer was not included until relatively late in the program which may

TABLE 1. *Rank order of topics according to frequency of request*

Rank/order	Tape number	Topic	Requests
1.	5	If You Want to Give Up Cigarettes	2,684
2.	3	Cancer of the Breast—And How to Detect It	1,391
3.	26	Effect of Cigarette Smoking on Non-Smokers	1,029
4.	2	Cancer's Warning Signals	883
5.	1	What Is Cancer?	758
6.	4	Lung Cancer	635
7.	7	Cancer of the Uterus	580
8.	20	Cigarette Smoking and the Pregnant Woman	576
9.	9	Cancer of the Colon and Rectum	561
10.	22	What Is the Pap Test?—How Can it Help You?	509
11.	10	Leukemia	484
12.	8	Cancer of the Skin	478
13.	19	Hodgkin's Disease	464
14.	16	Cancer of the Bone	426
15.	17	Cancer of the Stomach	406
16.	18	Cancer of the Brain	369
17.	13	Chemotherapy: Drug vs. Cancer	353
18.	11	Cancer of the Mouth	326
19.	6	Cancer of the Larynx	299
20.	14	Cancer of the Bladder	236
21.	21	Cigarette Smoking and Dental Problems	215
22.	15	Cancer of the Prostate	206
23.	27	Cancer of the Liver	169
24.	23	What Is the Roswell Park Memorial Institute?	139
25.	25	Words from a Hospital Chaplain	138
26.	24	Radiation Therapy in Cancer Treatment	125
27.	28	Cancer of the Pancreas	119
28.	12	Service and Rehabilitation Information for Cancer Patients/Families	80

TABLE 2. *Requested topic by age and sex*

Tape no.	Age/Sex unkn.	Male					Sub-total
		<20	20–39	40–59	60+	Unkn.	
1	31	144	39	11	3	44	241
2	56	118	67	18	1	45	249
3	65	76	38	9	1	40	164
4	28	84	43	10	5	39	181
5	72	230	324	98	23	127	802
6	12	20	25	10	2	20	77
7	27	29	16	6	2	10	63
8	16	34	40	26	6	18	124
9	25	25	36	34	6	35	136
10	20	38	12	9	3	33	95
11	13	34	14	3	3	20	74
12	5	13	4	3	0	7	27
13	15	31	10	5	1	18	65
14	9	9	9	10	3	9	40
15	12	18	24	19	15	17	93
16	13	32	17	6	2	10	67
17	14	27	24	10	3	16	80
18	17	58	17	4	1	28	108
19	42	38	32	15	3	25	113
20	25	34	30	0	2	16	82
21	10	25	14	3	2	16	60
22	27	30	12	4	1	19	66
23	6	27	6	1	0	7	41
24	12	16	9	2	1	7	35
25	10	16	5	5	0	12	38
26	38	142	71	21	5	58	297
27*	5	12	6	6	5	13	42
28*	4	11	2	5	1	9	28
Total	629	1,371	946	353	100	718	3,488

*Tapes 27 and 28 were not available before August.

		Female				
<20	20–39	40–59	60+	Unkn.	Sub-total	Total
148	47	17	0	18	230	502
133	98	35	15	59	340	645
219	258	93	12	159	752	981
73	67	41	5	33	221	430
293	452	146	19	201	1,111	1,985
22	51	34	2	21	138	227
63	139	44	5	69	320	410
61	77	28	5	41	212	352
21	86	68	35	51	267	428
88	56	30	2	45	216	331
39	47	17	7	29	139	226
15	12	10	1	11	49	81
21	28	29	11	31	120	200
19	42	21	6	31	119	168
11	20	10	2	14	57	162
43	38	34	2	31	148	228
30	76	35	5	31	117	211
58	48	20	4	46	176	301
68	86	26	16	52	248	403
117	132	6	2	55	312	419
34	23	5	7	17	82	152
118	94	15	3	57	287	380
29	14	5	0	17	65	112
9	15	6	4	16	50	97
16	9	10	3	14	52	100
156	92	39	4	65	356	691
20	42	19	5	23	109	156
5	20	16	5	11	57	89
1,929	2,201	859	187	1,262	6,350	10,467

account, in part, for its low popularity. The topics prostate and bladder, however, are probably affected by other factors such as age and sex. Both are mainly male problems, with prostate, especially, being a problem of old age.

It is interesting to consider our experience to date concerning the age and sex of respondents (Table 2). We have found that females exceed male callers in all age categories. This may be due to a greater health awareness or concern for health matters among females. It may also be due to the onus of breast cancer, especially since the recent experiences of prominent individuals. When age is examined, however, a slightly clearer picture emerges. Greatest response has occurred among the two youngest age groups. Contacts from those under 20 are due in large part to assignments of school projects. This is the largest category of male response, which seems to decline with an increase in age. By far the greatest response is received from females 20 to 39, after which it falls off rapidly. These findings indicate that our greatest success so far has been in disseminating knowledge to the populace under 40. Those who are over 40 are not utilizing the system to a sufficient degree. This is a cause for concern because these are precisely the ages when many forms of cancer begin to appear. Future efforts will be directed toward eliciting a greater response from these age groups and from males.

The system has been utilized so far in a fairly equal manner by all social strata (Table 3). The lowest stratum responds less frequently than all others, but the difference between highest response and lowest response never exceeds 10%. More data of this nature needs to be collected before we can be certain whether this is a significant difference. However, it has become evident that rural areas are using the system less than the Buffalo-Lackawanna urban area. We are now attempting to increase the response in those areas of low use.

CONCLUSION

Our initial impression is that Can-Dial has had a positive effect on the community, at least in terms of public education and increasing awareness about cancer. Such a conclusion is based on the high overall use of the system by the populace. Most of the high-incidence cancers are reflected in topic requests, with the exception of those occurring in older males. Use is also distributed fairly evenly among various strata, with use being highest in the metropolitan area and lowest in the rural areas.

At this stage we are unable to determine if the system has had an impact in changing behavior in a positive direction as far as health is concerned. We also do not know if the information disseminated by the system is being retained. We can, however, conclude that information about cancer is finding its way to the populace at large. Hopefully, at a later date, we will be able to demonstrate a positive effect in terms of the prevention and control of cancer.

TABLE 3. *Can-Dial response according to socioeconimic status*

SES groups		Population	Number of calls received	Rate per 10,000 population	Percent calls	Percent calls (Each area)	Percent total calls
Buffalo Lackawanna							
(High)	1.	80,455	490	60.90	17.44		9.2
	2.	79,512	485	60.99	17.26		9.1
	3.	80,311	447	55.65	15.91		8.4
	4.	81,453	462	56.71	16.44		8.7
	5.	77,153	457	59.23	16.26		8.6
(Low)	6.	87,888	468	53.24	16.66		8.8
Subtotal:		486,772	2,809	57.70		52.9	
First Ring Township							
(High)	1.	113,372	530	46.74	26.21		9.9
	2.	113,741	507	44.57	25.07		9.5
	3.	116,860	577	49.37	28.53		10.8
	4.	109,006	408	37.42	20.17		7.6
Subtotal:		452,979	2,022	44.63		38.1	
Outer Ring Township							
(High)	1.	45,195	131	28.98	27.63		2.4
	2.	39,296	119	30.28	25.10		2.2
	3.	40,234	140	34.79	29.53		2.6
	4.	44,361	84	18.93	17.72		1.5
Subtotal:		169,087	474	28.03		8.9	
Total by SES groups			5,305				

Subject Index

A

Adoption vs. diffusion concepts, relating to cancer control techniques, 243-254

Adriamycin, 187

Aflatoxins, 17, 19, 88

Air pollution, related to lung cancer, 86

Alcohol, carcinogenic effects of, 89

Ambulatory health care, remote medical-behavioral monitoring and, 361-367

American Cancer Society
  communication programs of, 179-186
  Science Writers' Seminar for, 181-182

Antimetabolites, 265

Antismoking projects, see Cigarette smoking

Anxiety
  as factor of participation in screening program, 36-37, 54-55
  postcurative therapy for, 5-6
  in public's conception of cancer, 147-148
  related to cancer in children, 6-7

Arsenic, related to cancer, 86

Asbestos, related to cancer, 86

L-Asparaginase, side effects of, 265

Attitude and behavior, media factors affecting, 211-213, 217

Attitude theory, to modify health behavior, 66-67

B

Bandura's theory of social learning, 64-66

Behavioral and medical information, through ambulatory health care, 361-367

Behavioral scientist
  American Cancer Society's use of, 182
  problem of funding, 112
  role in health care system, 168-169

Behavior modification
  in control and prevention, 118
  related to physicians' behavior, 167
  respondants' discussion of value of, 261
  social learning theory in, 63-73

3,4-Benzopyrene, 86, 88

Biofeedback, 284

Biopsy, patients' response behavior after recommendation of, 29-31

Birth control pills, fear of breast cancer and, 183

Bladder cancer
  Can-Dial response about, 375
  psychosocial epidemiology of, 12-14, 17, 20

Blood cancer, see also Leukemia; psychosocial epidemiology of, 12, 14, 18

Bone cancer, Can-Dial response about, 375